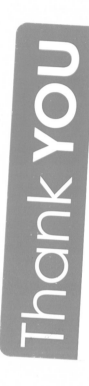

This book
purchased
with donations
made to the
GiveBIG
for Books
Campaign.

The
Seattle
Public
Library
Foundation

www.foundation.spl.org

D0952374

No More Diabetes

A Complete Guide to Preventing, Treating,
and Overcoming Diabetes

By Gary Null, PhD

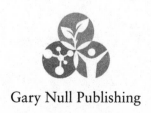

Gary Null Publishing

Gary Null Publishing books may be purchased in bulk at special discounts for sales promotion, corporate gifts, fund-raising, or educational purposes. Special editions can also be created to specifications. For details, contact the Special Sales Department, Gary Null Publishing, 307 West 36th Street, 11th Floor, New York, NY 10018 or info@skyhorsepublishing.com.

Gary Null Publishing is an imprint of Skyhorse Publishing, Inc.

Skyhorse® and Skyhorse Publishing® are registered trademarks of Skyhorse Publishing, Inc.®, a Delaware corporation.

Visit our website at www.skyhorsepublishing.com.

10 9 8 7 6 5 4 3 2 1

Library of Congress Cataloging-in-Publication Data Null, Gary.
No more diabetes: a complete guide to preventing, treating, and overcoming diabetes / Gary Null.
    pages cm
Includes bibliographical references.
ISBN 978-1-62636-155-3 (hardcover: alk. paper)
1. Diabetes—Popular works. 2. Diabetes—Alternative treatment. 3. Diabetes—Diet therapy.
4. Naturopathy. I. Title.
RC660.4.N86 2013
616.4'622—dc23
                        2013013718

Printed in the United States of America

CONTENTS

Preface

This book is to serve as a thorough resource manual about diabetes, its causes, prevention, and treatment. Throughout the text, scientific research on medical complications and the causes thereof when people suffer from diabetes—the majority having been published in peer-reviewed medical journals—was relied upon. The preventative and therapeutic approach that is provided is based on a natural systems approach. In addition to suggested nutrition and dietary regimens, this also necessitates lifestyle changes, including exercise, mental composure, and living habits. Invaluable information on particular superfoods and recipes are offered to help you begin altering the attitudes and ways in which we eat.

Having authored more than ninety books, I have discovered that personal testimonials by patients suffering from particular illnesses are very motivating for people. Therefore, a chapter has been included to offer individual stories by people who have beaten this seventh leading cause of death in the United States.

There are many people who contributed to *No More Diabetes*. Jim Feast, who has edited several of my other publications, performed his usual expert job in developing many of the more complex scientific data into a manner readable to the layperson. Special appreciation goes to my research assistants Mitzi Flade Sampson, Nadia Abdo, Porochista Khakpour and Jeremy Stillman who have devoted hundreds of hours individually to gathering the most current and past scientific data about diabetes and natural ways to prevent and treat it, and to my producer Richard Gale who provided insights from his medical background and coordinated the publication. Doug Henderson and Jennifer Shagawat gathered testimonials and recipes. Thanks also to my Art Director Jay Graygor for his excellent work on the cover design.

Chapter 1

Pushing Back Against Diabetes

"Thinking starts from doubt or uncertainty. It marks an inquiring, hunting, searching attitude."

—John Dewey, *Democracy and Education*

Americans love to make lists, but sometimes these lists are just too short. Take the list of the leading killer diseases. If I asked you which diseases were the primary causes of death in the United States, you would probably correctly identify cancer and heart disease, and stop there. It's more than likely you couldn't name the seventh top cause—in fact, you might even be surprised to learn it is diabetes.

This book is an in-depth study of diabetes, of the physical, behavioral and even mental causes that leads to its emergence, and of the practices that will block and reverse it.

Anyone familiar with my ideas can anticipate some of the points I will cover. Three things they could correctly put on that list are: 1) a presentation of the latest, cutting-edge research on the topic, including lengthy and fact-packed interviews with doctors who have made a study of and successfully treated the disease, 2) an emphasis on how you can be proactive in ensuring or regaining health through such practices as exercising and adopting a more natural, vegetarian or near-vegetarian diet, and 3) a list of mouth-watering vegetarian recipes, along with a vitamin, mineral, and herbal supplement protocol that has proven useful in helping to abate or forestall the illness.

There is much more inside, including some things that will not fit on any list of my favorite topics. Not many people realize that in my leisure moments I like to indulge my penchant for reading American literature and philosophy, and one philosopher who has proved particularly congenial to my way of thinking is John Dewey, a writer who was prominent from the early 1900s to 1950, and was long a fixture at Columbia University. Broadly speaking, in his whole life he made one argument: *We will destroy ourselves unless we see life whole.* This is the main reason I admire this man. That has also been one of my own driving thoughts and can be reformulated for this text along these lines: the scourge of diabetes will only be conquered through an *ultra-holism* that sees true bodily health as one component of natural living that includes not only a vegetarian or semi-vegetarian diet, exercise, and an aware lifestyle, but also the shape of our communities, our relationships, and our leisure and work habits.

All of that will be touched on here. However, don't be apprehensive. You will not suddenly come upon a lecture on metaphysics stuck in the middle of a talk on healthy living. That won't happen, but you will find, at key junctures, we are suddenly glancing off the thought of Dewey.

Now that you have some idea of what to expect in this book, let me begin with some facts about this disease, the illness that few people recognize as belonging on the list of leading killers.

Diabetes mellitus affects over 24 million children and adults in the United States, and each year the problem worsens. To put it in the starkest terms, ones provided by the CDC, every twenty-four hours, four thousand adults are diagnosed with diabetes and two hundred people die from it. If things continue as they have been, roughly one quarter of the American population is facing a future of diabetes. Furthermore, over 57 million American adults have a health condition known as pre-diabetes. "Pre" is something of a euphemism. Make no mistake, pre-diabetes is a serious condition, and those who suffer from it are well on their way to full-blown diabetes.

That's the US. If we think of the rest of the world, we find the problem is found almost everywhere. Partially as one of the unexpected byproducts of globalization, which has encouraged fast-food diets in countries where such eating had been previously unheard of, in 2000 throughout the world over 171 million people were diagnosed with diabetes. By 2030, The World Health Organization predicts that over 360 million people worldwide will have it. This is an increase of more than 40 percent in industrialized nations, where fast food and other unhealthy lifestyle choices reign supreme, and a 170 percent increase in developing nations, where diets are beginning to change for the worse, helping the spread of the illness.

Diabetes disproportionately affects certain ethnic groups. In Native Americans, Hispanic and Latino Americans, and African Americans, the disease is much more prevalent than in the non-Hispanic white population.

The disease is devastating, to put it lightly. If you have the illness, you can expect your life to be cut short on average by four to eight years. Diabetes can lead to blindness, renal disease, peripheral nerve damage, and non-traumatic amputations. Further, a person suffering from diabetes is also in danger for heart disease, stroke, cancer, inflammatory diseases, depression, and obesity.

Causes

When a detective arrives at a crime scene, the first question she or he asks is "Whodunit?" In the same way, when a doctor finds someone has a disease, the first question the practitioner should ask is "What is behind this manifestation?"

To continue with my metaphor for one more step, if the detective found four people dead at a restaurant dinner table and the only dish they shared was the dessert, the sleuth might well suspect the chocolate mousse of being the culprit. A similar suspicion might be cast on food and eating habits in relation to diabetes since it has been found that the incidences of both diabetes and heart disease skyrocketed when Americans began to change their diet. The late complementary physician Dr. Robert Atkins put his finger on this when he paraphrased something he had read in the book *The Saccharine Disease* by Dr. T. L. Cleave (who had been a surgeon in the British Royal Navy). Atkins noted that Cleave cited "'the law of 20 years,' which says that after you introduce refined carbohydrates into a culture, two illnesses emerge two decades later: diabetes and heart disease." Atkins elaborated, "We know a Third World diet without refined carbohydrates leads to substantially reduced heart disease and diabetes." However, once a Third World culture is "civilized" by its people being encouraged to eat refined carbohydrates, the levels of these illnesses increases. "More often than not, when one illness emerges, so does the other," Atkins goes on. So what is the connection between the three: refined carbohydrates, diabetes, and heart disease? To simplify matters, let's concentrate on just the first two.

Carbohydrates are made up of sugars, starches and cellulose. The body breaks them down so as to turn them into glucose (blood sugar). Refined carbohydrates are simply ones that through food processing have had many of their nutritional elements, such as iron, fiber and vitamin B, removed. However, let's put this difference between refined and unrefined carbs aside for the moment and just look at how the body deals with a situation where so many carbs have been broken down that the blood is overstocked with sugar. Under normal circumstances, insulin is released by the pancreas to handle this situation. Insulin helps direct the glucose to storage sites in muscle cells and various tissues, lowering blood sugar levels. In a diabetic, something is going wrong with the process either because of insulin deficiency, insulin resistance or insulin insensitivity. I want to examine these difficulties in turn.

Insulin Deficiency

For years, medicine ascribed diabetes to deficiency. It was thought the body didn't produce enough insulin to take care of any excess of blood sugar. Much recent research has established the result, one that came as a surprise to those who believed in the old model, that many diabetics *produce enough insulin*—it's just not being properly absorbed. The problem was not that they lacked for insulin, but their cells either were insensitive or resisted taking it up.

Insulin Insensitivity

So what would make a cell insensitive or resistant? Insulin enters the cells through receptor sites. When these sites are plugged due to an adherence of fat or cholesterol, not all the insulin seeking entry can get in and it bounces back into the bloodstream. Think of a mischievous child, caught fighting in the playground, who is told by the principal to go to the detention room. However, once there, he promptly climbs out the window and rejoins the outdoors scuffle instead of staying in the building.

When too much glucose gets in the blood because it has been turned away from the clogged receptors, this creates hyperglycemia (high blood sugar). Chronic hyperglycemia is the defining characteristic of diabetes.

If this uptick in blood sugar is caused by cells not being able to take in all the glucose directed their way, then the culprit causing the disease is not lack of insulin in the body but its inability to accomplish its mission of entering cells. And, so far as this is true, there must be a fundamental shift in how diabetes is treated. Doctors who have responded to this new understanding have changed their emphasis from increasing insulin production to enhancing insulin sensitivity.

Insulin Resistance

While insensitivity to insulin occurs when the cells are partially blocking the inlet of blood sugar, the closely related phenomenon of insulin resistance is found when allergic responses or other factors hinder insulin's activity. Again, there are adequate amounts of insulin available for the body but, most commonly, a particular food allergy is interfering. There is no one set of allergy-creating foods. These vary by individual. Wheat, for instance, may create symptoms of high blood sugar in one woman, while corn may affect another.

Types of Diabetes

Diabetes is generally classified into types I and II, with the more devastating form I having long been thought (until recently) to be confined to onset in childhood or during the teenage years.

Type I does involve lack of insulin. The pancreas, which produces insulin, is damaged. This could be because of a viral infection, extreme toxicity (from being exposed to poisonous chemicals, for example) or, according to some researchers, excess vaccinations. The pancreatic damage may also be connected to a genetic inheritance. In any case, this damage is tied up with a continued assault on the pancreas by a disturbed immune system. While the body's immune system usually functions by targeting and eliminating viruses and other types of germs, here it gets off the track and actually begins attacking and destroying the beta cells, which produce insulin, in the pancreas.

(One might imagine—this is only my speculation, not something backed up by my research—this type of scenario: the body is fighting an infection of the pancreas, and somehow in the course of this, the immune response is triggered to also attack the healthy pancreatic cells.)

With the pancreas undermined, there really is no insulin to process blood sugar. Therefore, someone with type I diabetes has to get the insulin from outside, perhaps by daily injection, for life. Usually type I is detected in patients before their twentieth birthday. This form of the disease though, is not the one responsible for the burgeoning increase in cases mentioned earlier. According to the American Diabetes Association, type I diabetes is responsible for only 5 percent of all diabetes cases.

Type II diabetes, also known as non-insulin-dependent diabetes or adult-onset diabetes, is the one whose numbers are getting staggering. This one, which occurs most frequently in adults over forty, and more often in women than men, is not tied so much to early infections or genetic factors as to lack of exercise, obesity, and lifestyle factors. However, it is now beginning to show up more and more in children and young adults.

Type II Diabetes in Children and Young People

This is a heartbreaking trend. Type II diabetes in children was practically unheard of until recently. Now, as the American Diabetes Association has found, nearly 4,000 children are diagnosed with type II diabetes every year, adding to the 190,000 adolescents who are already battling diabetes. The number of young people with this disease is not gradually growing but ballooning. Research presented at the 2012 annual meeting of the American Diabetes Association showed that from 2001—2009, the incidence of type II diabetes among American children and teens rose by 21 percent. In an interview with WebMD, Dr. Robert E. Ratner, chief scientific and medical officer of the American Diabetes Association, responded to the study results saying "these are harbingers of adult health problems. If the trend is not reversed, there could be an epidemic of heart disease, stroke, and kidney failure when this generation is age 25–35."

I mentioned Atkins's citing of the 20-year rule on the relation between a society changing from natural to processed food and the beginning of heart disease and diabetes. Maybe we should introduce another rule, one with a briefer time span. That would be the "five-year rule" that predicted the time lag between the introduction of computer video games, and other inventions that encourage children and adolescents to spend their afterschool hours sitting in front of a TV or computer rather than going outdoors to run around and play and the onset of type II diabetes in young people. For this to my mind is one of the major factors behind the sudden peaking of youthful diabetes type II. This disease is making its debilitating presence known in the overweight and inactive youth of America, afflicting them in astronomical proportions.

Of course, traditional medicine would laugh at the idea of a five year rule. They face this new crisis by directing their research into the discovery of the gene responsible for this meteoric rise of type II diabetes in children. They overlook the more obvious fact that simultaneously with the noted rise of this disease in youth, over the past thirty years the number of overweight American children has more than doubled. To my way of thinking, these two occurrences, a rise of type II diabetes in youth and a vast increase in youthful obesity, are linked by more than the fact that they happened at the same time. I believe American youth's carrying of excessive body weight has brought about the drastic rise in type II diabetes in this group.

Remember, obesity is a trademark of the disease. "A predisposition toward visceral obesity," to use a clinical expression—that is, adding fat around the midsection—has been linked to increased insulin resistance in research published in the *Journal of Endocrinology* (2006). That ties in with the report that 85 percent of children in the United States diagnosed with type II diabetes either carry some extra weight or are outright obese.

A moment ago I alluded briefly to the fact that certain American minorities were more prone to diabetes than the Caucasian majority. Let me draw that point out further in relation to youth.

It's been learned that African-American children are particularly vulnerable to diabetes and the conditions associated with this disease. Dr. Geoff Ball from the Faculty of Medicine and Dentistry at the University of Alberta made a comparative study looking at insulin problems in Caucasian children and African-American children at puberty. It turns out the levels of insulin in the African-American youth group worsened as they progressed through puberty, but in the Caucasian group the levels remained unchanged. There are physiological changes in puberty, and they seem to be particularly problematic in relation to insulin resistance for African-American youth.

Another significant study has also looked at insulin levels in youth, not as they are part of racial or ethnic minorities, but in relation to their mothers' conditions. If a youth's mother suffered from polycystic ovary syndrome (PCOS), a hormonal disorder associated with insulin resistance that affects women in their reproductive age, then during puberty the youth would tend to have excess insulin. Such were the findings of Dr. Richard Legro, professor of obstetrics and gynecology at Penn State College of Medicine. The study leads to the conclusion that children of PCOS mothers build up excessive insulin during puberty.

Another family factor that has an impact on a whether a youth will become diabetic is the health of his or her siblings. A study led by Dr. Sheela Magge, a pediatric endocrinologist at the Children's Hospital of Philadelphia, found that "overweight siblings of children with type II diabetes are four times more likely to have abnormal glucose levels compared to other overweight children." Magge also noted that "74 to 100 percent of children with type II diabetes have a first or second degree relative who also has the condition."

All of which should indicate that while all young Americans have to be careful and take steps toward healthy living, those that belong to certain groups, such as those with diabetic siblings, must be doubly careful.

Causes of Type II Diabetes

Though there is some evidence that a genetic predisposition is involved in type II diabetes, the fact that suddenly there is a mega-growth in the number of people manifesting the disease clearly indicates that something more than genetics is shaping the rapid spread of the illness. A growing volume of evidence indicates that a confluence of factors, from lifestyle to dietary and environmental causes, is behind this surge.

In type II diabetes, the beta cells in the pancreas are still producing insulin, but either not enough is being made or the body is not making effective use of what it has. So, the sufferer doesn't need more insulin, but a better use of the insulin he or she has.

Symptoms of Diabetes

Type I diabetes is characterized by the symptoms that have often been seen as "typical." These include frequent urination, especially at night, great thirst and hunger, fatigue, weight loss, irritability, and restlessness. As noted, those who suffer from this form of the disease need daily doses of insulin, and if they lack them, they can fall into a coma.

Type II diabetes can begin with fewer noticeable symptoms, although obesity often signals a pre-diabetic state, especially when the excess weight is concentrated at or just above the waistline. As the diabetes progresses, the eyes, kidneys, nervous system, and skin become affected, and infections and hardening of the arteries may develop.

The constant fluctuations in blood sugar that accompany both forms of diabetes are also debilitating. Remember, when insulin is in sufficient supply and working effectively, new glucose entering the blood through the breaking down of food is smoothly integrated in the body's overall architecture. On the other hand, if the insulin base is not there or not being used efficiently, blood sugar levels will fluctuate, leading to a wide range of disorders.

One particular accompanying problem is inner arterial wall damage. Weakened arteries contribute to cardiovascular stress. In fact, the incidence of heart attacks and strokes is five to eight times greater among diabetics than in the general population. Most deaths of diabetics, some 75 percent, are due to heart disease brought on by the hardening of major arteries.

Moreover, another negative effect on the circulatory system prompted by diabetes is damage to the vessels leading to the eyes, kidneys, and peripheral nerves. As these become thick and brittle, blood movement is impeded, making them less functional. Also, these vessels are put under pressure by sudden surges of blood sugar, which occur when insulin is not properly regulating the distribution of this glucose. For the sight, the repeated stresses that diabetics experience cause the vessels in the eyes to hemorrhage and break down. After several hemorrhages, a patient ends up blind.

Similar events brought on by blood sugar surges can weaken the kidneys, so that nitrogen wastes can no longer be eliminated efficiently and accumulate in the organ.

Interference with blood circulation in both large and small vessels is also responsible for the high incidence of neuritis (an inflammation of the nerves) and even gangrene, which results from insufficient blood flow to a part of the body, which, in the worst case, can end with amputation.

Having given a quick run-through of common symptoms and accompaniments of diabetes, let me spend some time going into a little more detail about the disastrous health problems that usually supplement the illness. These sections should bring home to you the frightening healthcare costs, both physical and financial, for which diabetes is responsible.

Diabetes is Blinding—Eye Disorders Are a Common Side Effect

A few paragraphs ago, I noted how the blood surges that are a characteristic of diabetes can damage the vessels leading to the eyes, eventually leading to blindness. In fact, many eyes diseases, such as cataracts, retinopathy, and glaucoma, are more common among diabetics than in the general population.

Let me say a few words about the prevalence of these different disorders. Among the working adult population in the US, retinopathy is the leading cause of blindness "with approximately $500 million spent on direct medical costs" for this disorder in 2004, according to a study in the *Archives of Ophthalmology*. Retinopathy is an umbrella term referring to a number of diseases that affect the retina. Another disturbance of vision is glaucoma, which comes from damage to the optic nerve. The most common form, which accounts for 60 to 70 percent of all glaucoma, is primary open angle glaucoma (POAG). This disease affects more than two million individuals in the US, and it is projected that by 2020 more than three million will have the diagnosis.

A number of studies have linked glaucoma with diabetes, but I will mention only one. A group of researchers at the Massachusetts Eye and Ear Infirmary, Brigham and Women's Hospital, Harvard School of Public Health, and Harvard Medical School got together and looked at detailed records of seventy-six thousand women, who had been enrolled in a study from 1980 to 2000. All the participants were at least forty years of age and without any diagnosis of glaucoma at the start of the study. Researchers found that, after controlling for age, race, hypertension, body mass index, physical activity, alcohol intake, smoking, and family history of glaucoma, they still learned that "type II diabetes was positively associated with POAG."

Physicians who have noted the diabetes/eye problems connection have emphasized that patients have to shift to a healthy lifestyle and diet to reverse or prevent the onset of diabetes before eye complications. Again to mention but one outstanding example, let me refer to physicians Thomas W. Gardner, MD, and Robert Gabbay, MD, of Penn State College of Medicine in Hershey. They have this to say about how to effectively treat these conditions: "Ophthalmologists must go beyond surgically treating late-stage eye disease and work with other clinicians to help patients control their diabetes before eye complications [begin or] worsen." They go on to remark on the need for physicians to acknowledge the diabetes/eye disease link so as to better treat the problem. "Ophthalmologists have a unique opportunity to influence patient behavior because vision loss is one of the most feared complications of diabetes. Helping patients make the connection between their eye disease and the ABCs of diabetes (high A1C, blood pressure and cholesterol [which are common markers of worsening diabetes]) can motivate them to improve their health."

Diabetes, Alzheimer's, and Cognitive Impairment

In my quick survey of symptoms, I noted that diabetes has been linked to nerve disease. Now one of the most terrifying of the neurodegenerative illnesses is Alzheimer's. Patients with this condition gradually lose normal mental function, Alzheimer's impairs an individual's ability to think, speak, and remember. As it progresses, the brain's executive functions are destroyed, resulting in the loss of ability to reason, plan, or organize thoughts, loss of language and inability to recognize objects.

Although the etiology of Alzheimer's is not well understood, it is known to be related to glycation. Let me say something about glycation, which is a primary component of aging. To explain it by a cooking metaphor, imagine putting a turkey in the oven. It is moist and pliable. Three hours later, the skin is stiff, brown and parchment-like. The process that changed the turkey is called glycation. To describe this in a more scientific way, let's say it involves glucose bonding with proteins so that the latter are disabled, leading to the undermining of a number of processes. Glycation is accelerated in the plasma of type II diabetics.

According to the National Diabetes Information Clearinghouse, which is part of the National Institutes of Health, "While many physicians recognize that nerve, eye, kidney, and heart damage are common side effects of diabetes, most are not aware that diabetes can also lead to the formation of damaging substances known as AGEs or advanced glycation end products."

While health-debilitating AGEs are encouraged by diabetes, so is the production of free radicals, which come from unstable molecules or atoms that release electrons, which may then cause cellular damage. AGEs become even more destructive when coupled with free radicals.

According to a study by P. L. Moreira and colleagues, who have looked long and hard at the genesis of Alzheimer's, the disease shows "a marked decline in the level of acetylcholine, the chemical messenger of the nervous system that helps to regulate memory." Not only do free radicals help prompt this decline, "new research indicates that advanced glycation end products may also initiate this dreaded condition." As we've seen, diabetes encourages both glycation and free radical creation.

Whereas this last study looked at the mechanics of Alzheimer's genesis, more anthropologic studies have observed the way in which those who have diabetes seem more prone to this mental disablement. For instance, a 1999 Rotterdam Study in the Netherlands tracked 6,370 elderly men and women over an average of two years, looking at subjects who became demented from Alzheimer's or had diabetes. According to a report by A. Ott, the researchers in the study "concluded that having diabetes almost doubled the subjects' risk of dementia." The conclusions of this report were backed up by research done in 2004 by J. A. Luchsinger and colleagues. It "examined the association between type II diabetes, high insulin levels, and Alzheimer's risk," and found, in line with what we would have expected, "that high insulin levels, which are intimately connected to type II diabetes, were significantly correlated with a higher risk of developing Alzheimer's." The conclusions of this report are supported by the results of a 2004 study which linked high insulin levels, type II diabetes with a significantly higher risk of developing Alzheimer's."

Clearly, the likelihood of developing Alzheimer's is significantly increased in people with insulin problems. It can be speculated that insulin fluctuations damage blood vessels in the brain and this may lead to memory problems associated with the disease. A few other links of diabetes to impaired mental functioning are found in the following research, selected from among many studies I could highlight.

Caroline Sanz, MD, at the French National Institute of Health and Medical Research in Toulouse, led a study that looked at whether people with Alzheimer's disease and diabetes have more rapid memory loss than those who have Alzheimer's disease but not diabetes, using as a base 608 mild to moderate Alzheimer's patients. As reported in the *Science Daily*, "Over the six month testing period, those with diabetes demonstrated significantly more decline [in memory] than their non-diabetic peers."

In another investigation, R. O. Roberts, MB ChB, MS, and his colleagues at the Mayo Clinic in Rochester, Minnesota, examined the associations between diabetes and mild cognitive impairment in patients ages 70 to 89. They reported "diabetes was significantly associated with chronic hyperglycemia (high blood glucose), which in turn [increased] the likelihood of cerebral micro-vascular disease . . . [which may play a role in the development of] neuronal damage, brain atrophy and cognitive impairment."

Lastly, research done by José A. Luchsinger, MD, and colleagues at Columbia University Medical Center suggests that "diabetes could be related to a higher risk for amnesic mild cognitive impairment by directly affecting the buildup of plaques in the brain, a hallmark characteristic of Alzheimer's disease."

Dr. Edward R. Rosick, DO, MPH, acknowledging the many studies that associate type II diabetes with an increased risk of developing Alzheimer's disease, says we may reasonably hope that strategies to prevent or manage insulin resistance and diabetes hold promise in also protecting against Alzheimer's disease.

The Skin Is the Largest Organ—Don't Ignore It

Now let's turn to the common skin disease psoriasis, a non-infectious disorder that leads to a rash and scaly red skin. Research into this condition has also found a link to diabetes.

Dr. Yi Ju Cheng and his colleagues at the Tiachung Veterans General Hospital and National Chung Hsing University in Taiwan make the connection by way of a third party. This is to say they find both diabetes and psoriasis have a common factor in that they both register high levels of leptin (a hormone that can lead to metabolic dysfunction and weight gain). This was why, in their study, when they found "associations among psoriasis and diabetes mellitus," both states showing elevated leptin.

A 2007 complementary study led by Dr. Michael David, a dermatologist at the Rabin Medical Center in Tel Aviv, didn't examine the causes of the two illnesses, but simply noted that there was a higher occurrence of diabetes in psoriasis patients compared to patients without psoriasis. Overall, their observations indicate that as psoriasis becomes more severe in a patient, the likelihood of finding that patient also has diabetes is higher.

When we consider that more than seven million Americans and up to 4 percent of the population worldwide suffers from this skin disorder, it becomes clear that the association of diabetes and the skin condition is an ominous one. This is especially so considering that in addition to its effects on the skin, psoriasis is associated with arthritis, depression and a lower quality of life.

Cancer May Be Just Around the Corner

In the opening of the book, I made mention of the fact that cancer and diabetes are two of the three most common diseases in the US Although people may not know the exact statistics, the majority appreciates that each is a devastating health problem. But most only consider them separately. They are seldom linked together;

however, the relationship between these two disorders is highly significant.

To speak generally, several studies demonstrate that cancer patients who already have diabetes when they get cancer have a greater chance of dying of the disease than cancer patients who do not have the blood sugar disorder. The reason for this increased mortality possibility rests in such factors as that high blood sugar can cause tumors to grow faster; that when a person has diabetes, he or she is automatically at risk for other health problems, such as kidney and heart failure; and the higher susceptibility to infections of diabetic patients may put people at greater risk of death after surgery.

There are many forms of cancer and many links between different versions of the disease and diabetes, so let's just look at a few examples that have been uncovered in recent research.

Pancreatic cancer is significantly higher among individuals who also have a diabetes diagnosis, according to a summary of research published in the *World Journal of Gastroenterology*, which preceded a report of the authors' own research. In this research, the investigators, led by Dr. Jamal at the Veterans Affairs Medical Center, Long Beach, California, looked at incidents of gallbladder, biliary and pancreatic cancer in patients discharged from VA hospitals from 1990 to 2000. They learned that "among patients with type II DM [diabetes], the incidence of pancreatic cancer was increased threefold compared to controls, and gallbladder and extra hepatic biliary cancers were increased by twofold compared to controls."

Another, more specialized study done by looking at pregnant women in Jerusalem from the 1960s to the 1970s, paid attention to those who had gestational diabetes (a situation in which women previously without diabetes exhibit its main symptoms, high blood sugar, during pregnancy). After following these women's histories, the conclusion was that they had a higher risk of developing pancreatic cancer later in life than those without diabetes.

Also looking at women, Dr. Marc Gunter and Howard Strickler, MD, of Albert Einstein College of Medicine in New York, found that breast cancer and high insulin hormone levels are significantly related. A sample of 835 women in the Women's Health Initiative Observational Study who developed breast cancer, contrasted to a randomly selected sample of 816 women in the study who did not develop breast cancer, revealed that women have a much higher risk of developing this cancer if their insulin levels are elevated—a typical accompaniment of diabetes—as compared to women with normal levels of the hormone.

Dr. Ann Cust, a researcher at the University of Melbourne, echoed these findings. Her research led her to the conclusion that women have a much greater likelihood of being diagnosed with advanced breast cancer if they are also type II diabetic.

I could go on and move through the connections of diabetes to other modes of cancer, but I think what has been said so far has already let you see that cancer is another disease which diabetes abets and promotes.

Your Kidneys Are at Risk Too

Where the links between cancer and diabetes are still being looked at—and some scientists might dispute certain of the findings in different areas—the link between diabetes and kidney disease, which is designated diabetic nephropathy, is well established.

According to Dr. Erwin Bottinger, MD, and professor of medicine, pharmacology and biological chemistry, and his colleagues Kaitlin Susztak, MD, professor of medicine at Mount Sinai School of Medicine, and Kumar Sharma, MD, professor of medicine at Thomas Jefferson University, "Diabetic nephropathy is the leading cause of kidney failure worldwide."

These doctors have been looking into how the disease takes action on the kidneys and found that in the cells of kidneys in both humans and mice the glucose binds with proteins there and triggers the death of kidney cells. This establishes another detrimental effect of high blood sugar levels.

Physician Dr. David A. Greenberg of the Columbia Presbyterian Medical Center in New York City and his colleague Maria C. Monti have acknowledged this danger from high blood sugar. They note that "getting blood glucose levels under control is essential for preventing complications from diabetes," such as kidney damage. They warn further that since women seem to be at greater risk than men of such kidney damage, females "need to be more diligent in keeping blood sugar glucose under control."

Pulling the Trigger on Inflammatory and Genetic Markers

We know diabetes is accompanied by inflammation and we also know that inflammation, when prolonged, leads to weakened body metabolism, but the connecting third party, tying together the two unhealthy conditions has not yet been discovered.

Researcher Kathrin Maedler and her colleagues posit that one link is that beta cells in the pancreas, which produce insulin, are failing due to inflammation in the body and this leaves individuals vulnerable to developing type II diabetes.

As we know, type II diabetes is caused by an inability of the beta cell production of insulin to meet the body's needs. Central to this is a loss of beta-cell function as a result of insulin resistance. The authors note, "The more common type II diabetes arises later in life when the body fails to produce enough insulin or grows unresponsive to the hormone. While scientists have floated many ideas, exactly what causes β cell loss in type II diabetes remains a matter of debate." Their team found that inflammation is an important trigger for β cells' destruction. In this, they are indicating a direct pathway from inflammation to diabetes, which gives us one clue as to why the two ill-health conditions appear in tandem.

A second area of linkage with diabetes has been found with some genetic conditions. In fact, as I will look at later, many scientists, those who tend to overlook the influence of lifestyle in the etiology of diseases, will overemphasize the genetic components of diabetes. By contrast, much of the research I look at below suggests that genetics may predispose an individual to get the disease, but only when this predisposition is combined with unhealthy choices, such as lack of exercise, does diabetes actually come to fruition.

Dr. Pamela Itkin-Ansari, professor at the U.C. San Diego School of Medicine; Fred Levine, MD, PhD, director of the Sanford Children's Health Research Center at Burnham, and colleagues in their research into genetics didn't find that certain genes push one toward diabetes, but that the presence of diabetes switches on genes that are normally turned off. In the adult pancreas, there are naturally occurring progenitor cells that have the potential to become insulin producing cells. They are active in a child's early years when the pancreas is in formation but normally inactive later in life.

Dr. Itkin-Ansari noted in the course of research that "Wnt signaling activity, which plays a critical role in the development of the pancreas, re-emerges in type II diabetes." These new cells then would create even more insulin to add to the overabundance of it already in the bloodstream with diabetes.

While this study looked at how certain genetic activity is ignited by diabetes, the new creation of insulin-producing cells, most work on the genetics of diabetes has looked at the ties between the possession of certain genes and a particular proneness to diabetes.

For instance, lead investigator Valeriya Lyssenko from Lund University in Sweden identified one of these genes as TCF7L2. When this gene exists in the pancreatic tissue, there was a decrease in insulin secretion in response to glucose exposure. This would appear to suggest that for people with this gene, insulin response in the pancreas is particularly disturbed by high glucose levels. It can be extrapolated, however, that this insulin disruption would not occur, and so help bring on diabetes, in individuals who guard against high glucose levels by lifestyle modifications, including good eating habits, exercise, stress reduction, and an overall healthy lifestyle.

A decrease in some genes in the skeletal muscle is also associated with type II diabetes. Again, this is an indication that genetic makeup does play some role in this disease. Charlotte Ling and colleagues at Lund University in Sweden "analyzed the expression of one gene NDUFB6 in muscle" and found that its existence did influence "susceptibility to type II diabetes." However, note the orientation of Ling's study. She was examining why not all individuals who are exposed to obesity and reduced physical exercise develop diabetes. In other words, the subjects were ones who had already made bad lifestyle choices, and the focus of her study was angled toward seeing why not all of them got diabetes. She was not looking at genetic influence toward diabetes on those who had healthy lifestyles.

We see that the association between inflammation and diabetes as well as the activation of a genetic potential for diabetes both are encouraged by poor lifestyles and mightily discouraged from expression by natural living.

Open Wide—Diabetes and Oral Health

So far, I have been drawing your attention to health problems that are instigated by or accompany diabetes, but let me now turn it around for a moment and look at a situation where a previous health problem often is a precursor to diabetes. I want to stress that while many people are aware that a few conditions, such as obesity, presage diabetes, few realize that individuals who have periodontal gum disease are also at a higher risk for diabetes. (With this in mind, dentists should consider offering diabetes screenings in their offices.)

Oral health symptoms of diabetics include dry mouth, oral and gum infections, gum disease, and cavities. Commonly with diabetes or pre-diabetes, bacteria in plaque can lead to inflamed gums, which destroy surrounding tissues.

The connection between dental problems and diabetes was zeroed in on by Dr. Shiela Strauss, an associate professor of nursing at NYU's College of Dentistry and Nursing. She reports that "93 percent of subjects [in her study] who had periodontal disease, compared to 63 percent of those without the disease, were considered to be at high risk for diabetes and should be screened for diabetes."

In a separate study led by Dr. Ryan T. Demmer, MPH, associate research scientist in the Department of Epidemiology at the Mailman School of Public Health, nine thousand participants who were free of a diabetes diagnosis at the beginning of the study were evaluated for twenty years. In total, 817 went on to develop diabetes and it was seen that "individuals with elevated levels of periodontal disease were nearly twice as likely to become diabetic in that 20 year time frame."

Similar findings were the result of research that targeted pregnant women and was led by Dr. Ananda P. Dasanayake, professor of epidemiology and heath promotion at NYU College of Dentistry, in collaboration with the Faculty of Dental Sciences at the University of Peradeniya, Sri Lanka. Dr. Dasanayake found that pregnant women with periodontal gum disease have increased risk of gestational diabetes even if they are in otherwise good health. These women did not smoke or drink, yet diabetes occurred significantly.

A couple of alarming findings in the area of oral health and diabetes, beyond what has been said already, are that gum diseases and other dental problems are being found more and more in youth, and that diabetics frequently ignore the need to get good dental care.

First, as to young people, research from Columbia University Medical Center has shown that the destruction of the gums can start in diabetic children as young as six years old. The principal investigators in this study, Ira B. Lamster, DDS, MMSc, dean of the College of Dental Medicine, and Robin Goland, MD, co-director of the Naomi Berrie Diabetes Center, commented that these findings indicate "programs to prevent and treat periodontal disease should be considered a standard of care for young patients with diabetes."

Their research clinically assessed dental cavities and periodontal disease in 182 children and adolescents, ages six to eighteen years old, with diabetes, and 160 non-diabetic control subjects. Goland, Lamster, and their colleagues found that "the children with diabetes had significantly more dental plaque and more gingival inflammation than children without diabetes." To be more specific, early signs of periodontal disease were found in nearly 60 percent of diabetic children in the six to eleven-year-old group, twice the percentage found in the non-diabetic children in that age range.

Common Complications

In discussing Alzheimer's, I mentioned glycation, which I defined as "a process that involves glucose bonding with proteins in a way that disables them." This is such an important activity and brings with it such a train of life-disturbing consequences, even without counting its role in Alzheimer's, that I want to spend a little more time talking about it and some other common complications of diabetes.

To expand on what I said about glycation and AGEs, let me look to the writing of R. R. Kohn and colleagues, who explain, "Glycation occurs when glucose reacts with protein, resulting in sugar-damaged proteins called advanced glycation end products (AGEs)."

They go on to link glycation, which we see is caused by glucose, and so encouraged by a glut of this substance in the blood, with inflammation, which we saw is a state that accompanies diabetes. Further, in this next passage, they show a possible pathway by which diabetes and inflammation may be tied together. "Glycated proteins cause damage to cells in numerous ways, including impairing cellular function, which induces the production of inflammatory cytokines."

Such damage can be cut short by slowing glycation, as has been shown in a number of studies, including research that found "in animal studies, inhibiting glycation protects against damage to the kidney, nerves, and eyes." One examination, led by I. M. Stratton, saw the same positive results with humans. As the researchers reported, "In a large human trial, therapies that resulted in each 1 percent reduction in HbA1c [a prominent AGE] correlated with a 21 percent reduction in risk for any complication of diabetes, a 21 percent reduction in deaths related to diabetes, a 14 percent reduction in heart attack, and a 37 percent reduction in micro-vascular complications."

I have already mentioned the danger of free radicals in the body and noted type II diabetes is linked to the overabundance of these radicals. Let me add that, according to A. M. Vincent and colleagues, "Glycation also produces free radicals that further damage cellular proteins."

On top of that, according to other research, "Diabetes encourages white blood cells to stick to the endothelium, or the thin layer of cells that lines the inside of arteries. These white blood cells cause the local release of pro-inflammatory chemicals that damage the endothelium, accelerating atherosclerosis."

To add to the woes of diabetics, as R. M. Luque and colleagues emphasize, "Insulin itself is a powerful hormone that, in high levels, can inflict damage." As we've seen, the high levels of blood sugar characteristic of diabetes prompt the body to emit into the bloodstream an above-average amount of insulin. This excess insulin has been tied to a number of physical problems, including that "increased levels of insulin contribute to the proliferation of colorectal cells, which suggests that high levels of insulin may be a factor in the development of colorectal cancer."

So far, I have painted a fairly grim picture, both here in describing some of the common complications of diabetes, and in the preceding sections where I looked at many of the other ills that diabetes brings in its wake, such as eye problems, kidney disturbance, and inflammation. Nonetheless, there are steps to be taken to avoid this disaster, which include a combination of improved diet, exercise, and supplementation, as will be explained in detail later on.

More Time in the Hospital

With this raft of side effects and direct effects that precede or occur with diabetes, it should be no shock to you to learn that diabetics have an above-average length of stay in hospitals and seem to fare worse once there than most other patients.

According to Dr. Rehan Ahmad, DO, and her colleagues at Penn State College of Medicine, patients with diabetes (versus non diabetics), who went to the hospital:

- Were more likely to experience complications
- Were more likely to require care in the intensive care unit (ICU)—38.4 percent vs. 35.9 percent
- Stayed in the ICU longer on average (7.6 days vs. 6.1 days)
- Required longer duration on the ventilator (10.8 days vs. 8.4 days)
- Developed more infections (11.3 percent vs. 6.3 percent)
- Were more likely to require home care or nursing care after being discharged
- Had higher mortality rates

These findings were based on a sample of 12,489 patients who were matched on sex and age across twenty-seven trauma centers between 1984 and 2002. According to the authors, "Results from this study confirm that patients with diabetes . . . require a higher level of care, which adds to the cost of hospitalization."

The study did not simply focus on patients who came to the hospital with diabetes or a complication from it, but who are being treated for other illnesses. According to the Ahmad-led research, "These patients develop complications more frequently and do worse after an acute illness than individuals without diabetes. Studies show that diabetics do worse after being hospitalized for stroke, heart attack and heart surgery."

Diabetes and the Latin American Community

Diabetes disproportionately affects certain ethnic groups. In Native Americans, Hispanic and Latino Americans, and African Americans, the disease is much more prevalent than in the non-Hispanic white population. The dubious distinction of the fastest growing ethnic group in America developing diabetes is the Latin American community. Hispanics are almost twice as likely (1.7 times) to develop diabetes as their white counterparts, with Mexican Americans the most affected. Further, Hispanic Americans are more likely to have end-stage renal disease from diabetes and to die from the disease. It appears that Hispanic children are the ones we most have to worry about. In 2010, 38.2 percent of Hispanic children between the ages of two and nineteen were overweight or obese, compared with 31.7 percent of all children on average, according to a study conducted by the Leadership for Healthy Communities in May of 2010. And, what's more alarming, the National Council of La Raza (NCLR) reported last year that one out of two Latino children born in the year of 2000 will develop diabetes!

Why is the Latin community so hard hit? The fundamental problems are obviously at play—eating too much of an unhealthy diet that is largely composed of refined carbyhydrates, fat, salt, and sugar combined with too little or no exercise. But there are other important factors making the situation worse, such as discrimination, poor access to affordable healthy foods, poverty, language barriers, and limited health care access. According to the Leadership for Healthy Communities, Hispanic neighborhoods have only one-third as many supermarkets as more affluent communities, and rely more on convenience stores and convenience foods. Foods that have the most calories per dollar are often "empty calories" that lack important nutrients and contain added sugars and fats. Lower-calorie, perishable products such as fresh produce provide less energy per dollar spent. Since they have eliminated physical education from most public schools and the typical school breakfast and lunch is calorie dense and high fat, parents have no help in trying to keep their kids healthy.

But there may be another reason that Mexican Americans seem to be suffering more than other Hispanic Americans. Thanks to years of globalization and the effects of NAFTA, Mexicans—formerly much healthier than their relatives who emigrated to America—now are experiencing soaring rates of obesity and diabetes is currently that nation's No. 1 killer. Public health experts blame changes in lifestyle that have made Mexicans more obese than any other country in the world with one exception—the United States. As access to healthy fresh vegetables and fruits has disappeared in favor of soft drinks, fat-laden snacks, and loads of sugar, the damage has been profound. Safe water, something we in America take for granted, is not always available in Mexico, so Mexicans usually have a sugar-filled beverage with meals. The average Mexican consumes 728 eight-ounce sugary drinks from Coca-Cola per year, which is even more than in the USA. A 2012 Federal health and nutrition survey found that obesity levels in the last three decades have tripled: 64 percent of men and a shocking 82 percent of women in Mexico are now overweight or obese! An expert in population studies at one of Mexico's most prestigious medical centers, Dr. Abelardo Avila Curiel states that

> "When we project the increase in diabetes and the costs associated with it, the Mexican health system will be overwhelmed. It can't be paid for. By the year 2020, it will be catastrophic. By 2030, it faces collapse."

While the US is still the fattest nation on earth, Mexico now has higher obesity rates among children ages five to eleven years.

As I will repeatedly emphasize through this book, one must take proactive measures to maintain and improve one's health that are based on *full knowledge* of the body and of threats posed to it. So, in laying out all the depressing information in the last few sections, I have not been thinking of making you downcast but of inspiring you by letting you see what you are up against. As one of the strategists in the old Chinese novel *The Three Kingdoms* puts it, "Know your enemy and know yourself. A thousand battles, a thousand victories."

In the following sections, we will see how you can begin obtaining these victories.

Chapter 2

Traditional Approaches to Treatment

The phrase "too much of a good thing" can almost be said of insulin as a medical prescription.

It's no wonder that it was proclaimed a miracle drug when it was introduced in the 1920s. Before that time, diabetic patients had a bleak prognosis. Sufferers saw the condition rapidly go from bad to worse as complications like blindness, gout, and gangrene developed. The overall life span was short.

Then insulin came on the scene. Now children with type I diabetes, who before probably would have only lived months, were living decades. Young people with the illness who might have expected endless time sick in bed, were now living normal and productive lives.

As we saw, insulin is still the primary therapy for type I diabetes. As we also saw, it does not make good sense to indiscriminately give insulin to type II diabetics, since some have sufficient insulin production in their bodies but are not using the hormone efficiently. Injecting insulin into a person who already has sufficient levels not only does nothing to correct the underlying problem—it only gives her or him more insulin that will be blocked from use by the cells— but may bring about unwanted side effects.

Too much insulin in the blood stimulates the development of antagonists in the body that counteract its blood-sugar-lowering effects. Even if it is not acting effectively, the body recognizes that the insulin is pulling all the glucose out of the blood and automatically increases the production of growth hormones and epinephrine, which lift blood sugar levels. In other words, there is a boomerang. Insulin is injected because the blood sugar levels are too high because, it is thought by the doctors, the body lacks insulin. However, since in reality this new insulin is being added to (poorly used) insulin already in the body, the blood sugar levels are brought down too far, so other bodily mechanisms react to increase blood sugar level. The result is the insulin, given to lower glucose, ends up boosting it higher. This is what I called "too much of a good thing."

However, don't get me wrong. Type II diabetes is not usually treated with insulin. Moreover, some cases of the disease do stem from lack of insulin production in the body and so a sufferer of this variation can profit from insulin. Even further, some people with type II are given oral medication, not injections. Some patients mistakenly think they are swallowing a form of insulin. Although insulin may be included in the medications, most of these pills are not a dose of insulin to add to whatever the body is producing, but rather drugs that help your body use the pancreas-created insulin more effectively or stimulate better insulin production.

Of late, new oral medications have been put on the market as treatments for type II diabetes. Unfortunately, as is so often the case with a profit-driven pharmaceutical sector, one whose malfeasances I have exposed on numerous occasions, the rush to get a seemingly

promising drug on the market, where it can generate a quick financial return, often causes a less scrupulous company to cut corners
when it comes to testing the drug. Some of these new oral medications, while beneficial in relation to treating diabetes, have been
found to or suspected of causing side effects—among them, side
effects as serious as heart attacks.

I am not idly speculating here. The drug Rezulin, which was being
used by 500,000 Americans, was pulled from the market in early
2000 after it was linked to 61 deaths and 89 confirmed reports of
liver failure. In my opinion, this was another case of profit trumping
safety.

Blood Sugar Control

So far, from what we have examined, it might be said that traditional medicine only looks at the *output* level of the problem. I'll
explain what I mean in a minute, but first let me mention a study on
levels of glucose in the blood that has direct bearing on my remarks.

Although diabetes can cause a wide variety of health problems,
many of them can be reduced by carefully controlling blood sugar.
We know that problems with insulin production and utilization
create ups and downs in blood sugar, but what about the average
amount of glucose in the blood? If a diabetic, on average, had a high
or low percentage of glucose flowing through her or his veins, will
this affect the disease?

A study completed in 1993, the Diabetes Control and
Complications Trial (DCCT), which was one of the largest studies ever conducted, showed that those diabetic patients with lower
"glycohemaglobin rates," that is, the amount of glucose carried by
the protein (or hemoglobin) in red blood cells, were at less risk for
eye disease than those with a higher amount. To give you the figures,
those with glycohemaglobin rates that averaged 7.1 reduced their
risk by 76 percent compared with the group with glycohemaglobin rates of 8.9 percent. Across the board, diabetics in the intensive

control group (with the 7.1 rate) had a 50 percent reduction in all serious diabetic complications. Although the trial was conducted just on type I diabetics, experts believe the findings are applicable to all diabetics.

Current Dietary Recommendations

Now what does this have to do with the subject of output, which I brought up at the head of the last section? Not using these terms exactly in their usual sense, I would say we can divide the treatment of diabetes into an *output* and *input* approach. Here's how I see it: a person eats food (*input*) and then, as that food breaks down, creating glucose, which insulin (the body's *output*) may have to shepherd through the body if there is too much in the blood.

The traditional practitioner looks only at the output of insulin the body employs to deal with an excess of blood sugar. So this doctor will be concerned with boosting or regulating the insulin levels. But what about *input*, the food we are eating? Is it possible eating the right mix of foods, ones that lower the blood sugar, will reduce the need for insulin? That would seem to be the major implication of DCCT study, which showed that lower blood sugar helped reduce symptoms.

A point I didn't bring out earlier is that the group with the lower blood sugar count in the study was one that was carefully monitored and directed to eat foods that would keep their blood sugar low, while the other group was not so closely watched. As far as the study's results can be extrapolated to other cases, as I believe they can be, we have proof that eating the right foods can help maintain proper blood sugar levels, thus boosting your immune system.

It is not as if traditional medicine was not aware of the importance of diet for diabetics, but greater attention to the subject recently has enabled us to understand the subject in a more nuanced way. In the past, there was one standard diet prescribed for all diabetics. However, that one-size-fits-all outlook has been abandoned and replaced with attention to the individual. Now the American Diabetic Association recommends that diabetics work with experts in diet and nutrition to personalize their diets.

Carbohydrates

New light has also fallen on some of the food groups. Traditionally, all carbohydrates, such as potatoes and bread, were restricted because it was believed that they caused moderate increases in blood sugar. However, it was not seen that a distinction has to be made between different carbohydrates. While some should be as restricted as they have been, others may actually be beneficial to diabetics.

Carbohydrates fall into two categories, simple and complex. The simple ones, found, for example, in candy, fruits, and milk, can be contrasted to the complex ones, found in bread, brown rice, and other foods. Both types of carbohydrates eventually convert into glucose. However, once ingested, simple sugars (from the simple carbs) immediately enter the blood while complex carbohydrates go through a longer process of digestion so they become glucose gradually. They *do not* contribute as radically to high blood sugar levels as simple carbohydrates, which rush into the blood soon after entering the digestive system. Complex carbs stabilize and improve health.

Fat and Protein

Another change in how diabetics' diets are looked at today is that fat and protein are more carefully monitored. It is now said that diabetics who are overweight should keep fat intake to no more than 20 to 25 percent of total calories. My own work would incline me to call for an even more drastic reduction to, say, between 10 and 15 percent of their caloric intake.

Protein intake is another important consideration for diabetics. Earlier I touched on the fact that surges in glucose can cause damage to the blood vessels leading to the kidneys. With these vessels weakened, kidney damage may result. Thus, foods that overtax the kidneys should be avoided so as not to add even more stress to the organ. Now the body cannot store protein, as it stores glucose, for example, so any that enters must be channeled to the kidneys. Too much protein going into the organ puts pressure on the nephron cells, which filter the body's toxins. These two stresses: a heavy protein diet and the damage to the vessels leading to the kidneys, either alone or together, often bring on kidney deterioration in a diabetic, which can only be addressed with dialysis or a kidney transplant. Studies show that the elimination of meat from the diet is often enough to reverse kidney damage since the kidney is no longer taxed with quickly processing all the protein meat puts in the pipeline.

Chapter 3

The Natural Approach

Having scrutinized the causes and symptoms of diabetes and even given some thought to counteractive measures, such as dietary changes, let me make a broader statement about the hope for those with diabetes.

One thing that often distinguishes traditional healers from natural ones is *where they locate their optimism*. Traditional doctors say there is great hope for eliminating or reducing the occurrence of this or that disease, but that hope is located firmly in the future. "In ten years," they say, "we expect a cure for AIDS or cancer, but, well frankly, right now, there's not much hope." Natural healers like myself like to shorten any given timeframe. I believe startling improvements can be made today.

Technically speaking we are repeatedly told there is no cure for diabetes; however, it has been my experience as well as that of many physicians that some patients are able *through a major change in their lifestyle,* including change of diet, to eliminate the symptoms of diabetes. A healthy lifestyle and alternative approaches to treatment in many cases can decrease the amount of insulin or oral medications needed (although type I diabetics will need to continue taking insulin).

The natural approach aims at making lifestyle choices—not medication—the center of the program, though this does not mean in every individual case drug use will be greatly reduced or eliminated. The goal of treatment is to build up the body's ability to function as independently as possible, so that, for example, blood sugar levels are kept low through proper diet.

This will not be accomplished overnight. Indeed, part of the natural approach is (generally) to avoid radical changes and opt for gradual transitions. A diabetic who moves from a totally traditional to an alternative approach should never immediately discontinue any diabetic medication. Instead, this patient should work closely with a physician, who would assist in a gradual transition. With this doctor's guidance, medication may be reduced or completely eliminated as the individual case permits.

The new program, which the patient making the transition will be entering, is one that combines exercise and dietary modification. These new regimens, aiming at better nutrition and at weight loss, will be the center of the plan, with medications as supplementary components, all helping the patient move to better health. This sort of program is less invasive than traditional ones that make drugs the major factor and put lifestyle changes in the background.

We need to acknowledge right off that this approach does not solve all problems or eliminate all traces of the disease. Still, while type II diabetics respond most dramatically to alternative approaches, even type I diabetics may be able to reduce their insulin dependency. More importantly, they are able to alleviate many of the dangerous complications that have come to be thought of as intrinsic to diabetes.

Diet

So let's get to work.

The rest of the book will give more information on diet, exercise and other important factors that play a role in an alternative approach to handling diabetes. You will get this data both via my own recommendations and by listening to the words of holistic healers who have made a special study of the disease.

I will begin by making some brief remarks on exercise and diet (to be expanded later in the course of the book) and then I will look at vitamins, minerals, herbs and other dietary supplements that have been shown to be efficacious in alleviating some of the effects of the disease.

Diet first. Years ago, Dean Ornish laid out a heart-right diet that was targeted at eliminating the bad foods that make one liable to develop heart disease. Since diabetes and heart disease are so closely related—both, for example, connected to a weakened circulatory system—many physicians, including Robert Atkins, have recommended that diabetics follow this Ornish program. The central tenet of Ornish's diet was to cut down on dietary fats. For him, the best diet would be one that emphasized high-fiber vegetables, either eaten raw, steamed, baked or stir-fried with little or no oil.

A moment ago I divided carbohydrates into simple and complex, underlining the difference in the body's use of the two. One thing that should have been taken away from that discussion, beyond what was explicitly said, is that, since diabetes is a disease caused by difficulties controlling glucose and all carbs break down into glucose, then the diabetic must be highly aware of his or her carb intake.

In line with this, many recommend completely eliminating, at least at the first stage of combating the disease, carbohydrates such as: bread, pasta, potatoes, rice, corn, parsnips, bananas, raisins, and other sweet fruits and vegetables. Note, I am simplifying for the moment, since some of the forbidden foods, such as bread, actually fall into different categories depending on the type. Moreover, many complex carbohydrates, including beans, grains, legumes, should be kept in the diet, and are contained in the recipes later in the book.

As to protein intake, I've already stated that gauging this is also extremely important given the negative impact excess protein can have on the kidneys. If I listened simply to my own inclinations, I would tell every diabetic, "Just go vegetarian," but I am aware that for the majority of diabetics this would probably pose a major challenge, something they may envision as possible in the future, but not now, since they can't wean themselves away from meat so drastically. Even so, these patients can take steps in the right direction by eating only organic, free-range animals, whether turkey, chicken, beef or non-farm-raised fish.

Having mentioned that monitoring carbs and protein in the diet are key to turning around your health, let me throw in a handy formula that many practitioners use as a way to think about the proper relation between food types eaten. This formula puts the acceptable ratio of complex carbohydrates to proteins to fats as 50:30:20.

I've been generalizing up to this point in discussing diet, but I haven't forgotten my earlier point that one of the hallmarks of new healing strategies is individualizing diet plans. A diabetic's personal eating regimen is something that has to be charted by the patient and a nutritionist working together. The way a healthy diet can be found for an individual diabetic is something that Dr. Atkins described in the following passage:

> It is important to know who needs carbohydrate restriction versus who needs fat restriction. To determine that, there are a variety of tests, including a cholesterol profile in which we look at the ratio between the triglycerides [a component of fats] and the HDL [high-density lipoprotein, which carry fats in the blood].

> By looking at this ratio, which tells the doctor whether the patient has high cholesterol, and at other tests, the physician can decide if there is more danger from glucose, thus demanding carb limitation, or from cholesterol, calling for fat reduction. After determining where changes have to be made, it is perfectly appropriate to spend five

or six weeks on one diet and then get all of your parameters checked again, and then spend five or six weeks on the other diet and then get them checked again. In that way, you can make an intelligent decision.

Atkins's comments should be taken not only as a presentation of how a doctor can work with a patient to arrive at the optimum diet, but should also alert the reader to a broader truth. As is the nature of a health book, this one will speak in generalities, making remarks that point you in the right direction, but it cannot lay out your individual path to wellness. That is something that, using this text for its wealth of pointers, must be arrived at as you (with a holistic practitioner working beside you) clear your own trail.

Allergy Testing

Since we are on the topic of food, let's return to my point, made in a discussion of the etiology of the disease, where I said the type II diabetes patient body's characteristic resistance to insulin may be due to an allergy. Testing for food allergies can help determine which foods are responsible for the insulin resistance.

To determine whether a specific food is causing hyperglycemia—a condition in which blood sugar is abnormally high, and which could be and is commonly brought on by diabetes, though it may have other causes—a doctor can monitor a patient's blood sugar before and after that food is eaten. The doctor will be on the lookout for sudden upward spikes in blood sugar, indicating the patient is allergic to the associated food.

Once allergy-provoking substances are identified and omitted, a patient with insulin resistance can often reverse his or her condition. Since the reactive food or foods are blocking insulin uptake, the patient who has dropped those foods can usually be weaned from insulin. This patient will also tend to lose weight, since he or she put on the pounds because of a craving for the allergy-producers. As with any addiction, such as that of cigarette smokers for their nicotine, after sufficient time has gone by, and a person's health improves, the desire for the once-craved substance abates. In fact, more often than not, the person who has dropped the food substance to which he or she was allergic, on now seeing a serving of that food on someone else's plate, says to him or herself, "What was I thinking when I ate that?"

Exercise

Now let's look at exercise.

Most people know exercise is good for your heart, since it gets the blood pumping, stimulating and improving oxygen intake and circulation. They also know that exercise is a weight-reducing strategy since the strenuous activity burns calories. What fewer people know is that exercise also heightens the body's sensitivity to insulin.

Remember earlier when talking about the causes of type II diabetes, I brought up that this often involves poor absorption of insulin by cells whose entrances are clogged. It may be cholesterol that is doing the clogging, and by lowering cholesterol, exercise makes cells more available for glucose assimilation. The exact mechanism that links exercise to this lowering is not fully understood, although it probably involves exercise increasing the production of certain enzymes that move cholesterol to the liver for excretion. What is established is that exercise brings down cholesterol levels, which helps with better insulin usage. This is why the insulin requirements of diabetic athletes usually drop while they are engaged in swimming, soccer, and other sports. Conversely, athletes notice an increase in their insulin requirements when they cease their physical activities for any extended period.

Athletes are not the only ones who can benefit from exercise. While we have seen that exercise reduces cholesterol, making insulin use more effective, a bout of exercise after meals will lessen the need for insulin by lowering blood sugar. Ten to twenty minutes of light exercise will have this effect. A brisk walk, for example, gets the body metabolism working a little bit faster so that the absorption of food becomes more efficient. That prevents blood sugar from rising too high.

Note though, an exception to the exercise-after-meals rule must be made for diabetics with heart disease. In these patients, the exercise immediately after eating may precipitate an angina attack, because blood needed for digestion in the intestines is too quickly transferred to the legs and other parts of the body that use it in the exercise.

Protocol

In addition to diet and exercise (already mentioned), and detoxification and stress management (to be touched on later), I would now like to lay out a vitamin, mineral and herbal supplement protocol, which is designed to improve blood sugar and take control of diabetes.

For type II diabetics, this plan of attack is to be accomplished, in part, through strengthening the thyroid, whose secretions regulate the overall metabolic rate (the speed of chemical reactions in the body); boosting the adrenal glands that need to work efficiently since they produces cortisone, which can raise or lower blood sugar; and detoxifying the liver, which we saw is often damaged in diabetics. By doing this, the long-term effects of chronically high blood sugar (which include high blood pressure, stroke, heart disease, neuropathies, eye problems, circulatory problems, and kidney disease) can be not only contained, but reduced.

I will begin by simply providing a list of the different vitamins, minerals and supplements I have found valuable. Then I will go through the list's varied components, one by one, noting each's benefits and effects. Here is the protocol:

Chromium Picolinate	200 mcg 2–3×/day
Vitamin C	1,000 mg 5×/day
Biotin	500 mcg
Vitamin B6	100 mg
Vitamin B12	1,000 mcg
Vitamin E	400 mg gamma tocopherol 2×/day
Calcium Citrate	1,000 mg
Magnesium Citrate	1,000 mg
Potassium	200 mg
Manganese	15 mg
Zinc	30 mg
Selenium	200 mcg
Quercetin	1,000 mg 2×/day
EFAs	3,000 mg/day
GLA	500 mg 2×/day
L-Carnitine	500 mg 2×/day
Inositol	500 mg
L-Glutamine	follow directions
Vanadyl Sulfate	follow directions
B Complex	50 mg
Garlic	1,000 mg 2×/day
Bitter Melon	100 mg
Gymnema syvestre	follow directions
Ginseng	100 mg
Aloe Vera	3 tsp/day
Alpha Lipoic Acid	600 mg
Grape Seed Extract	200 mg 3×/day
NAC	500 mg 2×/day
Coenzyme Q10	300 mg 3×/day
Turmeric	100 mg
Dandelion Extract	follow directions
Evening Primrose Oil	1,000 mcg
Sea Vegetable Powder	follow directions

Maitake Complex	follow directions
Proteolytic Enzymes	follow directions
Fiber Complex	Your diet should have 30–50 g of fiber a day; if not, have 15 grams with a beverage at night
R-Lipoic Acid	210–420 mg daily
Carnosine	500 mg 2×/day
DHEA	15–75 mg early in the day, followed by blood testing after 3–6 weeks to ensure optimal levels
EPA/DHA	1,400 mg ePa and 1000 mg dHa daily
Silymarin	containing 900 mg silybum marianum standardized to 80 percent silymarin, 30 percent silibinin, and 4.5 percent isosilybin b
Green Tea Extract	725 mg green tea extract (minimum 93 percent polyphenols)
Ginkgo Biloba	120 mg daily
Bilberry Extract	100 mg daily
Cinnamon Extract	125 mg Cinnamomum cassia standardized to .95 percent trimeric and tetrameric a-type polymers (1.2 mg) 3×/day
Coffee Berry Extract	100 mg (Coffee arabica) extract (whole fruit) standardized to 50 percent total phenolic acids (50 mg) and 15,000 micromoles per gram oraC, 3×/day

Supplements/Herbs

In addition to this protocol, also consider the following dietary recommendations:

- Chlorophyll drinks throughout the day
- Complex carbohydrates, such as lentils, peas, steel-cut oatmeal, whole grain pasta, and brown rice

- Raw and cooked vegetables. Carrots, beets, and corn are high glycemic foods; keep them to a minimum. Watermelon, blueberries and apples have a lower glycemic index.
- Consume 3–4 servings of protein/day (soy, fish, grains and beans, quinoa, protein shakes)
- Bean pod tea, which tonifies the kidneys and adrenal glands

This protocol was designed to utilize a range of supplements that improve blood sugar control or limit damage due to diabetes. Let's take them one by one. I will look particularly at scientific research that has linked the use of these varied substances to improvement in one or more debilitating conditions brought on by diabetes.

Chromium Picolinate

Chromium is an essential trace mineral that plays a major role in moving glucose through its metabolic processes, which include being broken down from an ingested food and transferred to a cell. Scientific studies have shown that chromium picolinate helps people with type II diabetes control blood sugar levels and enhances use of proteins, carbohydrates and lipids. Given in higher doses, it aids such patients by increasing insulin sensitivity, which helps glucose enter cells and so lowers blood sugar levels.

Vitamin C

The value of vitamin C and its remarkable powers in aiding the immune system and promoting health have been attested to so often that it will not come as a surprise to any health conscious person that I have put C in my diabetes protocol. What I want to call attention to now is, first, its value in counteracting diabetes-caused eye problems.

The aqueous humor of the eye supplies its adjacent areas with vitamin C. As we've learned, in diabetes insulin is not functioning properly to move glucose out of the blood. The excess glucose in circulation may inhibit vitamin C uptake, and so the aqueous humor's protective role, which depends on vitamin C distribution, may be thwarted. Supplementing with vitamin C will supply this missing element and improve eye health.

It should also be noted that taking vitamin C in mega-doses may lessen the negative effects of glycation (which I will discuss more thoroughly below in the section on vitamin B6). Vitamin C also alleviates other negative conditions through its enhancement of bodily activities. By improving blood flow and decreasing inflammation, for example, it is a blessing to diabetics with coronary artery disease. It also lowers blood pressure and improves blood vessel elasticity.

Biotin

As we've seen, diabetics have trouble moving glucose out of the blood into storage places in the cells. One place where glucose is kept is the liver. Here is where biotin comes in. Biotin boosts insulin sensitivity and increases the activity of the enzyme responsible for the first step in the utilization of glucose by the liver. This and other values of the vitamin have been shown in experiments on animals that indicate a high biotin diet may improve glucose tolerance and enhance insulin secretion.

Vitamin B6

A moment ago, in discussing vitamin C, its battle against glycation was mentioned without much explanation. For some reason, glycation is accelerated in the plasma of type II diabetics. Vitamin B6 is one of the most effective anti-glycating agents known. The main form of B6 is pyridoxine.

Vitamin B12

Another marker of disease that is present in diabetics is heightened homocysteine levels. Homocysteine is an amino acid whose presence in high levels in the body has been associated with cardiovascular disease. One example of this correlation was found in Japanese studies that reveal those with non-insulin-dependent diabetes, who have blood vessel problems, also have elevated homocysteine. When given 1,000 micrograms of vitamin B12 on a daily basis for three weeks, the patients in one study saw their homocysteine levels fall precipitously.

Vitamin E

While all the vitamins and minerals discussed thus far are effective in reducing the ravages of diabetes, vitamin E not only improves the health of diabetes sufferers but its lack in the body has been linked to the disease's occurrence. This last point was developed in a study in the *British Medical Journal,* which found that below-average vitamin E levels were associated with a 390 percent increased risk of developing type II diabetes.

This vitamin also registers a positive impact on persons who already have diabetes. A study in *Diabetes Care* demonstrated that just one month of vitamin E administration reduced protein glycosylation. Glycosylation, which is an enzymatic process of linking proteins and other compounds, can be benign, but can also interfere with normal cellular processes.

The most common form of vitamin E is alpha tocopherol. However, we have found that gamma, mixed tocopherols, and a full range of tocotrienols are more beneficial for diabetes.

Calcium Citrate

Another chemical, calcium citrate, which is a form of citric acid, is, like vitamin E, of value in reducing the likelihood of becoming diabetic. Scientists have found that the high intake of calcium citrate along with vitamin D3, and vitamin D3 especially from supplementation, can decrease the risk of diabetes by 33 percent.

Magnesium Citrate

Diabetics frequently are deficient in magnesium, either as the result of medications or disease. One double-blind, placebo-controlled study revealed the downside of this deficiency. When the patients took magnesium supplements, this helped with their control of blood sugar, so its lack in diabetics is part of the reason for their imperfect blood sugar control.

Potassium

We've seen that the keystone of diabetes is problems with availability of or the body's ability to use insulin. That is why potassium is so crucial. Studies show that potassium improves insulin secretion, sensitivity and responsiveness. And this counters the effects of insulin injection, which induces potassium loss. A high potassium intake also reduces the risk of heart disease, atherosclerosis, and cancer.

Manganese

In discussing the value of B6, I brought up its counteraction against glycation, a process that accelerates aging. Another key contributor to the deterioration normally associated with aging is the presence of free radicals, unbalanced cells or molecules that disrupt biological functions. Increased free radical production has been found in diabetics.

Manganese is a component of the antioxidant enzyme called manganese super oxide dismutase (Mn-SOD). All antioxidants destroy free radicals.

A second benefit of manganese is found in its reduction of the threat of arteriosclerosis. LDL cholesterol poses a great danger to the blood vessels, gumming them up with plaque, and thus promoting constricted blood flow, which can lead to heart attack or stroke. However cholesterol is a threat not in its natural but in its oxidized form. A study reported that diabetics with higher blood levels of manganese were better protected from the oxidation of LDL cholesterol than individuals with less manganese.

Zinc

I noted earlier that women are more susceptible than men to the dangers of diabetes. As far as studies have looked into this, they have shown that increased zinc intake is connected to a reduced risk of type II diabetes in women.

Selenium

A moment ago, in discussing the value of manganese, I alluded to the danger of free radicals, which interfere with organic processes and are viewed by many as key promoters of aging. The term "oxidative stress" refers to the results of an assault of an overabundance of free radicals on the body. One study of this stress in diabetics, though, in this case the subjects were mice not humans, found that selenium is a major factor in reducing the oxidative stress related to the disease.

Quercetin

I need to say one more thing about free radicals. mini Oxidation is a chemical reaction in the body that, like glycosylation, mentioned earlier, can be benign. However, it can also release free radicals. Antioxidants reduce oxidative reactions in the body and so forestall the creation of these radicals.

Flavonoids, organic compounds derived from plants, are antioxidants that reduce the harm associated with diabetes. Quercetin, a powerful flavonoid, decreases levels of blood glucose and oxidants. Thus it battles against a chief feature of diabetes, excessive blood sugar, and of more general bodily distress, the presence of oxidants, which promote free radicals. In addition, quercetin normalizes the levels of the following antioxidants: vitamin C, superoxide dismutase, and vitamin E.

EFAs (Essential Fatty Acids)

Anyone who has been reading closely through this annotated list will be getting further confirmation of the fact, brought out in the introduction, that diabetes is closely linked to many adverse states such as stroke and heart disease.

I mentioned earlier that manganese reduces the oxidation of LDL cholesterol, and that this oxidized form of cholesterol is the one associated with hardening of the arteries and related diseases. Another compound that has been tied to arteriosclerosis, along with LDL cholesterol, is triglyceride. Human studies demonstrate that omega-3 fatty acids decreased triglyceride levels, as well as reducing blood pressure.

It is also good to know that, according to animal studies, these worthy omega-3 fatty acids do not cause as much weight gain as other fats. They have no effect on LDLs, but do increase HDL, so-called "good cholesterol."

GLA

Since it has been established that diabetes and cardiovascular disease are closely linked, it is an especially encouraging note to see that GLA aids in combating both. The positive impact of GLA (and DHA) on the cardiovascular system have been well-documented, seen in modest, though steady declines in blood pressure and considerable decreases in serum lipids. It also has a beneficial role in decreasing cellular insulin resistance. While the first benefit mentioned, reducing blood pressure, relates to lowering the risk of heart disease, the last is more directly helpful to diabetics in that, as we've learned, insulin resistance is a major factor in the growth of diabetes.

L-Carnitine

Supplementation with L-carnitine is especially valuable as it can improve insulin sensitivity in those with type II diabetes. Carnitine, along with CoQ10 and NADH, also fights against heart disease by enhancing energy uptake in the heart muscle.

Inositol

A number of scientific studies have shown that inositol, a naturally occurring substance found both in the human cells and in vegetable fiber, is a powerful anti-cancer agent. More recently, however, it has been shown to also be an asset in the fight against type II diabetes. A large number of studies are suggesting inositol is key in regulating healthy insulin production, and, as we know, when this production goes awry, diabetes is the likely outcome.

L-Glutamine

Another study with mice looked simultaneously at diabetes and obesity. This study with rodents prone to obesity and diabetes reported that, after supplementing for one week with L-glutamine, the mice had a minimum 5 percent reduction in body weight and normalized insulin levels.

Vanadyl Sulfate

I noted earlier that insulin injection, while necessary for those with type I diabetes, when used by those with type II can sometimes be counterproductive. I discussed that this use of added insulin can often be reduced or avoided, but I didn't mention an interesting fact, which is that the chemical vanadyl sulfate mimics insulin.

Vanadium, the basic form of vanadyl sulfate, which works particularly with the muscles, and so is also of interest to bodybuilders, is believed to assist in the transfer of sugar in the blood (glucose) into muscles, just as insulin does. In addition, scientists believe it can increase insulin sensitivity in the muscles. These combined effects may show diabetics a natural way to lower blood sugar, decrease their insulin intake, and, perhaps, stop using insulin.

B Complex

The value of the vitamin B complex—a group of vitamins that includes thiamine, riboflavin, niacin, B-6, folate, B-12, pantothenic acid, biotin, and choline—in helping the body fight diseases has been so well documented in many books, that here I will simply underline its main features, which are that B complex reduces cholesterol and blood fat, both of great benefit to the diabetic.

Garlic

Throughout this book, we've seen that interconnectedness of diabetes with many other diseases. Garlic or, more precisely, its active ingredient allium, helps with a whole slew of these related health problems. Studies indicate it reduces the chance of cardiovascular disease as well as lowering oxidative stress and blood pressure. Animal studies have noted that allium promotes weight loss and insulin sensitivity.

Bitter Melon

Another all-purpose agent is bitter melon. In this case, it is not that it combats so many connected diseases, but that it works on both type I (insulin dependent) and type II (adult-onset) diabetes. For type II sufferers, bitter melon works by reducing insulin resistance, but it is beneficial to diabetics of both types due to its ability to lower and maintain proper levels of blood sugar.

Gymnema Syvestre

Obviously, animal trials with drugs, vitamins and supplements are a first stage of determining the efficacy of the substance. Once any chemical has proven its value in treating animals, it will ideally be tested on humans. Gymnema has been tested particularly on mice, and its results with them have been most promising indeed.

In rat trials, gymnema supported healthy blood sugar levels. These levels in normal and diabetic rats were lowered two hours after oral administration of a gymnema concentrate. Moreover, gymnema corrected hyperglycemia in mild diabetic rats, and considerably extended the lifespan of severely diabetic rats. Hopefully, studies with humans will confirm the importance of gymnema as an anti-diabetic agent.

Ginseng

A recent study by researchers from the University of Chicago that was published in *Diabetes* argues that an extract from the ginseng root could be an effective part of an overall treatment regimen for diabetes and obesity. They found that a ginseng extract normalized blood glucose levels, improved insulin sensitivity, and lowered weight.

Aloe Vera

Aloe vera, which many people will recognize as an additive to natural shampoos and skincare products, also has been shown to play a role in fighting diabetes. Studies indicate that it can lower glucose among type II diabetics. A particularly illuminating investigation reported that aloe vera, given to non-insulin dependent diabetics over a 14-week period, reduced blood sugar levels by 45 percent, on average.

Alpha Lipoic Acid

Like garlic, alpha lipoic acid combats many of the negative accompaniments of diabetes. It positively affects the control of blood sugar, lowering blood sugar levels, while helping fight off the development of long-term complications that can damage the heart and kidneys. As an antioxidant, it kills free radicals, helping to reduce pain, burning, itching, tingling, and numbness in people who have nerve damage caused by diabetes (called peripheral neuropathy). This last facet of the substance was established by a study that indicated treating diabetics with 600 mg/day of alpha lipoic acid for three weeks significantly reduced the symptoms of diabetic peripheral neuropathy. Lipoic acid also reduces fat accumulation, which will forestall the acquisition of diabetes in the first place.

Grape Seed Extract

In a landmark study, French researchers decided to see what would happen if they fed rodents a diet that contained 60 percent fructose. Not surprisingly, the rodents suffered a disastrous decline in health. Blood pressure shot through the roof, free radicals sped up, and the heart enlarged. However, the study was not conceived as a way to torment the animals, but to see what supplements could counteract these rapidly declining health conditions.

By study's end, all the negative effects of this diet were brought under control by a variety of the components of grapes. Anthocyanin, a part of the grape's skin, prevented heart enlargement and high blood pressure. Procyanidins, found in the seed portion, had a positive impact on triglycerides, and all the parts of the grape blocked free radicals. The application to the present subject is clear in that many of the rodents' symptoms of ill health, such as the presence of free radicals and high blood pressure, also accompany diabetes. This and other studies suggest the value of grape seed extracts in fighting the disease.

NAC

We must press forward into human studies with many of these compounds, but again with N-acetylcysteine, a powerful antioxidant, animal studies are the best we have. And they tell an encouraging story. In studies involving diabetic rats, NAC protected the heart from endothelial damage and oxidative stress, two conditions closely associated with heart attacks among diabetics. In another examination, NAC increased nitric oxide in diabetic rats, and this improved blood pressure and reduced oxidative stress levels in their hearts.

Coenzyme Q10

Coenzyme Q10 (CoQ10), like vitamin C, is another miracle worker. It is something of a Renaissance chemical in that it not only helps control blood sugar, but decreases blood pressure and reduces oxidative damage that is the result of diabetes.

Here human experiments have been done. In a trial involving type II diabetics, who took 100 mg of CoQ10 twice a day, there was a marked improvement in glucose levels. In another study, again of type II patients, CoQ10 increased blood flow.

Shifting to animal studies, in these we find CoQ10 again acting multi-purposely, killing free radicals, enhancing blood flow, decreasing triglyceride levels, and elevating HDL levels.

Turmeric

Where aloe vera is found in many beauty care products, turmeric is common in food. It is an Asian spice mixed in many curries, that is known to reduce inflammation, heal wounds, and ease pain.

Inflammation has not been mentioned thus far but, to say a word about it, it has come to the attention of scientists recently that type II diabetes interferes with cytokines, agents of the immune system that cause inflammation. Moreover, it has been seen that these imbalances and the inflammation they spur are particularly prevalent in the obese.

Animal studies have suggested that turmeric can both reduce the likelihood of the occurrence of adult-onset diabetes as well as the inflammation that is associated with it. Researchers from Columbia University found that mice treated with turmeric were less susceptible to developing Type II diabetes In addition, they came to learn that obese mice given turmeric reported considerably reduced inflammation in their liver and fat tissue as measured against the controls, who were not given the spice. These scientists hypothesized that the curcumin—the active, anti-inflammatory, antioxidant component in turmeric—interferes with the inflammatory response caused by obesity. With lowered inflammation, insulin resistance was also reduced and thus type II diabetes discouraged.

Dandelion Extract

While type II diabetics have too much glucose in their blood because cells are resisting the insulin that would shepherd the excess glucose into them and out of the blood, dandelion, with its active compound inulin, works against this effect of diabetes by trapping glucose molecules, stopping them from reaching high concentrations in the blood. Reports indicate that dandelion extracts reduce blood sugar levels by as much as 20 percent in a short period of time.

Evening Primrose Oil

Our brief examination of alpha lipoic acid noted that it counteracted the nerve damage associated with the progression of diabetes. Such nerve disturbance can hurt the feet, hands and other body parts. Evening primrose oil is also an effective agent in the battle to alleviate nerve injury.

An eye-opening study done to look at this particular problem looked at over 100 patients with mild nerve damage from diabetes. They were given six capsules of gamma-linolenic acid—this is the effective agent found in the evening primrose—twice daily for a year. The control group was given a placebo. Sixteen measures of nerve function were charted. The group on gamma-linolenic acid improved in every category. In thirteen of the sixteen measures, the improvement was significant. This is convincing evidence of the value of this supplement.

Sea Vegetable Powder

When you think of sea vegetables, probably the first one that comes to mind is kelp, which grows in giant "forests" under the sea. Kelp is a rich source of iodine, but so are the other sea vegetables.

In the lead-up to this protocol list, I noted that some of the items on it strengthen the thyroid, which is an important benefit in that the thyroid regulates the body's overall metabolism. Any dysfunction in the thyroid will mess up the body's functioning big time. Sea vegetables play a role here in that they are rich sources of iodine, and this substance works to prevent thyroid diseases.

Obviously, a body with a weakened thyroid will not be in an optimal place to combat diabetes and its related conditions, and so the iodine in sea vegetables is crucial here. Further, a diet that includes sea vegetables will benefit persons who have atherosclerosis or heart disease induced by diabetes.

Maitake Complex

Another medicinal food among the compounds on this list is maitake, a mushroom that has been used extensively in traditional Japanese and Chinese medicine. If the Asians got there first, in terms of learning of this plant's benefits, Western doctors now recognize it as a booster of the immune system. It has been useful in treating diabetes, high blood pressure, cholesterol, and obesity.

Proteolytic Enzymes

Enzymes are the body's catalysts, which promote specific chemical reactions, such as breaking down foods into usable components. The proteolytic enzymes, the major type, are ones that control reactions that govern proteins. Some natural health practitioners recommend taking them after meals to aid digestion. This is an efficient manner of getting enzymes into the diet. However, a lesser-known value of the proteolytic enzymes is that they reduce the inflammation connected with diabetes. That is why I am calling attention to them here.

Fiber Complex

Another substance that is well known in one of its properties is fiber. Older people are well aware that fiber promotes good digestion. However, like the just-mentioned proteolytic enzymes, fiber also has a less-known side. Taking sufficient amounts of fiber prevents and decreases the dangers caused by constantly elevated blood glucose. Its value in this respect was indicated by a study in which diabetics consumed 25 grams of soluble fiber and 25 grams of insoluble fiber daily. This high-fiber diet decreased blood glucose levels by an average 10 percent. Now, you've got another reason to put this in your diet.

R-Lipoic Acid

R-lipoic acid is another superhero among supplements, since it has a number of "superpowers." For one, it is a potent antioxidant. It enhances glucose uptake, the very thing that is wounded by diabetes, and resists glycoslylation, a process whose downside has already been noted. It also has anti-inflammation properties. The dangers of low-grade, constant inflammations in the body will be explored later in the book.

Carnosine

The antioxidant carnosine inhibits glycation, which we've seen disables proteins, and has demonstrated protective effects against diabetes-induced kidney damage.

DHEA

DHEA, a naturally occurring steroid that is produced by the adrenal glands, has some reported effects on reducing cholesterol and abating depression, although these effects are still under study. One valuable experiment was a six-month investigation of elderly people, who were given DHEA, with the end result that they significantly reduced abdominal fat and improved insulin action.

EPA/DHA

Earlier in this list, we mentioned the value of EFAs, essential fatty acids, which we saw decreased triglyceride levels and reduced blood pressure. We also learned in that section that EFAs do not cause as much weight gain, and they increase HDL, the "good cholesterol."

I now want to signal the special benefits of one particular fatty acid, DHA, which is helpful to diabetes sufferers who also are plagued by obesity. A study looked at overweight patients, who were started on DHEA, which they took daily for three months. Then this dosage was supplemented with DHA (docosahexaenoic acid), one of the fatty acids found in fish oil, and in many cases there was a significant improvement in the level of insulin sensitivity.

Silymarin

By this time, you may have seen through the method behind my protocol. Some of the recommended substances work all-around attacking diabetes and its accompanying illnesses, while others are poised to alleviate only one of the areas of stress. Silymarin is particularly pertinent in that it protects the liver. The extract from milk thistle, silymarin, has as its most active compound silibinin. It enhances the liver's control of glucose as well as decreasing the free radicals that could bring about liver damage.

Green Tea Extract

Without covering what I have discussed in other works, let me just say briefly that nature is a storehouse of invaluable medicines, and many of the most famous, scientifically "discovered" wonder drugs are, in fact, plant derivatives. In green tea, the special derivative is epigallocatechins, which may well have a major part to play in preventing diabetes. While all its effectiveness may not be due to this compound, we also know that green tea extract suppresses diet-induced obesity and acts as a potent antioxidant, while blocking processes that would injure the pancreas and liver.

Ginkgo Biloba

Studies of ginkgo biloba have progressed beyond experiments on rodents up to human subjects and produced encouraging results in both cases. In animal studies, it was learned that ginkgo improved glucose metabolism in muscle fibers. Other tests on animals indicated that the ginkgo biloba brought down post-meal sugar levels. Not only did it, thus, strike at the root of the diabetes problem, which resides in excess glucose in the blood, but ginkgo has been found to fight the symptoms in that it prevented diabetic retinopathy (an eye disease) in rats with diabetes.

Turning to human studies, let me note one in which type II diabetics were given 120 mg of ginkgo for three months. The subjects experienced enhanced liver functioning in relation to usage of insulin and oral hypoglycemic drugs, which was connected to a reduction in blood glucose levels.

Bilberry Extract

As with ginkgo, bilberry extract has been given a trial of its healing components with both animal and human subjects. Diabetic mice given a herbal extract with bilberry showed a significant lowering of their blood glucose. Humans with retinopathy (damage to the retina often caused by diabetes), who as part of a scientific study were given bilberry, were found to have decreased vascular permeability (blood leaking from the vessels) and reduced hemorrhage.

Cinnamon Extract

As with quite a number of the supplements profiled already in this protocol, a well-known substance, here cinnamon, contains within its chemical architecture one or more vital, health-enhancing substances. A study performed at the US Department of Agriculture's Beltsville Human Nutrition Research Center isolated insulin-enhancing complexes in cinnamon. These are involved in preventing or alleviating glucose intolerance and diabetes. Once again something from the plant world—cinnamon is obtained from bark—is revealing more about nature's medical bounty.

Coffee Berry Extract

I've mentioned tea so I also have to mention coffee, which also has health-enhancing properties. I'm referring to the entire fruit, not only the bean or seed. The fruit is chock full of advantageous antioxidants, which, as we know, forestall the creation of deadly free radicals.

Additional Supplements

While I have not made these part of my diabetes protocol, let me mention also a few herbs that contain phytochemcials, compounds that have a positive effect on health. All these herbs have either "anti-diabetic" properties or promote insulin production naturally.

Herbs

Cichorium intybus (chicory)
Rauwolfia serpentine (Indian snakeroot)
Thymus vulgaris (common thyme)
Arctium lappa (gobo)
Carthamus tinctorius (safflower)
Passiflora edulis (maracuya)
Opuntia ficus-indica (Indian fig)
Taraxacum officinale (dandelion)
Tetrapanax papyriferus (rice paper plant)
Canavalia ensiformis (jack bean)
Linum usitatissimum (flax)
Pueraria lobata (kudzu)
Hordeum vulgare (barley)
Inula helenium (elecampane)
Althea officinalis (marshmallow)
Oenothera biennis (evening primrose)
Avena sativa (oats)
Triticum aestivum (wheat)
Medicago sativa (alfalfa)
Panicum maximum (guinea grass)

Plants containing high amounts of phytochemicals and which promote natural insulin production in the body:

Cocos nucifera (coconut)
Plantago major (common plantain)
Dandelion root
Blueberry

Ginkgo biloba

Banaba and ampalaya

Cedar berry

Cranberry

Ginger burdock

Alfalfa

Goldenseal

Ginger

Pau d'Arco

Juniper berries

Fenugreek

False unicorn root

Onion

Goodness Is the Red Stuff—Resveratrol's Healing Effects

Having laid out my full protocol and added some further supplementation suggestions, let me refer to one last supplement, another found in grapes.

Just above, in my discussion of grape seed extract, I mentioned the curative powers of anthocyanin, a part of the grape's skin, and pro-cyanidins, found in the seed portion of grapes. The substance under discussion here, resveratrol, is also a grape product, found in the skin of red ones. It can be extracted from seeds, peanuts, and red wine as well. It is an invaluable aid against the problems caused by diabetes since it has been shown to protect against the cellular damage to vessels caused by the high levels of glucose in the blood.

Exactly how resveratrol delivers this benefit has been laid out in a study led by Dr. Matt Whiteman, senior lecturer at the Institute of Biomedical and Clinical Science, Peninsula Medical School. According to Whiteman and his colleagues, "The elevated levels of glucose that circulate in the blood of patients with diabetes causes micro- and macro-vascular complications by damaging mitochondria, the tiny power plants within cells responsible for generating energy. When they are damaged they can leak electrons and make highly damaging free radicals." We've already seen how destructive free radicals can be. Specifically, a multiplication of these free electrons can lead to kidney and heart disease as well as to retinopathy. When resveratrol steps in, however, it "stops the damage by helping cells make protective enzymes to prevent the leakage of electrons and the production of toxic free radicals."

Resveratrol also appears to produce positive consequences on the weight-loss front. A study done by Dr. Pamela Fischer Posovszky, a pediatric endocrinology research fellow in the Diabetes and Obesity Unit at the University of Ulm in Germany, and colleagues looked at the extract's ability to slow weight gain. Their encouraging findings were: "Resveratrol inhibited the pre-fat cells from increasing and prevented them from converting into mature fat cells. Also, resveratrol hindered fat storage."

Taking their discussion in a cultural direction, the authors add that "the new finding is consistent with the theory that the resveratrol in red wine explains the French paradox, the observation that French people eat a relatively high-fat diet, but have a low death rate from heart disease."

If I had time I might go through just about every substance in my protocol and cite the scientific studies that testify to the different health-enhancing properties these supplements, vitamins, minerals, and herbs have exhibited. But let's move on to a few final points about diabetes and its treatment.

Treating Ulcers and Wounds

In this long chapter, after looking at the etiology and different directions diabetes takes, including what other diseases it often brings in its train, I have studied natural ways of reversing it, including exercise, diet andproper supplementation. I want to end this section by bringing up a couple of other important subjects, the treatment of ulcers and wounds, and the necessity for diabetics and those in danger of getting the disease to closely monitor their condition and food intake.

Many diabetics suffer from severe ulceration, that is, open sores, which often lead to amputation. There are a number of therapies that have shown excellent results in clearing up these wounds. One is intravenous ozone therapy, in which an amount of blood is removed and mixed with ozone, then fed back into the body. Add to this a heavy application on the affected area of the highest potency topical vitamin E available, and you have a winning combination. Another suggested approach, supported by a number of studies, is to apply pure, unprocessed honey to the ulcerated region. Honey kills bacteria and therefore sterilizes wounds and ulcers. Lastly, some success has been registered with chelation therapy, which involves the ingestion of chelating agents, such as alpha lipoic acid (ALA), to remove heavy metals and other adverse agents, ones that may be encouraging the ulceration, from the blood.

Monitoring and Preventing Diabetes

In such matters as allergy tests and blood readings, a patient has to rely on a doctor, but in many other ways, when it comes to keeping track of your personal health, the responsibility is in your hands.

Let's look at this from two perspectives, that of the person who is in danger of getting diabetes and that of the person who has it.

A person who does not yet have the disease but who, if the individual is closely monitoring her or his own state of wellness, notes certain telltale signs of the incipient appearance of diabetes, can then take resolute steps to change lifestyle and health patterns before diabetes fully sets in. This doesn't mean a doctor's aid should not be solicited. If you may be a candidate for diabetes and are unsure of your health status, see a physician who is trained in testing for pre-diabetes or metabolic syndrome.

If you already are a diabetic, monitoring will play an even more important role since it will be one clear guide to practices that are helping or hindering the improvement of your condition.

One of the key indicators of the state of your disease is how foods affect your body. If a food causes nausea, dizziness, hyperactivity, lethargy, stomach pains, headaches, or any pulse changes, your body is notifying you that it is not happy with that sustenance. The reactions indicate the food is troubling your system in some way. Stop eating foods that elicit these reactions, and alternate the foods in your diet so you can be aware of what is healthy for you.

That's only one part of awareness and throughout this book you will find other aspects of your life of which you need to be conscious. But don't think of this just another *list* of things you have to but would rather not do. Monitoring will open you to a fuller contact with yourself, so that your body doesn't appear as a bundle of aches and pains, with occasional joys thrown in, but an intelligently functioning companion that has a lot to communicate if you open your (inner and outer) ears to hear.

I have included in this book resources to help you do just this. Throughout this book you will find the tools to educate you on what to eat, recipes to make, what to avoid, how to diet and exercise to lose weight. These are the tools to change your life and find happiness. All of this is premised on increasing self-knowledge and awareness, in building, as in Dewey's quote at the opening of this text, a self that "will be more inclusive than the one which [now] exists."

Author's Note

In order to provide up-to-date information from the finest peer-reviewed journals on the subject of diabetes, we have reviewed thousands of studies. I have chosen not to include references and footnotes at the end of each section, but, rather, place the references and additional reading materials, as well as abstracts, at the end of the book.

Chapter 4

The Experts Speak Out

I believe one becomes a good doctor or health practitioner not so much through oneself as through others. Paradoxical? Let me clarify. Over the decades I have had the opportunity to interview many of America's leading medical authorities on diabetes. One thing I found was that even though each had a unique, carefully thought out perspective on the illness, it was one all of them had arrived at, not from sitting alone in their studies and spinning ideas, but as an ongoing reflection of their interactions with patients and other health workers. These were women and men who constantly developed and refined their ideas in dialogue.

It is often believed that people like this, ones with highly personal outlooks, are cranks, the types who bore everyone they meet by detailing their own idiosyncratic thoughts. For the doctors I am profiling here, the opposite is the case. Each of these women and men, with their own definite but flexible ideas on the disease, were always ready to give a listen to other points of view, for they had a refreshing willingness to look in all directions for promising therapies.

Perhaps this attitude comes from the fact that they wanted to see all sides of the medical issues. What distinguishes these individuals from your regular physician, clinician and scientist is that each has adopted comprehensive, integrative approaches to preventing and treating diabetes. Collectively they have worked with thousands of patients, many with full-blown diabetes along with the additional complicating conditions and diseases. Among those they have served, people that started out in such a dire state of health, quite a few are now living healthy, normal lives.

These are the types of experts that are worth listening to, ones who have gotten results. These are the men and women I sought out so I could hear their ideas on the causes and means of reversal of diabetes.

In this section these medical experts will "speak out," giving you a credible account of what works and what does not in the treatment of diabetes. They do not all come from one camp or all champion one therapy or each peddle some new drug. Instead, their insights are representative of interrelated disciplines that are proving to be enormously beneficial. Moreover, in the course of these coming pages, we will also listen to diabetics themselves in order to hear their own words of advice. For this was part of the dynamic that led the medical experts to their own creative explorations of healing. They listened to, drew feedback from, and were inspired by patients with diabetes, whom they helped to naturally regenerate their health.

Dr. Jill Baron

Dr. Jill Baron is a board-certified family physician who practices integrative medicine in New York City. She combines conventional primary care medicine with mind-body therapies, including nutrition and weight management;

lifestyle counseling; stress management; visualization and imagery; and energy medicine. Dr. Baron is also a certified menopause practitioner from the North American Menopause Society. As a doctor, her primary objective is to get to the root of patients' health issues.

One of the most frightening aspects of diabetes is that many people are unaware that they have it. These people have a condition known as pre-diabetes, and are unknowingly continuing a lifestyle that will end in full-blown diabetes, a stroke, or heart disease.

Pre-diabetes is usually seen in people who tend to be overweight and have visceral or abdominal obesity, but it can be symptomless.

When I see patients, I recommend blood tests. I feel all patients should have three tests, to assess whether they have pre-diabetes. Pre-diabetes is a condition where the fasting blood glucose is between 100 and 125. Diabetes has a fasting blood sugar of 126 or more, and a normal blood sugar level is less than 100.

After looking at their fasting blood glucose levels, the second test I recommend is called fructosamine, a blood test that averages a person's blood sugar over two to three weeks. The third test is called a hemoglobin A1C. This useful test measures a patient's blood sugar over three months and, if it is over a 6.0, that person could be at risk for pre-diabetes or diabetes.

Being aware of where we are on the diabetes spectrum is essential to altering our lifestyles so that we can not only improve our health, but live a happier, longer life.

Much like pre-diabetes, there is another condition called metabolic syndrome, which is the clinical name for several risk factors that increase your chance for diabetes. Metabolic syndrome serves as a huge health warning, and, unfortunately, due to our unhealthy diets, many people have it and are not heeding its warning.

We can look around us and see a lot of people who have abdominal obesity, and likely several of the other indicators for metabolic syndrome. Metabolic syndrome is characterized by having three or more of the following traits:

1. Abdominal obesity—If a man's waist circumference is over 40 inches or a woman's over 35 inches, that person has abdominal obesity.
2. Blood pressure—Blood pressure over 130/85, which is high blood pressure.
3. Triglyceride Level—The triglyceride is a type of fat in the blood, and if a person has a triglyceride level over 150, his or her health is suffering.
4. Fasting Blood Sugar Value—An elevated blood sugar level (after an overnight fast) above 100 means there is a strong risk for metabolic syndrome, and a blood sugar level over 140 indicates diabetes.
5. HDL Count—Having an HDL count under 40 is another indicator.

A lower-than-normal level of HDL (high-density lipoprotein cholesterol) increases your chance of heart disease, and is a sign of metabolic syndrome. If three out of these five traits are present, the individual has metabolic syndrome.

Inflammation is another significant condition to consider when discussing diabetes. While inflammation is a protective mechanism in the body—we need inflammation when we fight infection and the body rallies white blood cells—inflammation provoked by an immunity response from an unhealthy lifestyle leads to insulin resistance and type II diabetes.

Various causes can lead the body to become needlessly and consistently inflamed. A diet very high in animal fat, including red meats and saturated fats, like butter and whole milk, causes inflammation. And there are many other dietary sources of inflammation, including an acidic diet or one high in sugar and deep fried food. Eating things like pizza, hot dogs, hamburgers, and French fries is also pro-inflammatory.

How does a person know that he or she has inflammation? People who are overweight usually suffer from inflammation. There are also blood tests that measure inflammation indications. These tests look for cardiac C-reactive proteins in the blood. These are proteins that increase when inflammation occurs. If you have a cardiac C-reactive protein level of less than 1, that's optimal. If it's between 1–3, you have average cardiovascular risk. If your cardiac C-reactive protein count is between 3 and 5, you have a high risk of heart disease.

How can we prevent inflammation and treat inflammation? Of first importance is to have an anti-inflammatory lifestyle. This includes reducing stress, for this decreases inflammation, and having healthy eating habits. A plant-based diet that is rich in whole grains (such as legumes) and fish will combat inflammation. Conversely, red meat encourages inflammation. If it is consumed, it should be done so infrequently and in small quantities.

Many supplements decrease inflammation. Omega 3 fatty acids, such as DHA and EPA, two essential fatty acids, are very important in reducing inflammation. The only place in which you can get the vital combination of both DHA and EPA is in fatty fish or fish oil.

Vitamin D is also helpful in reducing inflammation. Getting back to testing for a moment, let me emphasize that it is important to have your vitamin D levels checked, specifically for 25-hydroxy vitamin D. This should be at a blood level between 50 and 80. Vitamin D deficiency has been associated not only with inflammation but also with cancer, multiple sclerosis, depression, and heart disease.

Exercise and maintaining an ideal body weight is also conducive to preventing inflammation. To speak more philosophically, ending diabetes would be simple if humans were, well, not human. It is very human to want to overeat; it is very human to crave sugar; it is very human to feed our emotional needs, and, sadly, it is very human to feed them with foods that do us the most damage. It requires discipline to eat healthfully. It is frequently easier to give in to our cravings and eat foods that endanger our bodies.

But, it is also human to reverse bad patterns. It can be done. By following a proper diet and taking the proper supplements, by exercising and listening to our body's needs (not cravings, but *needs*), and by having our health monitored and staying aware of our physical indicators, we can not only fight inflammation, but reduce metabolic disease and reverse pre-diabetic conditions, thus keeping out of the clutches of the dreaded silent killer, diabetes.

Luanne Pennesi

Luanne Pennesi is a registered nurse who has practiced for nearly 30 years in both conventional and integrative medicine. She was a supervising nurse for 18 years at a major New York City hospital.

I'm a holistic nurse. What most people don't know is that just about every nurse practicing today was taught to be holistic. What "holistic" means is that we look at every facet of the person's lifestyle and explore what could be creating the imbalance in her or his life. Therefore, we learn about psychology, biology, and physiology. We take into account the impact of our environment. In nursing school, we look at energy medicine. We also look at what things from the past as well as from the patient's personal constitution could be contributing to an imbalance. Sadly, once many nurses get out of school, the majority work at hospitals or for physician's practices where their job is essentially to administer drugs and write up documentation. While most still do some physical assessment, overall they lose that holistic piece, the piece that considers every facet of the person before diagnosing him or her.

What I love about my work is that I can have four people come in with diabetes, who can each be best worked with using a different approach, because every individual has a different root cause of the disease. I don't seek to cover up symptoms or get them to turn to drugs as the one cure. Instead, I focus on the causes of their health imbalance.

With diabetes, the first thing I look at is constitution. Next I examine physiology. Most people are very dehydrated because they are not getting enough fluids. To maintain a proper balance, we must ensure that we are hydrated and drinking healthy fluids. Soda and coffee do more damage than good, whereas filtered water and green tea (which is loaded with antioxidants) not only hydrate but improve our health.

I also look at my patients' diet and, when it is unbalanced, I try to understand what led them down the wrong dietary path. I've noticed that as a society, we have become carefully conditioned to believe what we see on television. All of our media is infiltrated with information on what is "healthy." We are also affected by what we see being done by people around us. Thus, if everyone is drinking soda, it must be okay. If they're serving us pizza in public schools, it's okay. Instead of questioning, we just go along with it, and we eat so that we're not hungry anymore, not paying attention to a food's value. The problem is that the standard American diet is, in my opinion as a registered nurse, killing us and our children.

I work with people to help them integrate a healthy diet. A healthy diet does not require giving up every sweet thing. Agave, which is cactus nectar, and stevia, a herb that can taste sweet, does not raise your blood sugar, and yet provides natural sweeteners. And these sweeteners do not have the side effects associated with aspartame and other artificial sugars. These have terrible affects on our nerves. I know, I used to be on them.

Other sweeteners people overlook are fruits and berries. When people start their morning with a smoothie that contains healthy protein powder, along with blueberries, strawberries, raspberries, and pomegranate, then add lecithin and glutamine, natural ingredients that help our bodies process sugar better, the smoothie drinkers are not sacrificing taste for health. That breakfast is sweet and filling. Moreover, when you start your day with something that contains protein that will stabilize your blood sugar for four to six hours, you reduce those pesky cravings and urges to snack.

But it's not just at breakfast that people are likely to err in their food choices. Think of the things on offer in the traditional, commercially pushed lunch and dinner menus. We are hungry. What do we have? Pizza. Fast food. Hot dogs. Hamburgers. Fatty sandwiches.

If you want a healthy body, those are not for you. I help people understand there are healthy foods to eat, like beans and grains, squash, yams, and all the green leafy vegetables. Also, seeds are great to snack on when the cravings hit.

Another important option is green vegetable juices. Now to most people drinking them sounds peculiar. They think, "I'm going to mow my lawn and drink it." Let them taste a well-prepared juice and they'd be surprised to find it is absolutely delicious. When green vegetables are put through a juicer, you get a powerful, concentrated drink that oxygenates the body, which is exactly what we need.

Let me go at this from a different angle. As a nurse, with the long hours we are sometimes asked to put in, I have had plenty of experience combating fatigue, sleep deprivation, and lack of energy. You know what I mean, that afternoon time between 3:00 and 7:00 when you need a little pick-me-up, that you expect to get from caffeine and/or sugar. I used to have such expectations. Every afternoon on the job I had a big cup of coffee and some kind of chocolate bar to keep my energy levels up. Now I substitute a big green juice. It picks me up, but it doesn't later put me down as do the unhealthy foods and beverages that lift the energy levels temporarily.

After examining diets, the next thing I look for in diabetic or pre-diabetic patients is how they are moving. Most of us are sedentary. We are driving or sitting on public transportation to get to work where we sit at a desk or stand at a counter for long hours. In other words, we are not moving our bodies much and not getting exercise.

So developing a healthy, *individualized* exercise regimen is the next step in treating diabetes. I emphasize individualized. When I meet a patient who is 200 pounds overweight (which I see a lot of), I help that patient plan an exercise schedule that is worlds away from what I would work out for someone who is 20 pounds overweight.

Along with exercising, managing stress is important. One part of a fuller program to handle this is to take quiet time every day, for at least 30 minutes, and perhaps listen to beautiful music or do a meditation or relaxation exercise.

As I continue to work with a patient, I make sure to examine environmental aspects of each patient's life. One often overlooked element of our lives that can cause stress is clutter. We have clutter in our environment, we have clutter in our minds and clutter in our bodies. A way to approach that triangle of three clutters is to organize our physical environment, decluttering and cleaning with natural products. That ensures we inhabit a peaceful environment and are limiting the chemicals we bring into our bodies.

By looking at all these facets, among them health, exercise, environment, stress, and decluttering—that is, taking a holistic approach—we can avoid putting on a health band-aid and actually solve problems.

My joyful discovery is this: when I give people the right tools— the practical ways to integrate a healthy lifestyle—and help them find a balanced way to live their lives, they get amazing results.

Dr. David Edelson

Dr. David Edelson is the founder and medical director of Health Bridge. An assistant clinical professor of medicine at Albert Einstein College of Medicine and an associate attending physician at North Shore–LIJ Medical Center, he is widely recognized as one of the nation's top weight-loss experts. He is board certified in both internal

medicine and bariatric medicine, and a two-time recipient
of the Faculty Teaching Award at LIJ Medical Center.

When talking about diabetes, it is first necessary to distinguish between two different types of diabetes and recognize that the form people most frequently suffer from is type II diabetes, in which there is too much insulin in the system. It is helpful to look at diabetes as a timeline, rather than a singularly occurring event.

Starting off, many people have a genetic predisposition towards developing diabetes, but they have not yet gotten the disease or shown any of the symptoms. Over time, with the addition of environmental problems, poor lifestyle, sedentary activity, poor diet with lots of high glycemic carbohydrates and inflammatory types of trans fats, we see the first stages of insulin resistance.

As doctors, we test to see if the patient has reached these stages using several markers, including C-reactive proteins and fasting insulin levels. We may start to see the beginnings of the changes that underlie diabetes. From the initial point when the patient begins experiencing insulin resistance, the glucose levels begin to climb and the hemoglobin A1c or fructosamine levels, both indicating the amount of glucose in the blood, shoot out of the normal range.

This leads the patient into the next step, which is metabolic syndrome. Metabolic syndrome is a constellation of symptoms, which traditionally we describe as appearing when the patient has three out of five of these factors: 1) elevated blood pressure, 2) low HDL [good cholesterol] levels, 3) high triglyceride counts, 4) high fasting blood sugar, above 100, and 5) abdominal obesity. [More details on this checklist appear in Dr. Jill Baron's remarks.]

When we see these signs, we know the patient has crossed a threshold from the early stages of pre-diabetes to the midpoint of the disease process. If there are continued problems with lifestyle, diet, and environment, and we move further along the spectrum, we go past the midpoint to where we can finally call the patient fully diabetic.

This is not the end, however. Once they've reached this point, *people can still progress in either direction.* That is a key point to realize when approaching diabetes.

Understanding it as a spectrum helps us to not only take the people who have reached the end of the line and push them back towards the starting point, but also, *more importantly,* the spectrum helps us look for the earliest signs of insulin resistance, warning us the patient is on track to becoming fully diabetic unless steps are taken immediately. Early prevention makes it easier to halt and reverse the progression so they will be able to avoid taking daily medications and suffer the complications that are so prevalent with diabetes.

So as physicians and healers we have our work cut out for us: getting people not just to treat the condition once it's established, but to start much earlier and prevent the disease from coming to fruition.

In order to understand my approach to treating diabetes and obesity—I like to use the term "diabesity," which I think really adequately describes the problem—it is helpful to look back at my own personal journey.

I went straight from high school into a six-year medical program at Northwestern University. From there, I began a traditional internship in internal medicine. I was promoted to chief resident, and then completed a fellowship in diabetes research in Israel. Finally, I returned to New York to start my own practice.

After I hung out my shingle and started seeing patients in a primary care setting, I began seeing things from a different perspective. Day after day I was seeing patients with chronic illnesses: heart disease, hypertension, obesity, and diabetes. I got to feel more like a fireman than a doctor: putting out fires all day long by throwing medications at them, trying to move people through the office as quickly as possible since so many people needed help.

After about ten years of this, I found myself feeling very unsatisfied with what I was doing, because I couldn't convey the value of my own lifestyle practices to my patients. I believed in a healthy lifestyle; I ate as healthily as I could; I exercised. I ran marathons; I did triathlons. *But I couldn't convey the value of this to my patients.*

As a result, I joined a group called the American Board of Bariatric Medicine. I became board certified in weight loss and bariatrics, the form of medicine that focuses on the causes and treatment of obesity. My new approach began.

Let me tell you about my inaugural case. A woman came in with her daughter who was about 240 pounds and five feet four inches. At age sixteen, she had already developed diabetes. She plopped down in the chair in front of me and started eating a bag of Twizzlers. The mother looked at me and said, "I need you to help my daughter."

I realized I was completely unprepared. As a primary care doctor, working alone, I didn't have the tools to give her real, sustaining help. I saw there had to a better way. So I decided to work with others to build an "integrative medical facility" where we would bring together healing practitioners from many diverse life approaches.

Now at this new facility, we have nutritionists and psychologists, along with exercise and fitness trainers. We even built a gym in the facility so people could exercise under supervision. We brought in physical therapists and chiropractors to help the injured. We added a sleep medicine facility, because so many overweight people had developed sleeping disorders. With that, we discovered sleeping problems were one of the underlying reasons they became overweight.

As a team at our facility, we developed a model called "puzzle theory." This theory holds that there is never a single problem that leads to obesity. Rather, it is a compilation of many different pieces. Little things begin to go wrong, problems begin to tangle together, and, eventually, the patient responds in a negative way and develops dangerous conditions, obesity and diabetes.

So, starting with this puzzle model, we try to break everybody apart into related pieces. Our team of specialists then evaluates each individual area. The nutritionist looks at a person's diet, the exercise people look at fitness, and the physical medicine team looks at the patient's injuries. We conduct sleep evaluations, as well as blood testing, including full lipid profiles, insulin levels, C-reactive proteins, and hormonal profiling with thyroid imbalances. We look for menopausal hormones, as many women after menopause gain weight. Growth hormones and Leptin levels are also reviewed.

From this, we better understand the person and the pieces of the puzzle. The goal is to catch diabetes signs early, before the individual has reached 300 to 350 pounds, and has full-blown diabetes. We hope to get to them at the earliest stages, so we can intervene with lifestyle changes, such as healthier diets that reduce the amount of low glycemic carbohydrates and remove trans fats from their lives. Teaching people about exercise also has a huge impact on combating diabetes.

Similarly, helping individuals with psychological issues, which often are associated with weight problems and diabetes, are intrinsic to resolving their health issues.

The problem with medicine today, as I learned in my first years in private practice, is that too many times the focus is on curing the symptoms rather than getting to the source of the illness. And this can backfire.

Interestingly, one of the problems with the diabetes medications frequently prescribed is that they actually cause weight gain, which then causes more insulin resistance. Insulin shots for type II diabetic can often result in disaster. While there are some cases where these shots are necessary, 90 percent of the time I see a patient on insulin or drugs called sulfonylureas, it is not only unnecessary, but the medications are raising insulin levels by causing weight gain.

Here's the cycle. As the body begins to store fat around the midsection, the fat makes them resistant to insulin. More resistance calls for higher insulin levels, in the eyes of the traditional doctor. The medications given to help this situation cause weight gain, and so this creates the need for even more insulin. It's a classic vicious cycle, which tragically results in the worst outcomes.

By interrupting this cycle and removing the offending agent, and by reversing the underlying causes of diabetes with natural therapies, we've seen tremendous results.

My goal as a doctor is to help people understand their issues and to be part of a group that forms a holistic medical team with a changed approach to treating diabetes. This is the wave of the future for medicine. Not sick care, but real healthcare!

Dr. Chris Cortman

Dr. Christopher Cortman has been a licensed psychologist in Florida for the past twenty-three years. He has facilitated more than 80,000 hours of office and residential psychotherapy and provides psychological consultation services at five local hospitals. He also serves as a consultant to government and law enforcement agencies, and frequently testifies as an expert witness in civil and criminal courts.

Why is diabetes such an issue today? Why is the current generation overweight? Why is there such a prevalence of type II diabetes? The answers have everything to do with lifestyle and priorities.

The average child today is watching more than thirty hours of television per week. So who is the storyteller in our society? The media. And what kind of story is the media telling us? 1) That we need to have things, 2) that we need to have them fast, and 3) those things need to be gratifying now, in the short term.

Children are taught that what they see or desire they deserve. In their minds, they are entitled to be gratified now. When we think about who's putting the food ads on children's TV programs, we see it's the fast food industry.

True to its name, fast food is instantaneously gratifying and you can get it in a second. It's easy to grab and gulp. You just drive to the window, pick up the bag and your kids are fed in a matter of minutes. With today's fast pace, when people have no time on their hands, this becomes the easy answer. For a lot of parents, it's difficult to put together a well-balanced meal. It's easier to stop by the fast-food restaurant.

Unhealthy food plays a large part but is not the only cause of the sudden rise in type II diabetes. Another point to bear in mind is that children today are sedentary.

A generation ago, we were kicked out of the house and told not come home until the street lights clicked on. We were out there playing and, consequently, would burn thousands of calories a day in sports and running around with our friends. We didn't get rides everywhere, we walked to school. The last thing we wanted to do was park in front of the television.

It is a different generation now. Instead of being outdoors, the average kid is indoors, seated or prone in front of a TV or computer monitor. I have parents telling me—with a straight face—that they're doing a pretty good job parenting because they are now limiting their kids to *only* four or six hours of video games per day. And that is during the school year!

In the summertime the kids are left home while their parents are working. The young turn to their electronic devices. They may play sixteen hours of video games a day. That does not burn a lot of calories, and it hooks children on a very passive form of entertainment.

It's not hard to figure out, then, how the diabetes problem came about. Children have stopped being active. They stopped eating well. They stopped being healthy.

If this is where we are now, what leads people to change? Many doctors say the best thing we could do for diabetes is promote early detection and prevention. That looks good on paper, but there is a psychological barrier, namely, people usually don't do anything to change until it's nearly too late.

I've done more than fifty thousand hours of psychotherapy, and I am still waiting for a patient to come in and say, "I want to talk about improving my life." Nobody does that! They come because they are in crisis. They have trauma. They don't come in because they're afraid that twenty years from now they're going to have an illness; they are coming in because they *have* diabetes.

That's when they are willing to change. It takes a doctor telling a patient, "If you want to be here for next year's physical, you better lose 100 pounds. If you don't, you're not going to make it." That gets a person to finally start making changes.

Even when people have the desire to change there are many obstacles, some external, some internal. Yes, internal. I believe we all have a saboteur inside, a wily character who will try by any means to block any changes that we try to make. Why would we create a part of ourselves to stop us from improving our lifestyle? Fear.

It can be terrifying to change things, even to change what one eats. It seems ridiculous, right? It might be inconvenient or demand creativity, but what could be scary about changing one's diet?

For one, many people look to food for much more than nutrition. Some seek consolation from what they eat. I have had more than one person tell me that food is not only a comfort, it's a best friend. One woman I treated put this humorously by saying, "My two best friends are Ben and Jerry." Those are the guys that she counts on. To give their ice cream up is like losing two good buddies.

However, even if a patient has firmly decided to face his or her fears and make a change, there are still pragmatic struggles. The patient typically asks something like this, "Where do I fit all this exercising into my busy life? I'm working full time. I've got children. I'm trying to do the best I can to make ends meet in a tough economy. Where and how am I going to add this exercise in?"

And even if time is found to start the new routine, the individual still has another hurdle. He or she has to break with old habits. The easiest way to change habits is to have a plan, and the plan has to be something that's built into the schedule.

I'll tell my patients that after work today, I'm going to lift weights. It is not contingent upon how I feel. It does not matter what's going on in my life. I'm going to lift weights. And you know why? It is not an option. It is mandatory. In order to make the difficult life changes required to fight a disease like diabetes, we need to start now, and we need to create a solid, consistent, and determined plan.

When I arrive at work, if I don't plan in advance to eat a healthy lunch, I won't. I need to plan enough ahead to make that healthy lunch happen. A successful eating plan has to take into account every day of the week. I need to decide what I'm going to eat for breakfast, what I'm going to eat for lunch, and what I'm going to eat for dinner.

So what kind of a mindset is needed to make lifestyle changes? First, the individual must believe changing for the better is a possibility, and that she or he can evolve a plan that is going to help.

Next, the person needs a sober perspective that allows her or him to say, "Okay, I can do this." And there has to be the realistic sense that it can only be accomplished gradually. A person does not gain two hundred pounds overnight and, consequently, will not lose them overnight. It will be hard, and it will take work, but it is something that can be achieved.

Thirdly, if we are going to make any kind of significant changes in our lives, we need a support system. In assembling it, the individual has to carefully distinguish between people who he or she can turn to for help, and those who have been part of the problem.

In this context, we can think of diabetes as a family illness since it is highly likely family eating habits led to diabetes initially. So, the fight against a person's diabetes ought to be something taken on as a family, with everyone on board to help the diabetic.

Finally, it is important to deal with the underlying issues, such as psychological scars. That's where counseling or psychotherapy can come in handy. I'm currently working with a woman who has come to realize that she seeks to be overweight because when she was a child she was abused. To avoid that again, she doesn't want to be attractive to men. She feels like she's not desirable as long as she's heavy and so no one's ever going to hurt her again.

I am saying that there are issues that underlie eating disorders, reasons why people do what they do. Even when actions seem irrational on the surface, such as bingeing on a food, generally speaking, that behavior make sense as a response to certain feelings or situations. Everything that a person does is often because it meets some kind of a need. Counseling can bring out what a need is and suggest more self-enhancing ways to meet it.

Let me end by getting back to where I began, the topic of children. Many of our public spokespeople are either shills or charlatans because, while out of one side of their face they say we need to emphasize athletics for our children, out of the other, they tell children to refresh themselves after a workout with a sports drink that's loaded with so much fructose and so many calories, drinking it will counteract many of the health gains that came from the exercise.

In response to my earlier characterization, where I noted America was raising children who are ill-nourished and sedentary, I would offer this alternative route. We have to give children a good solid diet from the very beginning, and lots of exercise and active play time. Children can and will learn to eat healthy things from an early age, and they'll learn to like the things, like exercise, that are good for them.

To move our children onto this path, we, too, have to change our lifestyles. And change is hard. It often requires a great deal of pain and fear, even to initiate behavioral change. But, above all else, change is worth it.

Dr. Harold Shinitsky

Dr. Harold Shinitsky is in private practice in Florida. He is a board certified psychotherapist and currently consults for several countries, states, counties, and schools on the development, implementation, and evaluation of adolescent prevention initiatives. He was previously the director of the Assessment/Intervention Team Prevention Services at the Johns Hopkins University School of Medicine, Department of Pediatrics.

Why do we make poor choices? It's not just some type of a surprise that happens at night. If you have type II diabetes, you probably arrived there through a long series of permission-granting acts that have brought you to this position.

There are many people with type II diabetes. More and more in this country. Why? The reality is we are eating ourselves into this situation. Our sedentary lifestyles have led to this.

Let me give you some background. I was on faculty at the School of Medicine at Johns Hopkins University and was the Director of Prevention Services in the Department of Pediatrics. When I was working in the adult world, we kept seeing all these adults who were displaying medical problems, behavioral problems, social problems, and when we evaluated them we found out that actually earlier in their life they were doing just fine. There was something that happened in the transition.

So I decided to do an elective rotation in pediatrics and try to catch what happened. An ounce of prevention is better than a pound of cure, I thought. What we ended up doing then was setting up a number of prevention programs for youth in the Department in the School of Medicine.

We didn't just address the situation from a child's point of view. As we saw it, the child isn't the patient. The family is the patient. And from this experience, I could draw conclusions about how people end up giving themselves permission to do these types of behaviors, such as overeating.

We can begin to understand this by looking at self-justification. People justify their behavior. They give themselves rationalizations, excuses, alibis for why they deserve this extra cupcake or this day off from exercising, etc. As you keep talking yourself into allowing yourself this one unhealthy opportunity, you establish a cycle or what is often referred to as compulsive behavior.

But why did the person first find a rationalization? When we look at this behavior, we see an individual who is probably trying to do his or her best to get through life, and then some stressor appears, an emotional strain that the individual seeks to cope with by granting the permission to bypass a healthy norm. Strangely enough, this stressor could be a fear of success. The person finds success difficult to face because she or he has low self-esteem, so the person's life is incongruent. The individual's self-worth doesn't match up with what they're achieving. The unhealthy behavior not only is allowed because the person feels he or she needs it to cope with the stress, but it may directly sabotage achievement of the positive goal.

Another question. How did they get this negative self image? This brings me back to the family situation. This low self-esteem clearly comes from the way they were raised. I've seen families that would bring their infants into our waiting room and they would be feeding them French fries as their meal. A child whose parents were this careless about its nutrition might easily develop feelings of low self-worth.

So, how do we work with a youth who has been hobbled with low self-esteem? You need to show individuals that they have potential and that there are goals that they can achieve. Most important, they have to understand that there are capacities that either they possess or the ability to find where those skills are. It's called *self efficacy*.

For example: I know behavior A leads to outcome B, and I either possess the behavior or I know where to find that behavior. If I just know a behavior leads to something, but I don't have the behavior, I'm stuck. If I have the behavior, but I don't know that it actually leads to something, I'm stuck. I need to have both of these. And parents need to recognize them, so they can provide this lesson to their children early on.

Let's go back to the situation of meeting a stressor, which is leading to dysfunctional behavior. The case we first dealt with in relation to this was one where there was a mismatch between esteem level and achievement. A youth feared success. But there are many other stressors besides this fear, which affect people and drive them in the wrong directions.

We have an individual who faces some type of *perceived* stressful situation in his or her life. To other individuals that same situation may not be stressful, but to this individual it is. The effected individual reacts by engaging in the behavior that is bad for him or her.

Counseling and therapy can teach us alternative ways to deal with these difficult situations. One way to approach a stressful situation is to talk and think it through. If we know that there's going to be a stressful situation ahead, we can plan for it. That's called anticipatory guidance. Counselors use this approach by asking their patients to think about what to do "if this were to happen." They help the individual plan a new outcome, other than using the stressor as a rationalization. They may ask, "What are you going to do at that time? How are you going to handle it so you don't do what you did before?" This pre-planning of responses is necessary so that individuals don't lapse into negative coping behaviors.

That's not all to be said about stressors. If we don't understand why we did something, especially a self-undermining behavior, we are more than likely to repeat it, so we need to understand the underlying dynamics. Our role as counselors is not just to tell someone "Don't do that." We have to help them understand why they did it. That's where in-depth counseling and guided self-searching come in.

Now let's follow the compulsive behavior cycle a little further for there is a further step so far not mentioned. Here's a typical scenario. There is a stressor. There is a thought. The thought leads to a behavior and that behavior oftentimes is inappropriate. Let's say after the behavior, say, after bingeing on a food, negative guilt appears. The person starts abusing him or herself emotionally for making that lapse.

Let's use for our imaginary example an adolescent girl. She is so fed up, she says, "I'm never going to do that again. I'm going to change my behavior!" On the surface, this is very positive. And, let's say, even more positively, for a period of time, she is not doing the wrong thing. However, if she has not developed coping skills, such as the self efficacy discussed earlier, when a strong life stressor happens to her again, she will probably suffer a moment of weakness, and return to the bad behavior.

So, it is this point, the moment of weakness, which we need to be able to figure out. Any proper fitting solution that will enable an individual to change compulsive behavior must, when push comes to shove, enable the individual to turn away from the "temptation" to fall back into old, comfortable, but counterproductive behaviors.

How do I work on helping them face that moment? I know there are a variety of things to do with patients. With weight management, for example, which is a big issue with diabetes, I ask people where they are right now and where would they like to be. Then we figure out how to break down the route to what the patient wants into objective, measurable, and quantifiable steps that increase the probability of success. This has to be planned so that each step along the way is one that increases the probability of success. In essence, no one plans to fail, but many people fail to plan.

Another side of the issue to address, given that the stressor triggers a bad choice in our patients, is the emotional issues that create stress. Remember stress itself, even before it elicits the reactive action, is bad for the body. When an individual is hyper-stressed, overwhelmed with anxiety or depression, it leads to an increase in toxins. Under stress, the adrenal glands produce the hormone cortisol. An overabundance of this hormone in the blood has been linked to obesity. Again counseling can help the individual channel and lessen anxiety.

Looking more globally, and returning to my point about the need for a plan that proceeds to move toward health by means of calculable, incremental actions, I would say there are five stages a person passes through if she or he is going to move from a compromised system to full health.

The first stage is pre-contemplative. The patient is not thinking about the issue. It's as if this individual needs something or somebody to awaken him or her. For example, the doctor might say, "You're morbidly obese. You eat poorly. You don't exercise. You have a family history of this condition. You might want to consider changing your life." In response, that person might say, "Me, not eating well? I had no idea."

That individual at least is willing to entertain new ideas about health. Other patients are hyper-resistant. It is as if they have perverted the idea of free choice. Choice in its better sense is shown when an individual selects the best alternative to living a fulfilled life. For the hyper-resistant, there is another, more willful version of choice. I've seen this in patients who, when I try to shake them out of the pre-contemplative stage, say, "I can do whatever I want to my body. You're not going to tell me anything about it."

If a person is able to awaken from this stage, the next is the contemplative one. People in this mode have grasped that they have serious health issues. They have begun thinking about what's best for them, looking forward to what they know would be the best outcome for them, and conversely, also imagining the worst. After a greater or lesser time, the person is suddenly able to make a decision to change their habits.

This is the preparation phase, when people get their ducks in a row. They make sure that they have friends and family for support. They may clean junk food out of the refrigerator. However, while seeing and knowing what they have to do, these people are readying themselves without action.

Then the individual enters the action phase. He or she is doing things differently, accumulating new and more responsible ways of living. There may and will be setbacks and relapses, but a new stage of life's journey has been embarked on.

After a couple of months of doing the right thing, a person enters the maintenance phase. Now the health-enhancing behaviors become part of a lifestyle. It is at this phase where we have changed our lives for good. This is the stage we all need to seek and attain. Those with diabetes or individuals on the road to diabetes can all achieve this stage.

Certainly, it's hard, and people can either get stalled at the first three stages and relapse from the fourth or fifth, but I've seen countless patients reach the fifth and continue on it. Reaching that stage is hard, for all change is challenging, but it is possible and necessary for those who want to live longer and to survive.

Dr. Chris Calapai

Chris Calapai, DO, is board certified in anti-aging medicine as well as family medicine.

Let me get straight to the point and, first, lay out my understanding of how young people become unhealthy. Diet and our attitudes towards what we eat have a great deal of bearing on why more and more young individuals are becoming diabetic.

Typically, with a young diabetic, we see that carbohydrate intake as a child was overwhelming. When those sugars and carbohydrates get into the bloodstream, they raise the blood sugar. As the glucose elevates, it starts to damage the lining of the blood vessel. Meanwhile, insulin is released to try to keep the blood sugar in an appropriate range.

This might not be so bad if it was an occasional or rare occurrence, but it's happening with every meal, three or more times a day, adding up to 300 or more grams or so of sugars and carbs per day. Now, I'm coming to the heart of the matter. With these massive amounts of carbs, there is an overproduction of insulin. This upped insulin knocks down the blood sugar, perhaps to an even lower level than it would be in a normally functioning metabolism, and that makes people crave sugar.

This is the crucial point. Hypoglycemia, a state in which blood sugar is below normal rates, makes a person want to eat carbohydrates, which, when broken down into sugar, boost the blood sugar back up. So, people continue to eat more and more sugars. The drive to eat sugar and continue to keep your blood sugar up is occurring over and over again, though, since the years of high carb diets have created a situation where too much insulin is being produced, and this keeps bringing down the boosted sugar levels, which are then replenished by more carbs.

When we talk to patients and ask them what their parents had them eat when they were young, and we then ask the parents what they ate when they were children, we start to see a tradition of overabundance of carbohydrates. This is what sets the stage for diabetes.

So, let's say I have a patient, a man who has been sick, weakened by years of high carb intake. How would I approach him? I would tell him we need to do comprehensive testing.

The first thing here is to look at blood sugar. I would also want to do a chemistry CBC, a complete blood count that looks at the distribution of the different types of blood cells. But, most importantly, I would do a blood test for vitamins and minerals.

Your nutrients protect every single cell and tissue of your body. If you're taking a handful of nutrients, almost at random, but you've never been tested to see what your B vitamin levels are, vitamin C levels are, and so on, you don't know the areas where you may be deficient and what those deficiencies could be doing to your health.

I would also tell the patient, I want to look at hormone levels, particularly those produced by the thyroid. If your thyroid level declines, I'd tell him, it becomes harder for your body to burn sugar, burn cholesterol and fat. That is, harder to convert food stuffs into products usable in the body's metabolism.

When we doctors examine the thyroid, we typically do a TSH and a T4 test. The TSH (thyroid-stimulating hormone) is a secretion that regulates the thyroid. The T4 test measures thyroxine (or T4) one of the hormones produced by the thyroid to regulate body functions. Even if the thyroid is producing adequate amounts of T4, there are other thyroid tests worth doing. You have to look at T3 (another hormone produced by the thyroid), and study the uptake of T3 and T4.

In other words, the thyroid has to be evaluated in the most thorough manner. Over my twenty-one years in this field, I've seen thousands of patients that have a normal TSH and T4, yet the T3 is low. The thyroid is still not working well. Appropriate and thorough testing is essential to understanding the health status of every patient.

When we look at hormone levels, we can't stop at examining thyroid function. We also should test testosterone levels in men and women. Testosterone is important for many reasons, one being that it helps burn fat and sugar, streamlining the body's utilization of these substances. An imbalance here can contribute to a decline in the body's ability to maintain appropriate blood sugar levels.

Besides testing for vitamins and minerals, looking at the hormones and blood sugar, I would want to examine my patient's different cardiovascular risk factors. A couple can be mentioned here, among fifty that are influential. One is homoscysteine levels. High levels of this hormone in the body have been correlated with increased risk of cardiovascular disease [as mentioned earlier in this book]. Now they're linking homocysteine with Parkinson's and Alzheimer's disease. C-reactive protein should also be tested since they are created when there is inflammation. Moreover, they will also occur in heightened amounts when excess sugar has damaged the lining of the blood vessels.

Along with all these tests, I will look for the presence of bacteria, viruses, and parasites. One notable bacteria, helicobacter, has been implicated in weight gain. It can irritate the lining of the stomach, making people feel hungrier.

Fasting blood sugar, which is simply the presence of glucose in the blood after the patient hasn't eaten for a spell, is something else to examine carefully. For one reading, I will look at a patient's blood sugar level two hours after he or she ate. For another reading, I will first take the level of the person's fasting blood sugar. Then, if it's a little bit elevated, I ask the individual to go out for a half hour and exercise. Then I recheck the sugar to see how much the patient has brought the sugar down with that activity.

The more information we gather, the better. This is often an important educational tool for the patient as well.

To continue with my imaginary patient, after testing him, I would ask him to write down what he's eating every day: breakfast, lunch, dinner, snacks. Then I would sit down with him and point out the bad foods that are high in carbohydrates as well as those that have lots of free radicals. I would work with him to set goals to get the carbohydrates intake down, initially to 60, then 50, then maybe 30 grams per day. The body would then be able to smoothly burn the sugar produced by the carbs. Meanwhile the triglyceride level would be plummeting. Triglycerides are fats that are a significant heart risk by themselves. With a low carb diet, your body is burning sugar and triglycerides quickly. Not only do your cholesterol and LDL levels drop, but your weight also comes down.

Having worked out this schedule with my patient, he must become proactive. It's not all uphill. Psychologically, as he begins to make progress, it will empower him to continue on the new diet as he charts his progress, sees his waist narrow, and feels more energy. I've seen that as people document the positive changes that come from improving their diets, this further reinforces their willpower to continue making positive life changes.

Let me move from this imaginary case to a real one. I've got a terrific case. He was a longshoreman, now seventy-five, a very big, strong, stocky guy. He was diabetic for thirty years, and his cholesterol was high for many, many years. He came to me, saying he had high blood pressure and was at least fifty pounds overweight, and he wanted to change. We did the blood work and tested his sugars. I had him come back in a week because I wanted to see what he was eating over the course of the week.

We then looked at his diet and discussed his protein, carbohydrate, fat, and oil intake. To him, this was very educational and eye-opening. I started to put together the plan for him and explained what I wanted him to do and that I'd walk him through it. He began bringing his sugar down and losing weight. Over the course of about a month, he was non-diabetic. It was astounding. After thirty years of being diabetic, he was non-diabetic. By the third month he lost fifty-five pounds. There's a story for you.

Patients like this one are better able to make choices because they are educated about the outcome of those choices. I don't just write out prescriptions and tell the patient what to do. I explain things to them, so, for example, they learn the importance of the B vitamins, vitamin C, magnesium, potassium, and all the minerals.

To take an example, I will mention to a diabetic patient that chromium is ideal because it helps to stabilize blood sugar. Vanadyl sulfate also seems to have this effect. I will also underline that intravenous vitamin C can reverse the damage on the lining of the blood vessels that is a byproduct of diabetes.

Once the patient has fashioned a new diet and has been educated about rebalancing his or her vitamin, mineral, and hormone levels, we also have to get onto the topic of exercise habits. For those that are in relatively good shape, I recommend they walk a little bit every day. If patients have problems with their legs, I recommend they try using an exercise bike. The important thing is that they complete at least one physical activity a day. As long as they are doing that, we can move forward. To progress, I have my patients add an additional five minutes to their exercise regime every week. Soon, they are able to complete more strenuous work-outs and the results start getting dramatic.

From hearing about my methods, you should see that true success relies upon using a combination of therapies. These must be carried forward while results are carefully monitored and observed, so that, if the patient's health is not improving, the necessary changes can be made so their conditions can be alleviated. To walk you through the steps one more time, I have found success in this way: I learn about the patient, test his or her health, and then work with the individual to put together a comprehensive diet, exercise and lifestyle-change plan. Then, after the program has been underway, retest to make sure we are getting the desired results. That is how we can beat diabetes.

Dr. Patricia Gerbarg

Patricia L. Gerbarg, MD, is an assistant clinical professor in psychiatry at New York Medical College and has maintained a private psychiatric practice for 25 years. Dr. Gerbarg has held numerous academic positions.

I am an integrative psychiatrist, which means I am both classically, traditionally trained as well as being educated in complementary treatments. As a psychiatrist, I seek to improve my patients' health and minimize their need for medications. One of the areas I take particular interest in is looking at the stress response system and how stress affects us psychologically and physically.

So what is stress? When people are under stress, they feel anxious, worried, frightened, and often they are overwhelmed. Their feelings can be summed up by saying, they feel *unsafe*.

Let's keep in mind that everything in our body is balanced. There is a kind of yin and yang to everything, including the body's stress response, which can be divided between the actions of the sympathetic and parasympathetic systems.

The sympathetic system responds to threat or danger, that is, to a sense of being unsafe, by getting us ready to either fight or run away. There is increased adrenaline release, upped heart rate, and faster respiratory rate. This preparation was one humans evolved for survival when they faced intermittent, short-acting threats, as when the saber tooth tiger came bounding out of the jungle and the early human had to run like hell. Once the danger has passed—you climbed up a tree and the tiger ran past—the sympathetic system calms back down.

A problem in our culture is that the system doesn't have sufficient time to calm down, because a person sees threats on all sides, as if a saber tooth hid behind every tree.

The counterpoint to the sympathetic system is the parasympathetic one, which goes into action when the threat has passed. While the sympathetic system speeds the heart up, the parasympathetic system slows it down. The same with respiration, the sympathetic system speeding it up, the parasympathetic slowing it. This is the body's balance I mentioned.

Our modern day lives do not have occasional, life-threatening stresses, such as our ancestors faced due to the existence of hungry prehistoric predators. But, we have different kinds of stressors, particularly, threats of stability. We worry about the loss of our jobs and of loved ones and have fears about our health. Any of these can be suddenly heightened by an event, such as the company one is working for announcing there will be layoffs. Such sudden sharpening of one's fears, which are constant occurrences in many people's lives, ratchet up the sympathetic system. When this keeps occurring—imagine, for instance, the state of nervousness among workers at a company that is having financial problems and may close down, meaning everyone will lose their jobs—the sympathetic system is chronically over-activated. A sympathetic system that is constantly alarmed will inhibit insulin release and adversely affect glucose metabolism while increasing blood pressure.

If the parasympathetic and sympathetic systems are set up to work in harmony, then if one goes out of balance the other soon follows. With the sympathetic system over-activated, to compensate the parasympathetic system actually becomes underactive. Everything is out of balance.

Let's examine the parasympathetic system more closely for this will bring us to see the key role it can play, when not functioning properly, to the production of diabetes. Now it might seem this system, which is something like a damper that lowers the body's excitement level, is less crucial than the sympathetic one. After all, it is the latter that takes charge when a person has to outrun a saber tooth.

However, as the discussion thus far should have suggested, each of these stress control systems is equally crucial.

A word on how the parasympathetic system operates. The two vagus nerves are the main pathways of the parasympathetic system. They exit the brain stem and travel down through the chest into the abdominal cavity, branching out to all our internal organ systems and tissues. The word vagus is Latin for "wanderer," an appropriate designation because these nerves "wander" everywhere, making connections throughout the body.

In the service of bringing the body back to a calmer state, these nerves both bring messages from the brain down into the body and information about the state of our body up into the brain, which processes this knowledge and uses it to make decisions on our internal and external reactions. From this it can be seen, the parasympathetic system is of critical importance.

If, in a state of excitement, the body has excess glucose in the blood, then when that excitement is over and it's time for the body to calm down, that glucose has to be removed. The calming is controlled by the parasympathetic system and, in keeping with this, the vagus nerve innervates the pancreas. When you activate the vagus nerve, you trigger a release of insulin, whose function, as we know, is to help move glucose out of the blood. Furthermore, aside from dealing with times when the body needs to cool off after a period of high stress reactions, the parasympathetic system and the vagus nerve are critical to optimally managing the level of glucose in your body after you eat.

The next part is easy to figure out. A good, robust parasympathetic system is required in order to have a healthy insulin response and proper glucose management. When the parasympathetic system is under-active or overshadowed by the sympathetic system, as in the scenarios we discussed earlier, you have disturbances in insulin metabolism, which contribute to obesity, cardiovascular risk factors, and diabetes.

So let's see how one approaches repairing this imbalance between the two stress response systems. There are sympathetic system medications used in psychiatry, anxiety anxiolytic drugs, which function to temporarily dampen down the sympathetic system. There are, sadly, no known medications that will strengthen or boost the parasympathetic system. Nevertheless, there are non-drug-based ways we can strengthen and activate the parasympathetic system, an area of research I have been focusing on for over ten years now.

Certain activities boost the parasympathetic system. Not surprisingly, these activities involve bonding, love, and our close relationships. For example, cuddling with someone you love and sharing loving feelings will actually activate your parasympathetic system. These are the type of things that traditionally make a person feel better for, after all, if one feels loved and accepted, it is easier to endure the buffets to one's self-esteem, such as loss of a job or a less drastic event, that are such common occurrences nowadays. This is why signals of love, closeness, human bonding, and safeness aid our parasympathetic system. And I might add, it is hardly an unpleasant treatment, like so many health remedies. Instead, it is pleasurable and fun.

Beyond these practices, which might be called "home remedies," my research has brought me to examine a series of mind-body practices, some of which I feel can aid in rebalancing an out-of-whack sympathetic/parasympathetic system. I am not a lone researcher, by the way, for other scientists have also gone in the direction of looking at the benefits of yoga and mind-body practices. Over seventy studies of these practices were reviewed by researchers at the University of Virginia, who concluded the practices can significantly reduce the risk factors in people with metabolic syndrome, insulin resistance, and cardiovascular problems. Add to that twenty-five studies that have shown the positive impact of these practices on people with type II diabetes.

My own research has led me to sort through the different mind/body disciplines, searching for various practices that will provide the greatest impact in the shortest period of time in terms. I have done this because I realize people today, who want to practice yoga, for example, cannot sit for eight hours a day as the Indian teachers used to do in their ashrams. I've found that, even in a more restricted time frame, certain practices, in particular movement, breathing, and meditation, can offer multiple benefits.

I will concentrate on breathing here. Now, it so happened that I had the privilege to work on a study of people who survived the 2004 Southeast Asia tsunami. And let me say, if we can study people who have extreme stress disorder and find things that can help them, then those same valuable practices will benefit individuals who are suffering from less severe, everyday stress.

In our study of the 183 refugees, we learned that with an eight-hour breathing program we had 60 percent reduction in symptoms of posttraumatic stress, and a remarkable 90 percent reduction in symptoms of depression.

We also did a study with Vietnam veterans who had treatment-resistant, posttraumatic stress disorder, and they showed a remarkable response to mind-body practices, especially breathing programs. More recently, over the last couple of years, we've been working with people affected by the World Trade Center attacks. Here again there were reductions in many of the parameters of posttraumatic stress and anxiety, following workshops that taught breathing methods and other mind-body practices. These studies are certainly very encouraging.

Most obviously, when a person who is feeling stress stops and concentrates on breathing, he or she is listening to the body, and not engaging in distressed and distracted activities such as running to the refrigerator to eat some unhealthy comfort food.

However, there's more to it than that. Of all the automatic activities of the body, such as heartbeat and digestion, the only one that can be voluntarily controlled easily is your breathing. When you purposefully change the pattern and the rate of breathing, you change the messages that are being sent from thousands of receptors in the lungs, the chest cavity, the pharynx, and the throat, all of which feed into the vagus nerve and the parasympathetic system. A relaxed, smooth, deep breathing pattern will convey a message up the vagus nerves to the brain that says, "You know, it really is safe. You really can relax now." Ideally, this can override other messages your body may be conveying that run in the other direction.

Breathing is powerful. What we as scientists would like to find is a sort of Rosetta Stone, the archeological find that allowed Egyptian hieroglyphics to be translated. What is the language of the breath, in the sense of what rhythms and speeds communicate what messages to the brain? If we could get some understanding of what breathing patterns engage the brain so that it responds by moving our physiological patterns forward in the most therapeutic, soothing way, so that we feel safe, this would have incredible and multiple health benefits, including a reversal of the parasympathetic derailment that contributes so greatly to the origin of diabetes.

Dr. Richard Brown

Dr. Richard Brown is associate clinical professor of psychiatry at Columbia University. After receiving his MD in 1977 from the Columbia University College of Physicians and Surgeons, Dr. Brown completed his residency in psychiatry and a fellowship in psychobiology and psychopharmacology at New York Hospital. He is the recipient of numerous awards and has authored over eighty articles and book chapters on pharmacological treatments, clinical studies, and complementary approaches in psychiatry.

Stress is a factor in most illnesses. Stress comes in reaction to any change we experience, both those happening inside us or around us. The greatest stresses I see come from emotional separation and loss, but any change, even a positive one, will engage the stress response system. For example, getting married can be a great stress for people. Moving to a better home than you had before or taking a new job that you wanted to get can be a great stress.

The stress response system, when it's turned on too long, as it often is in our society, burns a lot of energy. In response, we often put food in as a source of energy—carbohydrates are quick energy—but food is only one of the places from which we can gather energy. It also comes from sleep, the proper balance of rest and exercise, and breathing. I question whether people are always drawing the replacement energy they need from the right sources. You can go thirty to forty days without eating and we can go maybe five or six days without sleeping. Yet, in our society, a lot of people don't get the necessary sleep, but, at least in New York, they can't go a half hour between snacks. We seem to have it backwards.

Breathing is even more essential. You can only go a few minutes without breathing. Indeed, the quality of your breathing plays a big role in determining the balance of your stress response system. If it is calmed and relaxed, this will aid the parasympathetic system. This, in return, is soothing and recharges your anti-inflammation system.

Now when a person is under stress, she or he often becomes much more focused on the outside world. Not a shock in a society likes ours where we are bombarded with ads for products that will supposedly solve all our problems. Someone influenced by this pervasive propaganda will immediately look outward for a solution. In this mode of outer direction, you're not aware of the signals from your body and rarely ask yourself, when picking up a sugary soda, for instance, "Do I really need this? Am I thirsty or am I reaching for this bottle because I'm feeling lonely or emotionally empty and need some comfort?"

What my patients are learning is that instead of using that soda, similar anxiety-lessening results might have been achieved by simply . . . breathing!

The average person is breathing about fifteen to eighteen breaths per minute. When you take about five or six breaths per minute, your system changes its balance. It communicates calm to the body, and begins to balance your stress response system and your soothing recharging system. [In the previous section, Dr. Gerbarg called these the sympathetic and parasympathetic systems.] They are harmonized by slowing your breathing.

Let me cite a case. A 300-pound woman was dragged to one of our breathing and meditation courses, which combine yoga techniques with Qigong from China. Let me tell you, she was terrified of coming, but there was no way she could participate in a walking or bicycling program. She forced herself to come and looked very frightened when she got here.

By the end of the several-day course, she said, "I'm so aware now of my body after this course. And I love my body again!" I talked to her about this new sense of herself, and she, being a very thoughtful person, had a very articulate explanation. She continued, "I had grown to hate my body and avoid thinking about it. One way I avoided thinking was to use food as a distraction. All the time, I wanted to stay separate from people because I thought no one could like me the way I am. This made me feel lonely, another thing I tried not to think about."

With a new body awareness, that was prompted by the workshop but developed over time, she became aware of signals from her body telling her not only whether it was the right time to eat, but how much to eat and when to stop. You see, normally when she would eat, she wasn't paying attention to body signals. It was as if she weren't really present as she ate. She was watching TV or gossiping with friends. It is difficult to control portions or watch what you are putting in your mouth when you are not paying attention.

This woman became almost a role model. As she became aware of her body's messages, which told her, for instance, how the food she ate was affecting her, she was better able to discriminate, differentiating between foods that were satisfying over time versus those that gave a quick burst of energy.

All this meant she developed a very different relationship with her mind-body-spirit complex, and felt empowered to continue the changes she was making in her life. Every day she practiced better and did a little bit of movement. It didn't take much time. She also started implementing peaceful meditation and prayer. She wasn't eating as much, didn't need to eat as much because she was more content with her life, which was finally moving in the right direction, and more connected to the signals from her body. So, she lost weight, as a matter of course. It all started with breathing.

Young babies breathe in a very relaxed way that balances their systems, but as adults we have to strive to regain that kind of in-touch breathing. Even scientists have been studying this relaxed drawing of breath, which they dub coherent or resonant breathing. Its goal is to breathe in a way that helps synchronize the brain, heart, and lungs, using blood flow as one of the regulators. The forward-looking research of modern scientists into this topic is also linked backward since this type of breathing was recommended in ancient Chinese medical texts.

A simple way to work toward better, resonant breathing patterns is to practice breathing about five breaths per minute. In this exercise, the point is not just to slow down but to bring one's attention inward. It is important to sit comfortably and easily, but with the spine erect. With eyes closed, pay attention to the feeling of the breath moving in your nose, throat, chest and belly. Try and replace mental chatter with this awareness of the breath's movement through the channels of the body.

This, by the way, is the breathing routine my once-300-pound patient followed. Doing so, she became so attuned to her bodily signals, she could give up craving things her body didn't want, turning away from using food as a comfort. Instead, she found other comforts, connecting to people, restfully sleeping, going for a walk, or just getting in touch with her body with some gentle movement. She was using the breathing time to listen to those bodily signals that she had gotten used to ignoring.

She came to our class frightened and emerged to become a model, both for me, in showing the way people can make positive, cumulative changes that move them from a depressed state, and perhaps for readers, who can follow her in the way she coordinated mind, body, and spirit, in the process of becoming more aware of her inner world, as the royal road to personal growth and health.

Dr. Sabina Grochowski

Sabina Grochowski is an internist who has been in private practice for the past thirteen years. After graduating from medical school, she completed an internship and residency in internal medicine and a fellowship in pulmonary medicine. While building her practice, she worked as an ER physician for several years. She believes that traditional medicine does not deal with the whole patient. It is a black-and-white model that says you're either healthy or you're sick. For her, there's something in between—a place of movement toward better health when the patient modifies or changes diet and behavior to maintain youthfulness, vitality, and happiness.

Today, many people place the responsibility for acquiring debilitating diseases firmly on the frail shoulders of the patients, but nobody speaks up about the healthcare practitioners. I'm thinking not so much of these practitioners' interventions, as of their mindset.

In a typical case, a patient has a normal blood report, so the doctor tells him or her everything is fine. Strangely, it turns out a couple of years later, everything isn't quite so fine. The patient has diabetes, cancer or a heart attack. That's because of a medical mindset that considers people as being in only one of two states: sick or healthy.

I ascribe to a different model. I think there is an in-between when a person doesn't yet have a disease but is moving toward acquiring it. Certainly, it's difficult to diagnose a disease in its earliest stage, but, nonetheless, when caught at the beginning, it is very easy to heal. Conversely, it's easy to diagnose but difficult to cure a disease in its later stages. The doctors I mentioned above wait till the disease reaches its late stage before they intervene, and it's then that there is very little we can do to cure it.

To catch diabetes in its early stage, comprehensive testing is necessary. I like to test for adrenal fatigue (when the adrenal glands are functioning below par), leaky gut (in which the intestine lining is damaged), and gut dysbiosis (a bacterial imbalance in the intestines). I focus on the gut because it plays a significant role in most illnesses. In fact, with the diets in our country along with the toxins we're exposed to, including heavy metals, all of which are processed through our intestines, most of us have problems with leaky gut.

Because of these digestive tract problems, I start by checking for gut dysbiosis. I like to do a comprehensive stool analysis to see if my patient has bacterial overgrowth and/or yeast overgrowth, which are negative features, and also to check, on the positive side, if their lactobacillus and their other probiotics (healthy micro-organisms) are in balance. If complications exist, I start with repairing the digestive system first.

Following these digestive system exams, I look at the possibility of the patient having the metabolic syndrome [which, as we saw earlier in the book is the name for several risk factors that increase your chance for diabetes]. This fits with my philosophy of identifying the disease in its early stages. Weight gain, for instance, is a possible sign of a patient moving toward the illness. I haven't seen many skinny, type II diabetics.

I look at the glycohemoglobin (amount of glucose in the blood) and the post-prandial glucose (blood sugar level in a patient after he or she has eaten a meal), which should be less than 110. All of these measures can be used to determine whether the patient has the metabolic syndrome.

The testing has to be thorough so, while inspecting obvious things like insulin levels, I also look for endothelial dysfunction—the endothelium is the layer of cells lining blood vessels—and at such indicators as the presence of interleukin 6, which indicates inflammation.

Another thing. Everyone who has diabetes probably also has hypertension, so I look for the telltale signs of this disease. Therefore I look for evidence of left ventricular diastolic dysfunction, which occurs when there is a disturbance in the ventricle that is filling with blood (the diastole phase). This is often brought on by high blood pressure (aka hypertension).

After testing, conclusions are drawn, and I begin treatment. In the beginning, I primarily address lifestyle issues, including diet and exercise. I also institute a course of supplementation.

I am acutely aware at this stage of the danger of heavy metals, which can displace an individual's nutrients. So, I do heavy metal detoxification. With some patients I have used chelation therapy, putting nutrients and supplements in the body to leech out the heavy metals.

With one patient, I used a combination of n-acetyl cysteine, alpha lipoic acid, milk thistle and a few other nutrients. For further supplementation, I prescribed fish oil, CoQ10, chromium, and quercetin. His glycohemoglobin count, the measure of glucose in the blood, came down from 11.5 to 6.5. We were all proud of this achievement.

Successes like this arise when a person's disease progression is noted and checked at an early point. Being aware of potential dangers before they become real dangers is the best way to combat disease.

Dr. Martin Feldman

Dr. Martin Feldman is a pioneer in complementary medicine, having developed natural therapies over a medical career spanning more than twenty years. At his office on

*Manhattan's East Side, he applies his wide experience to
a broad patient base with problems related to digestion,
energy, immunity, allergies, skin and arthritis.*

When people say, rightly, that there is a diabetes epidemic in America, they are generally looking at the topic too narrowly. The broader problem is an epidemic in bad glucose levels in the blood. If diabetes, which is high blood sugar, represents one side of the problem, the other is hypoglycemia, meaning glucose is low. Hypoglycemia is also found in epidemic proportions in this country. The body has a thermostat which controls the glucose in the blood minute by minute, and the glucose has to be maintained at a certain level. If it goes either too far up or too far down, the individual is in trouble.

Hypoglycemia is easier to overlook than hyperglycemia (excessive levels of sugar in the blood) because it is episodic—that is to say, the blood sugar count may fall too low for part of the day but then resume normal levels later that same day. Even the symptoms, such as headaches, are episodic. Many people learn that if they eat a little bit their symptoms go away.

Both these factors, the transient nature of symptoms and the temporary drop of blood sugar, make hypoglycemia easy to miss. Take when a doctor tests for blood glucose level. The level is determined for only one moment: when the needle goes into the arm and draws some blood. The glucose taken at that one point is generally all the physician takes into account. That would be fine if blood sugar level was unchanging, but, as we've just seen, this is not the case with hypoglycemia.

The only way to really get to the bottom of things and see if a person does suffer from low blood sugar would be to administer a glucose tolerance test. If it is done properly, that runs over for four or five hours, because glucose level may be relatively normal the first hour or two, and then, in say, hours four or five, the hypoglycemia is apparent.

If a doctor wanted to take the testing further, she or he could examine some of the blood issues, by, for example, looking at the HgbA hemoglobin (the part of the blood that carries oxygen) and giving a A1c test (to measure blood sugar over a prolonged period of time).

Since few people take and few doctors offer the glucose tolerance test or assess these other parameters to check if a person has hypoglycemia, a patient who suspects he or she has this problem should start with a self-diagnosis. How? By being aware of personal behavior and certain symptoms. Hypoglycemics will often carry around food, because they know when they feel badly enough they must eat something. Such a person tends to crave carbohydrates. Also he or she will feel the need to have caffeine. If an individual is doing these things, packing "emergency" food or craving caffeine and carbs, the person is likely to be hypoglycemic.

In a self diagnosis, the key symptoms of which to be cognizant of are brain related, because if the glucose level falls too much or goes down rapidly, the brain is affected. The brain runs on glucose. So a hypoglycemic will experience episodic headaches, which come and go as the glucose level fluctuates. Such a person will also suffer from periodic fogginess in thinking as well as dizziness.

Self diagnosis is extremely useful, self treatment of the disease less so. Many people think that they can alleviate hypoglycemia simply by eating frequent, small, protein-filled meals. That will help, but does nothing to fix the problem.

Why does a person's sugar drop too low? A moment ago I referred to the body's sugar thermostat. This thermostat controls the pancreas's production of insulin and glucagons, the adrenal glands' production of hormones, and the liver's role with glycogen. These three components are all significant. In order to fix hypoglycemia, the thermostat needs rebalancing. This is the root problem, which eating frequent small meals neither addresses nor ameliorates.

Let me go through these three components in turn, suggesting therapies that will aid in tuning up each organ.

The pancreas likes the following nutrients very, very, very much. First is chromium. A good beginning dose is 200 micrograms. For some individuals, this may need to be doubled or even tripled. Chromium picolinate and other types of chromium are also very effective as well as being inexpensive and safe to take. Next is zinc. Hypoglycemia patients should start at 20 milligrams, and may have to lift their dose to 40 or even 60 mg to get the pancreas shaped up. Next would come manganese. Commonly, 10 milligrams are needed to help the pancreas to rebalance. Vitamin B complex (50 milligrams per tablet or more) three or four times a day will also be of tremendous help here.

Let's shift the focus to the adrenal glands. While complications with the adrenal glands can often be more complex than those related to the pancreas, they are very amenable to treatment.

Before jumping into taking therapeutic measures, it is necessary to carefully investigate the state of this organ. One can begin with the DHEA-S assessment, a simple blood test for adrenal function. If the adrenals are low or weak, DHEA-S will be low.

Another thing to look into is cortisol, a hormone produced by the adrenals. Cortisol is best tested in the morning when the cortisol level is the highest in the body. It is difficult to test this in a doctor's office, in that the optimum time to measure the hormone, when cortisol peaks, is about thirty minutes after waking. It wouldn't be an easy task to wake up, dress, get down to the doctor's in a half hour, but it is possible to get around this difficulty by collecting saliva thirty minutes after you wake up. This saliva can be put in a vial and mailed to the lab in a regular envelope. For an even more thorough screening, an individual can take samples of her or his saliva every few hours during the day, storing it in labeled vials, later to be sent to the lab.

A final useful assessment of the adrenals is the Ragland's Blood Pressure Test. A patient will take a first reading while lying down, then he or she stands up quickly and does a second reading. In normal circumstances, when an individual stands up like that, the brain needs a sudden increase of glucose flow and blood pressure should rise. However, when people have low adrenal function, they often see no blood pressure change from lying down to standing, because the blood sugar is being inadequately regulated by the gland. The blood pressure may even fall, leaving the person feeling a little dizzy.

Once the tests are completed, we can move to the healing process. Here I have found vitamin C of the utmost value as are pantothenic acid and rhodiola herb.

The liver is the third part of the glucose-regulating thermostat and, as with the adrenals, one has to test carefully to assess its state. One pitfall here is that, when a doctor suspects the liver is off balance, he or she will look at two liver enzymes, AST and ALT. However, the liver has to be in a deplorable state for problems with those enzymes to show up. Other tests that will reveal liver problems before things have reached a near-crisis state should be tried. One of these is to have an acupuncturist check the liver meridians. This will help catch the difficulty early on.

As with the other two elements in this system, the liver can be rebalanced. I would prescribe milk thistle as an excellent healing herb to use for this problem. However, the central action is to accomplish clearing the body of its poisons, the mind of clutter and anxiety, and one's environment of noxious influences. In other words, carry out a complete mind/body/environment detoxification. The individual and therapist can work together to create a program to bring this into being.

Even though it might seem hypoglycemia, having low blood sugar, is at the opposite end of the spectrum from diabetes, which is characterized by high blood sugar, any disruption of the blood's optimal glucose rate will lead to the disease. After a person has been hypoglycemic for many years, she or he ends up with diabetes. I've seen this in hundreds of patients.

The reason for both hypo- and hyperglycemia have been laid out briefly. There is a triangle of organs: liver, adrenal gland, and pancreas, that work together to regulate blood sugar, forming, as I've said, the body's glucose thermostat. Those in danger of diabetes, especially those who by their self-diagnosis have been alerted to a possibility of hypoglycemia, should test all three organs to see if they are functioning well. And if there is a reduced functioning in one or all of them, the appropriate, healthy steps should be taken to re-invigorate them and ensure the thermostat is in prime working order so as to yield a healthy, well-balanced life.

Chapter 5

Do Vaccines Contribute to Diabetes?

At this point, I'd like to shift the discussion in two ways. For one, let me talk about the causes of diabetes somewhat differently. So far, in examining these causes, I have looked at habits, such as a sedentary lifestyle and bad eating, which, while part of an individual's lifestyle, are certainly encouraged by the media and many institutional social practices. But I haven't brought up the possibility that some diabetes is caused by *unwitting* medical ignorance

I have also given most attention thus far to type II diabetes since this is the one contracted later in life and most associated with lifestyle choices. This is the form of the disease that, on the surface, is most amenable to treatment. Type I (juvenile diabetes), on the other hand, sometimes seems as if predestined in that a young child can get it from (as is theorized in one scenario) a viral infection that permanently damages the pancreas, disabling it so it is not able to deliver adequate insulin.

My departure in this section will be that I will turn my attention to type I diabetes and consider if some of its occurrence has been provoked by bad medical practices.

In other works, I have considered how unsafe and ineffective many vaccines are, but the focus in this book will be on the vaccines that some evidence links to the occurrence of diabetes in animals or humans. What the researchers I will highlight argue is not that there have been a few, statistically insignificant cases where the disease follows vaccinations, but an epidemic of vaccine-prompted juvenile diabetes.

As I noted early in the introduction, type I diabetes is considered an auto-immune disease. In such a disease, the immune system, whose role is to fight off viruses and other invading entities, mistakenly perceives some of its own molecules as foreign invaders and attacks them. For type I diabetes, what the immune system is going after are the pancreatic cells producing insulin. This is why, as I mentioned, juvenile diabetes sufferers will probably have to take insulin injections their whole lives to make up for what the pancreas can't produce. I also underlined some of the complications likely to be encountered by those with these conditions. The disease can lead to blindness, loss of hearing, heart and kidney disease, strokes, cataracts, nerve damage, paralysis of the intestinal tract, and gangrene requiring amputation.

To say a little more about the calamitous effects of this form of the disease, let me add that while, as mentioned on our first page, diabetes overall is the third leading killer in the country, diabetes type I (which I noted only accounts for 5 percent of all diabetes cases), by itself is the seventh leading cause. On top of that, it is the number-one cause of blindness and renal failure. Lastly, another sobering statistic, half of the amputations performed in the United States are done on diabetics.

Obviously, with death and disability numbers like this, diabetes will be making a dent in our country's healthcare spending. In 1997 it was estimated that diabetes cost the US a staggering $85 billion for medical treatment and an additional $47 billion for lost work time, disability payments, and premature death.

To expand on the array of figures presented in the introduction, the Centers for Disease Control announced in 1997 that the incidence of diabetes had increased six-fold since 1958. Approximately sixteen million Americans are suffering from this disease and five million more may have it but have not been diagnosed.

So let's get back to my statement about vaccines, which some readers, who haven't yet heard the evidence, may consider a trifle inflammatory.

The first reports of a possible link between diabetes and vaccination go back to 1949 when studies showed that children receiving pertussis vaccine had difficulties in maintaining normal blood levels of glucose. Further investigation done on animals showed that pertussis vaccine disrupted blood sugar and could cause diabetes in mice.

I noted earlier a theory drawn from diabetes research over the next four decades, which was the hypothesis that viral infections may be a co-factor in the development of diabetes. These infections damaged the pancreas and may have led to autoimmune responses. Now where do these viruses come from?

As we know, a vaccine's operational principle is to infect a person with a very weak form of the dreaded illness, so the body develops an immunity, building up a storehouse of targeted antibodies, which will fight off any infection with a robust form of the disease. Yet even a very weak form of a disease, administered to a very young child, may not be that safe.

Thinking along these lines, some medical researchers have asked whether the introduction of live attenuated virus vaccines, such as the MMR vaccine, could be a co-factor in causing chronic diseases such as diabetes I. Note, I say co-factor, not sole cause, in that it is believed some individuals have a genetic predisposition to auto-immunity, such as those with a family history of auto-immune disease. So—I am now speculating—if you combine a genetic tendency to get auto-immune illnesses with a live, if weakened, virus that may attack the pancreas, an easy route to juvenile diabetes has been laid out.

Think about the following four points for a moment and consider whether they might be connected. The rubella virus has been shown to persist in the body up to several years after a rubella vaccination. The rubella and mumps virus have been shown to infect pancreatic cells and cause a marked reduction in levels of secreted insulin. Children with congenital rubella syndrome, which is not acquired from vaccination, but from a rubella-infected mother, often develop type I diabetes. There have been several reports in the medical literature on the occurrence of diabetes following live rubella and measles vaccination. These facts certainly give one a pause for thought.

Now let's look at a particularly damning study. In 1996 Dr. Classen, a former researcher at the National Institutes of Health, did a study that linked New Zealand's initiation of a massive campaign to inoculate babies with the hepatitis B vaccine to a 60 percent increase in type I diabetes.

The study (cited in the bibliography) revealed that among a cohort of 100,000 children followed since 1982, the incidence of diabetes increased from 11.2 cases in the group per year before the hepatitis B vaccination program started in 1988 to 18.2 cases per 100,000 after the vaccination campaign.

Classen then looked further into the possible connection of vaccinations with diabetes, still using the method of examining the disease statistics before and after vaccination was inaugurated in a nation or following changes in a country's inoculation program.

He noted that in 1974 Finland started experimenting with a HiB vaccine, giving it to 130,000 children aged three months to four years. In 1976, the Scandinavian country made a second innovation in its health program, adding a second strain of bacteria to its pertussis vaccine. Following these changes, Finland experienced a 64 percent increase in incidence of juvenile diabetes.

As said, the HiB vaccine was brought into Finland on a trial basis, but in 1988 it was added to the vaccination schedule, thus making it compulsory. A few years before, in 1982, live MMR vaccine was added to this schedule. Not only was there an increase of diabetes in the zero to four-year-old group of children, but a 147 percent increase in the incidence of IDDM (insulin dependent diabetes mellitus). IDDM is an older name for type I diabetes.

Note this next set of statistics since as these vaccines were newly introduced they were only given to younger children. As noted, the youngest group took the two vaccines (with a 147 percent rise in incidence of diabetes) while the five- to nine-year-olds only received one of the vaccines. Their incidence of diabetes rose 40 percent. Ten-to-14-year-olds, who got no new vaccines, saw a rise in the incidence of IDDM by only 8 percent between the intervals of 1970–1976 and 1990–1992. Classen's conclusion: the rise in IDDM in different age groups correlated with the number of vaccines given to each group.

We've already underlined that the rates of type II diabetes have been going through the roof, but a similar process is taking place in relation to type I. In many European countries, during the past twenty to thirty years, the rate of juvenile diabetes has doubled. Typically such a doubling was seen in England in the period from 1985 to 1996 in relation to IDDM rates in children zero to four years of age. A smaller, but still significant, increase was also seen in children five to nine years old and ten to fourteen years old. In the US, according to a published study, "an exceptionally large increase (in cases of IDDM) in the youngest group (0–4 years of age) was observed."

As it's highly unlikely that there would be a sudden appearance of many more individuals genetically predisposed to diabetes I, the spiking incidence rates are probably due to environmental influences encountered very early in life.

Classen's research points to vaccines as the disturbing influence, and other studies have furthered this thought. Bear in mind, the appearance of more cases after the introduction of a vaccine does not prove the vaccine brought about the sky-rocketing disease incidence. There could be another, unknown factor responsible. Still on the face of it, such statistics as those of Classen and others about to be considered do make one question the possibility that these vaccines have very deadly, never-considered side effects, such as promoting diabetes I in some of the inoculated.

One of the other statistics to examine concerns England. The introduction of the HiB vaccine in 1985 was followed by an 11 percent annual increase in the incidence of diabetes among children aged zero to four, who commonly receive the vaccine by age fifteen months. Older children, between five and nine and between ten and fourteen, experienced a lower increase, 4 percent and 1 percent, respectively.

I've just remarked that evidence thus far only suggests but hardly proves any causal relation between vaccines and type I diabetes. This is the type of suggestiveness Classen and his fellow researchers try to move beyond in a new article where they argue that, in a particular case they look into, there is a causal association between immunization against H influenza type B and type I diabetes. In a letter published in the *British Medical Journal* (October, 23, 1999), the authors present preliminary results of their study (submitted for publication), which evaluated the incidence of diabetes among 116,000 children randomized to receive either four or one dose of the influenza vaccine, and compared it to the incidence in 128,500 children who did not receive any vaccine, since they were born in the two years prior to release of the vaccine.

They found by the age of seven, the incidence of diabetes per 100,000 individuals was 261, 237 and 207 among those receiving four, one or no doses of vaccine, respectively, while the incidence in the same cohorts when they had reached the age of ten had increased to 398, 376, and 340.

Averaging out these numbers and assuming the higher diabetes figures were caused by the vaccine's effects, Classen and his fellow researchers say this means we should expect at least 58 extra cases of diabetes for every 100,000 fully vaccinated children. The cost of treating these added diabetes patients greatly exceeds the potential benefits claimed to flow from vaccination (i.e., the prevention of seven deaths and 7–26 severe disabilities per 100,000 vaccinated children).

According to the authors' conclusions, "Research into immunization has been based on the theory that the benefits of immunization far outweigh the risks from delayed adverse events, and so long-term safety studies do not need to be performed. When looking at diabetes—only one potential chronic adverse event [since vaccinations may cause other diseases beside diabetes]—we found that the rise in the prevalence of diabetes may more than offset the expected decline in long-term complications of H influenza meningitis. Thus diabetes induced by vaccine should not be considered a rare potential adverse event. The incidence of many other chronic immunological disease, including asthma, allergies, and immune-mediated cancers, has risen rapidly and may also be linked to immunization."

Perhaps one of the more troubling points made in that conclusion, aside from the link between this vaccine and increased juvenile diabetes, is the thought that such possible links have never been scrutinized because they were *presumed* to be negligible. Earlier, in a number of remarks from the featured health professionals, it came up that some patients with health problems would refuse to look at their unwise lifestyle choices till it was nearly too late; in other words, when they had diabetes. Unless we wake up and carry out the needed studies, it seems the use of vaccines will follow a similar path. The deleterious effects that it appears some vaccines are producing, in upping the rates of juvenile diabetes, will not be looked at as they continue to increase until their occurrence become so alarming that the possible causal effect of vaccines must be faced, analyzed, and, to the degree they exist, eliminated.

Chapter 6

It's Not Your Fault You're Fat

I want to talk about the connection between obesity and diabetes, but I will begin from an unusual angle, by saying a few words about choice. As noted in the introduction when I brought up the American thinker John Dewey, I said he strove at all times for an integrated perspective. When discussing how people make decisions, he developed the idea of the *holistic choice*. In *Human Nature and Conduct*, Dewey divided between a spur-of-the-moment, off-the-cuff, unthinking choice and an intelligent, integrated choice. What distinguishes them?

In an unthinking choice, "the object thought of may simply stimulate some impulse or habit to a pitch of intensity, where it is temporarily irresistible." Consider, for example, the impulse buying of a sugary soda. This desired object "looms large in the imagination; it swells to fill the field . . . it absorbs us, enraptures us, carries us away, sweeps us off our feet with its own attractive force." So we buy and consume without further thought.

But there is another way of choosing. To appreciate it, Dewey says we must accept that all of us are made up of a mix of desires. For instance, let's say a woman wants to live healthily, but she also wants to drink something sweet at the moment, and she may also be an environmentalist, who doesn't want to, say, buy something in a plastic container that will be discarded and add to the earth's burden of pollutants. This woman, when she wants a sweet drink, makes a holistic choice to use a home juicer to produce a fresh fruit beverage. This choice is one that works by "unifying, harmonizing, different competing tendencies." All three of her desires (for something healthy, sweet, and environmentally benign) are bundled together, instead of, as in our prior example, the desire for something sweet taking precedence.

This holistic choice "may release an activity in which all [the person's desires] are fulfilled, not indeed, in their original form, but in a 'sublimated' fashion, that is in a way which modifies the original direction of each by reducing it to a component along with others in an action of transformed quality." This integration makes the choice deeply satisfying.

Two earlier points made by experts who voiced their opinions have direct bearing on the idea of holistic choice.

Dr. Shinitsky brought up health-compromised patients who were in a pre-contemplative state. In such cases, he said, "The patient is not thinking about the issue. It's as if this individual needs something or somebody to awaken him or her." One way of thinking about this is to say the patient is ignoring his or her own body, which is giving out unheeded distress signals.

If awakened, the patient begins perceiving the body's messages. Dr. Brown reported on one of his successful patients, who did listen to her inner voice. To recall his words, "As she became aware of her body's messages, which told her, for instance, how the food she ate was affecting her, she was better able to discriminate, differentiating between foods that were satisfying over time versus those that gave a quick burst of energy."

With these thoughts in mind, we can reinterpret Dewey's idea of integrated choice. A poor choice is made not just because one impulse overrides all the others, but because a person has not considered the full range of his or her desires, not listening to the body, for instance, when it is signaling that it is, say, "fed up" with a person's reliance on fast foods. Only when one knows the options can she or he practice holistic choice.

I will return to a discussion of choice below, but here and throughout I will also take on the broader topic of knowing your options, something extremely important when it comes to dealing with weight loss.

Take the simple caloric restriction diet. It seldom works because people think their only option is a blanket curtailing of calorie consumption. They don't realize the other option is a reduction of *select* calories. This second option differentiates, for example, between calories from the sugar of an apple (as it naturally occurs) and white granulated table sugar. Nor does the blanket condemnation make a distinction between the fiber in a laxative tablet and the naturally occurring fiber in roughage, such as in whole grains, legumes, beans, fruits and veggies. Without knowing about the option of choosing a selective calorie reductive diet, a person wanting to lose weight is often drawn to a diet that is failure prone.

Another point to consider is the question of competing desires raised at the head of this section. The typical diet considers only one desire of an adherent, to lose weight. But that means other desires and feelings, such as the loneliness that may be compelling a person to binge on a junk foods, doesn't enter the picture. But will a weight-reduction program be successful if it only considers this single desire? Maybe the fact that so many diets, ones which tens of millions of Americans have gotten on, ones that *look good on paper,* have had only marginal success. They have not tried to work with the whole gamut of issues related to losing weight, which involve emotional and physical needs.

It is highly unlikely that someone will make the best lifestyle choices when she or he is stressed out by such woes as loss of a job, unpaid bills or strained relationships. So if we do not speak about better ways of coping, we will undermine the most carefully crafted, anti-diabetic diet. To guard against this, part of this section will address the issues facing many Americans that create the stress and encourage them to use unhealthy "comfort foods" as a way of sublimating anxieties. One aim of this chapter is to help individuals at an emotional level so that they have the inner strength and stability to respond in a sustainable way at the dietary level.

In the chapter, we will first look at the causes and consequences of being overweight. Special attention will be given to overweight youth and children. Next, we bring up dieting, a practice that is seldom successful, versus a lifestyle change in eating habits, which is usually quite helpful. The importance of more exercise, detoxification and deep relaxation techniques will also be addressed. I will then look at some health problems that commonly accompany obesity, including depression and thyroid dysfunction. Eating disorders will also be examined.

No doubt about it, if we continue on the current path of increasing obesity among youth and children, the future looks grim. Extrapolating from childhood obesity rates in 2000, Dr. Kristine Bibbins-Domingo of the University of California, working with colleagues at San Francisco General Hospital and Columbia University, estimate that by 2020 as many as 44 percent of American women and 37 percent of men at age 35 will be obese—obese and, therefore, ill. By 2020, she writes, "we found, not unexpectedly, that the prevalence of heart disease will rise by as much as 16 percent, and heart disease deaths by as much as 19 percent between the ages of 35 and 50 years."

This increased incidence of obesity in the US has paralleled the growing number of cases of diabetes. For at least the last forty years,

Americans in all age groups have been gaining weight, and for the first time we have an epidemic of adult diabetes (type II) in children and teenagers. I doubt if you would be surprised to learn that the majority of people with type II diabetes are overweight, obese, and do not exercise.

Let me say a few more words about this linkage. According to the Centers for Disease Control and Prevention, "Compared to adults of a healthy weight, obese adults had twice the risk for high cholesterol, three times the risk for asthma, and four times the risk for arthritis. The strongest correlation was between obesity and diabetes: obese people exhibited over seven times the risk for diabetes compared with people of normal weight."

Much earlier in this text I gave a hint of one possible physiological connection between the added weight and the disease. I mentioned that sometimes insulin is blocked from ferrying glucose into storage cells because the cell receptors are clogged with cholesterol. I should add now a second problem with glucose uptake. As fat cells get bigger, especially the visceral fat, the number of insulin receptors declines, leaving less of them available to take up glucose. This also can lead to diabetes.

One may well ask what catastrophic change in our society has brought about these epidemics of obesity and diabetes. Previously in the book, Dr. Chris Cortman provided part of an answer by fingering a greater consumption of the "empty calories" of junk foods and sedentary lifestyles, encouraged by computers and other electronic playthings as two major culprits.

He could have expanded on his later point by saying that the electronics, from the Internet to cell phones and other new technologies, are time bandits. Individuals devote untoward amounts of daytime to being online, and when the sun goes down children, teenagers, and adults often stay up late twittering, connecting with friends on Facebook, and talking on cell phones. Valuable sleep time is traded for distractions. Moreover, since the users of electronics are so absorbed with their toys, they can't be bothered to cook a meal and turn to junk food for energy. Moreover, as these devices leech away time, little is left for such essential activities exercise. An individual often ends up with this health-threatening combination: lack of quality sleep, high levels of stress (because, for one, essential tasks are being neglected), inadequate exercise, and a highly processed, fast-food diet.

What I have just tried to do is render an integrated portrait of the problem. I didn't just say the factors involved are sedentary pursuits + junk food + lack of sleep, and so on. Rather, I tried to show these components synergistically work together to deplete your health. In other words, my presentation could be visualized: sedentary pursuits/ junk food/lack of sleep.

One problem with current recuperative strategies in our society is that they do not strive for such an integrative, comprehensive view, thus missing inner links and connections. A patient's problems are parceled out rather than taken as part of one package. If you are overweight, you will see a bariatric specialist. If you are stressed, you see a psychologist. High blood pressure puts you in the hands of an internist or cardiologist.

Think about this. Before a person is diagnosed with diabetes, he or she will normally 1) be overweight, 2) will have some form of inflammatory response, 3) will frequently have high blood pressure present with regular chronic infections, and 4) show symptoms of depression. If the person with these interconnected problems is seeing four specialists, one treating the weight, one the inflammatory response, and so on, then it's likely the underlying pathology is being missed. We'd have to get the four together in one room for them to figure out the patient had pre-diabetes.

To solve the problem, this dispersal of medical attention will not do. For true healing, you have to connect the dots and see how each of these conditions ultimately either leads to or exasperates diabetes. With this way of thinking, keeping the whole syndrome in mind at all times, then by preventing or treating one condition, by extension you are helping prevent or improve all of the conditions. Further, holistic diets and exercise regimens are designed not to cope with a single condition, but to condition the body to resist multiple possible health underminers. For instance, the diet that I am recommending for diabetics will help prevent:

- Heart disease
- High blood pressure
- Elevated cholesterol
- Arthritis
- Cancer
- Obesity

This diet relies on the Super Foods defense, utilizing a number of foods that are packed with immune-system boosters and natural energizers. These foods will be profiled in a separate chapter. Another section that takes a holistic view is "No More Excuses." There, I bear down on the question of choice, raised at the beginning of this chapter, and show how if we make the wrong choices each day—choices on any front from what to eat to how to deal with a new stressor—we end up engaged in a negative cascade that only makes our health conditions worse.

Our country's health and welfare delivery systems have been too long immersed in a compartmentalized view of the human condition. The integrated view presented here is the one that has empowered many alternative health practitioners searching for a better way. In my own work, I must say, thousands of individuals from my own health support group have reported that conditions as different as eczema, acne, psoriasis, fatigue and pain as well as respiratory conditions such as asthma and emphysema, and many other conditions including Alzheimer's, dementia, and Parkinson's disease, have been alleviated or completely rolled back seeking health the holistic way.

How Our Food and Environment Impact Us

Bottom line, even the healthiest eater in this country is being poisoned. Many of the foods we eat contain pesticides, herbicides, dyes, preservatives, flavoring, growth hormones, and antibiotics. And even a scrupulously careful vegetarian who seeks out food grown without pesticide use will inadvertently take in the poisons contained in air and water pollution. From these sources, environmental toxins enter our bodies through the lungs and skin. With all this bad stuff coming in, the organs responsible for detoxification, mainly the liver, the kidneys, and the skin, are working overtime. In the worst case, they are overtaxed and a person ends with a weakened immune system.

Bedeviled by all these incoming toxins, some of which (such as those in the air) are unavoidable, it is wise to at least avoid the ones you can, such as those contained in unhealthy foods, and eat health-giving ones. To find these life-enhancing foods, you have to patronize health food stores, which give access to high-quality materials, among them foods that are low in calories, high in fiber, contain quality proteins, and some that are gluten and sugar-free.

If you are going this route and eating non-toxically, avoid meat, dairy, processed sugar, artificial sweeteners, white bread, canned meats, alcohol-processed foods, cereals, coffee, and white rice. These all contribute to an overall acidic state.

An overly acidic condition is unhealthy, and is brought on by eating acidic foods, such as those listed above, which when they break down leave a residue of acid (as opposed to leaving traces of alkaline). This has adverse effects on the blood pH, which optimally needs a balance between acids and alkalines, and on the state of the fluids circulating between our cells. Chronic acidity will contribute to or exacerbate disease. An alkaline state is better for health and can be cultivated by eating a diet founded in whole, raw, organic plant-based foods.

And, if the danger of over-acidity and the growth hormones and other additives found in milk and meat weren't enough to steer you away from consuming them, think a moment of the environmental impact.

The meat and dairy industries harm us from two sides. For one, as few people know, they are devastating the natural world. These combined producers are major creators of water pollution in the United States using about 50 percent of the country's water supply to run their industries. Deforestation around the world, such as the denudation of the Amazon jungles, is also partially caused by the need for more room to raise animals for food.

In America, the cows, pigs and other animals are warehoused, raised in small pens and constantly injected with hormones and anti-biotic chemicals just to keep them alive long enough to kill them for their meat. With this treatment, the animal's meat is well laced with disease-causing organisms, including pesticides and herbicides, growth hormone, and tranquilizers.

From the other side, the consumption of this "diseased" meat con-tributes to illnesses in the eater's body.

Cow milk is no less harmful than meat, for one, because it is overly stocked with protein. Human breast milk is about 5 percent protein; cows' milk about 15 percent protein. That's overkill, given that, as mentioned, too much protein in the body strains the kidneys. Consuming dairy also raises the acidic environment in the body. If there is too much acidity, then in order to rebalance the pH level, the body will withdraw calcium from bones. The loss of this bone calcium contributes to osteoporosis. Add to that, the toxic ingredients mixed in the cow's meat, such as growth hormone and tranquilizers, are also are found in milk. For all these reasons, I encourage replacing cows' milk with soy, rice, almond, coconut, and/or hazelnut milk, which are delicious, nutritious alternatives.

To end this section, having suggested some of the dangers and pitfalls of eating meat and drinking milk, let me show the other side of the picture by enumerating some of the benefits of a plant-based diet that is further enhanced by taking supplements. Rather than give an exhaustive list, I will just mention a few supplements and foods off the top of my head, leaving a fuller exposition to the super foods section.

Take the supplement chlorella, which is derived from green algae. It contains much more chlorophyll than green leafy vegetables and it is also a detoxifier, binding with heavy metals, pesticides and carcinogens, which it escorts out of the body. This algae also holds high levels of nucleic acids, DNA and RNA, which are crucial for cell growth and repair.

Two other valuable supplements are acidophilus and bifidus, which are probiotics. The probiotics are the friendly bacteria, making up four hundred microspecies, that inhabit the small and large intestine, aiding digestion. Acidophilus is like some of the other Renaissance players named in my protocol. Not only does it help prevent disease, but also aids in the production of vitamins, increases the absorption of calcium, helps normalize cholesterol levels in the blood, and promotes the production of digestive enzymes. Bifidus also takes many roles, including ensuring regular bowel movements and stimulating vitamin B production. These two are real multi-taskers.

Flax seeds are also invaluable, for one, because they provide essential fatty acids, namely the omega-3 and omega-6 varieties. All cells contain these fatty acids as components of their membranes, and if the acids are lacking the membranes become damaged. In consequence, the cells fall out of balance, losing both their ability to communicate efficiently with other cells and to regulate hormones. Any diet high in omega-3 foods will help lower cholesterol, blood pressure, and diabetes risk; help prevent heart attacks and cancer; protect against allergies; and turn down inflammation. Flax oil is the best way to keep a steady flow of high omega-3 fatty acids in the body.

Other things to get into your body are enzymes. These energized protein molecules assist in the regulation of all living cells. In both plants and animals, they provide the energy for biochemical reactions, such as those involved in the absorption of nutrients that goes on in food digestion. Note that while fresh, raw or lightly steamed foods vegetables are chock full of enzymes, cooking foods above 100 degrees Fahrenheit will destroy many of these enzymes. This can be taken as another fact that points to the "wisdom" of mother nature or, perhaps, to the way our bodies are adapted to the foodstuffs in the natural environment, in that the closer an eaten vegetable or fruit is to its natural state, the more health-giving it tends to be.

As noted, I've mentioned these few foods and supplements only to give you a "taste" of what is to come later when I bring up super foods and related subjects. The point is again double. I want you to begin to move to eating a vegetarian or semi-vegetarian diet. But also, I want you to do so in an informed manner. I agree with what Dr. Calapai said earlier: "I don't just write out prescriptions and tell the patient what to do. I explain things to them." In short, as long as you act on what you know, the more you understand, the more you heal.

Obesity Classified

"Obesity" should not be taken as an insulting term given to overweight people, but part of a classification drawn from a rough and ready measurement called the Body Mass Index (BMI). It is commonly used to give an approximate measure of obesity, although, as I will indicate below, it is not to be substituted for more refined ideas to determine how dangerous to health the added weight is. The BMI is calculated by dividing weight by height squared with the formula: BMI = kg/m^2. It was originally developed by a Belgian thinker and so is formulated in metric figures. To translate it to feet, inches, and pounds use the formula: weight in pounds/height in inches squared × 703. Using this calculation, a classification of normal and abnormally light or heavy-weighted people has been developed:

Obesity range	BMI kg/m²	Health status
Underweight	18.5	Increased risk
Normal	18.5–24.9	Normal risk
Overweight	25–29.9	Increased risk
Obese 1	30–34.9	High risk
Obese 2	35–39.9	Very high risk
Extreme obese	≥ 40	Extremely high risk

I mentioned that this chart is not an be-all and end-all determination of health in that certain types of fat are more harmful to the body's functioning that others. Visceral fat in the midriff, such as that found on a man with a beer belly, is dangerous because that fat closely surrounds organs like the heart and liver. This kind of obesity is associated with heart disease and diabetes. Peripheral fat, on the other hand, fat lying right under the skin but not protruding further into the body, is less hazardous, being less related to the mentioned illnesses. Sumo wrestlers have this kind of peripheral fat.

What Type of Fat Are You Carrying?

Yet, some researchers have pointed out that visceral fat, bad as it is, is not the type to be most worried about. Senior investigator Samuel Klein, a Danforth professor of medicine and nutritional science at Washington University's Center for Human Nutrition and Geriatric Science, points his finger at fat in the liver as even more dangerous.

He notes that when individuals carry an excess of fat in the liver, this leads to insulin resistance, a precursor or accompaniment of diabetes. He argues that the greatest hazard the body faces is from this type of poundage, saying, "Those [whom he studied] without a fatty liver did not have markers of metabolic problems. Whether shaped like pears or apples, it is fat in the liver that influences metabolic risk." (By his allusions to fruit-like bodies, he is referencing a common medical shorthand, which contrasts apple-shaped people with fat around the waist to pear-shaped people, who carry weight in their thighs and backsides.)

It is particularly disheartening when fatty liver disease, brought on when the liver is swamped with fat, is found in young people. Dr. Klein elaborates, "Multiple organ systems become resistant to insulin in these adolescent children with fatty liver disease. The liver becomes resistant to insulin and muscle tissue does, too."

This doesn't mean that abdominal fat can be discounted as an indicator and provoker of illness, which Klein himself acknowledges. He points out, noting some of the facts noticed in the last section, a fat belly is an important marker for inflammation that is present in heart disease, diabetes, and high blood pressure. Moreover, as testified to by numerous studies, fat around the belly and abdomen indicate a defect in the body's response to insulin.

Overall, excess weight is always bad, but as these researchers make evident, not all fat is created equal.

The Multi-factorial Etiology of Obesity: Genetics, Environment, Psychological, Behavioral, Emotional, Lifestyle, Media, and Socioeconomic Factors

When we began this chapter, I laid out a couple of what should be evident factors behind the increased incidence of obesity in our society. These were a sedentary lifestyle and junk food consumption. I say "should be" only because people tend to deny their influence, and certain interests, such as those who sell soft drinks and French fries, do their best to foster such denial.

That wasn't the whole story however, since a number of other factors have been identified as playing a part in the etiology of obesity. Indeed, the inclusion of a whole host of contributing factors that go from the deep internal genetic ones to the seemingly external larger socioeconomic ones, such as the effect of lower economic status on exercise time, which will be noted below, is one thing that differentiates *integrated healthcare* from traditional medicine.

Interestingly enough, Dewey made this same distinction in contrasting progressive education, which he helped found in the 1920s, from the old pedagogical techniques. The older model never went deeply into the factors that determined what needed to be understood in a child's background for an educational process to be successful. It relied only on what was already accepted. Progressive education tried to be multi-factorial in analysis. As Dewey puts it forcefully in *Experience and Education:*

> Traditional education did not have to face this problem [of looking at all the factors that determined whether an education is effective]; it could systematically dodge this responsibility. The school environment of desks, blackboards, a small school yard, was supposed to suffice. There was no demand that the teacher should become intimately acquainted with the conditions of the local community, physical, historical, economic, occupational, etc., in order to utilize them as educational resources.

From this passage, you can see that though his subject matter is different, quite like practitioners of integrated healthcare, Dewey was concerned with examining every available component of a situation in order to move ahead with the utmost clarity. This type of as-thorough-as-possible examination is what I want to carry out here in looking at the roots of obesity.

One additional factor we have to consider is genetics. Six genes have been identified as contributing to obesity. It has been found that 8 to 10 percent of obese patients have a genetic disposition to gain weight, something that seems to be rooted in metabolism difficulties.

A word about how this genetic flaw may play out in the body, which will require a brief elucidation of how hormones regulate food intake. When a person's stomach is relatively empty, the hormone ghrelin is released, telling the brain it is hungry and needs to eat. Once food has been consumed, leptin, a hormone made by fat, goes to the brain and tells the body to stop eating. From the brain's end, this is controlled by a number of integrated entities, including the hypothalamus, which, reading the hormone intakes, tells the body when to eat and when to stop eating. For instance, towards the end of a meal, ghrelin stops being released, and the brain calls for a slow down. It has been theorized that some individuals with a genetic disposition to obesity do not have enough leptin or they do not have the receptors to bind to the leptin, so their brains are not getting a proper message warning them that they are full.

Turning to other factors that encourage obesity, let me go back to something said in the introduction to this section. There I talked of how people find it easy to grab a sugary or salty snack while they are tuned into their electronic playthings. I didn't add the fact that commercial interests involved in the fast-food industry do everything they can to discourage thought about the costs to the body of eating too many of their products. These interests also rarely consider such costs when they roll out a new commodity or addition to a commodity that looks to be lucrative. In the 1980s, for example, soda manufacturers started putting fructose in soft drinks. This significantly increased their sugar and calorie load.

And these commercial interests make their voices heard. Billboards, advertisements, and commercials proclaim the virtues of stacker combos, and speak of bonuses for eating more. The way these interests see it, the more you eat, the greater their revenue, so roll out the value meals, kids' meals, and jumbo portions.

The interests hyping these foods represent one of the economic factors at play in the promotion of obesity. Another is found in the financial pressure many people are under, particularly when our economy itself is under stress. This affects the poor disproportionally. For instance, individuals with only a high school diploma report almost no time to exercise. One reason they are feeling this time crunch is due to the need to put in long hours to make an adequate paycheck. Working several jobs to pay bills is the priority, and exercise is put off till better times. You can see this by states. Those with lower income levels lead the pack in obesity rates. By state, Louisiana and Mississippi vs. Colorado and Connecticut represent the highest and lowest obesity rates respectively. The way these figures tally with economic figures can be seen by checking the 2000 census. According to its findings, the percent of people who made under $10,000 a year in Louisiana and Mississippi were 15 and 16 percent, in marked contrast to Colorado and Connecticut, who both showed around 7 percent in the lowest bracket.

Note, too, that if overwork keeps people from the gym or other places of exercise, the schools are also dropping the ball. While physical education classes were a requirement before 1991, between 1991 and 2003, these courses became an elective in many schools. This is ironic on many fronts, not only because there is also an emphasis on student athletics just as many PE classes are being cut, but because much research has shown that youth who are fit are more alert in class and more apt at learning.

As a number of the experts whose voices we heard earlier remarked, emotions play a big role in connection to food. Remember the patient who counted on her "friends," Ben and Jerry, when she was feeling down. This is emotional eating, the kind engaged in, not to fill one's stomach, but assuage such feelings as sadness or anxiety or fear. There is also a mirror image situation in relation to friendship. If one is with unenlightened friends, for example, who are going out to eat their favorite burger and fries, to be part of the crowd one eats the same. On the other hand, if one is lonely, the individual, like the pal of Ben and Jerry, eats to alleviate feelings of being unwanted.

Putting it all together, we see that obesity is tied to a whole host of factors, possible genetic predisposition, a society that has many sedentary pursuits and junk-food delights on offer, along with a commercial structure of ads and an instant gratification philosophy that encourage bad eating. Add to this economic factors, such as abnormally long hours at the workplace, and the elimination or cutting down of PE classes in public schools, often because of budgetary constraints. Plus, the fact that unhealthy foods often have a compensatory emotional uplift, craved by many in an emotionally impoverished society. These multiple factors are the force behind today's tidal wave of obesity.

Am I Full?—Body and Brain Messenger Players Need to Communicate

In the previous section, I brought up the role leptin takes in regulation of food intake. As I put it, "Once food has been consumed, leptin, a hormone made by fat, goes to the brain and tells the body to stop eating." For some that explanation was probably sufficient, but since so much work has been done recently on leptin's place in the etiology of weight gain, I thought I might say a few more things about it.

Scientists at the Oregon National Primate Research Center looked at the workings of leptin and made the surprising discovery that obesity in mice correlated with excessive leptin levels. On the surface, it might appear that leptin, which tells the brain it's time to stop eating, should be scarce not abundant in the overweight. However, the research showed that "high levels of leptin can lead to leptin resistance. Leptin resistance means that the body no longer responds to the hormone's weight-suppressing effects."

As Dr. Michael Cowley and associate scientists in the Division of Neuroscience at ONPRC, who were studying the reaction of brain cells, ones that normally respond to leptin by sending signals to the body to stop food intake, explain, "Eventually the cells behaved as if there was no leptin present, even though levels were forty times higher than in normal animals."

Noting the problem caused by excess leptin, researchers at the University of Florida College of Medicine, led by professor of pharmacology and therapeutics Dr. Philip Scarpace, wanted to see if there was any way leptin could be used to prevent weight gain, even though its chances of being of value would seem to be diminished by the fact that the obese seemed to have become unresponsive to its signaling function. As the researchers put it bluntly, "Scientists had [once] hoped to wield leptin as a weight-loss weapon. Studies in lean animals were promising, but overweight animals and people don't respond the same way, likely because their bodies already overproduce leptin, causing them to develop resistance to the hormone."

However, Scarpace's group found that while, as expected, obese rats given leptin showed no reduction in weight, if overweight rats were put on an exercise regimen as well given the leptin, they did achieve weight loss. "What the act of running [the rats' exercise] appears to do is allow the leptin to work again. It's a demonstration that this simple act can reverse leptin resistance. The obese rats that ran and took leptin kept the extra weight off."

As of yet, scientists can't pinpoint exactly why overweight people develop resistance to leptin and what role the hormone really plays in obesity. The research reported here goes part of the way toward an understanding of this hormone and also gives powerful encouragement to those, like myself, who see regular exercise as one of the paramount parts of a weight-loss plan in that the obese's resistance to leptin was overcome in individuals who exercised.

The Globalization of Obesity

While the previous paragraphs focused on ill health in the US earlier in this text I brought up the spread of diabetes around the globe. There I talked of the 20-year rule, the concept that heart disease and diabetes appeared in non-Western countries twenty years after a Western diet, heavy on the junk foods, is taken up. Here, let me add that obesity is also undergoing this form of "globalization."

Some of the healthiest people on earth are the citizens of Okinawa, which are a set of islands off the coast of Japan. The residents of these islands are of Japanese descent, yet they live much longer and are healthier than Japanese living in Japan. Why?

Traditionally, the diet of the Okinawans is low-fat, low-salt foods, such as fish, tofu, and seaweed. Such eating not only keeps them fit but grants them longevity. Five times as many Okinawans live to be 100 as compared to the Japanese on the mainland, and the Japanese are longest-living people in the world! It is not just eating, of course. Several studies have shown that the Okinawans have not been compromised by high levels of stress, a fast-paced existence or by succumbing to a fast-food Westernized diet.

Sadly enough, those in mainland Japan, who used to have lifestyles or at least eating styles not that different from those of the islanders are now succumbing to the same diseases and, significantly, the same obesity as found in the West because they have adopted many of the West's disgraceful dietary habits.

The same faulty moves are being made in China and in India where the same overweight problems and attendant diseases are appearing. Both countries have approximately 1.2 to 1.3 billion citizens. The vast majority are dirt poor in both countries. Obviously there are numerous downsides to extreme poverty, but traditionally these did not include an addiction to junk food or high-meat diets since these were pricey.

The traditional diet in India, with the exception of the deep frying of some foods and the adding of large amounts of sugar to others, is very healthy. The Indians rely extensively upon legumes and basmati rice, as well as potatoes and starchy vegetables as a center of their diet. The traditional Chinese diet, although it varies widely by region in this big nation, put grains, such as rice, at the center, and also gives big play to vegetables.

In both these countries, in some sectors, there has been a shift to a heavy meat, pork, cheese, and processed food diet. Suddenly and predictably, now obesity is epidemic in both countries. Also predictably, these results are being seen among the better-educated, higher income earners for it is they that can afford the meat and junk diets. They are less likely to be physically active and more likely to spend much time stationed in front of a computer.

On a personal note, I have several friends who are physicians of Indian origin. They are disheartened by this growth of obesity and its related diseases in their home country. Such bad eating styles were simply not an issue when they were growing up or in their earlier years of medical practice because there was no cachet to eating Western foods or gorging on meat.

Even in the Mediterranean countries known for their healthier diets, such as Spain, Greece, and Italy, things are beginning to change. Broadly speaking, they traditionally had a lifestyle where food consisted of whole grains, lots of fruits and vegetables, red wine, and fish, and existence was centered on an extended family, laid-back living, and being physically active throughout one's life.

Again, things are changing, at least in the more affluent groups, where suddenly obesity in children and adults is common, fueled by junk food. As a sign of the latter, France, long considered a center of haute cuisine, expensive but healthy eating, a country whose citizens would have once turned up their noses at the foods consumed by Americans, is now the host to numerous McDonald's, ones usually bulging with customers. This is another mark of the impact of globalization, which in many ways has proven a health disaster.

The Symptoms, Stigma, and Human Toll of Diabetes and Obesity

This last section has revealed that obesity is a global epidemic, and its downsides are many, not the least of which is that it is very common for observers of the situation, overlooking the multi-factorial origin of an overweight condition, put total blame on individuals for the obesity epidemic.

If an unenlightened youngster sees an obese kid coming, he greets him by calling out "fatty" or "supersize." Adults, who usually are a little less crude, judge obese people as weak willed and lazy. The result, since how a person looks at you has so much influence on how you look at yourself, is low self-esteem for obese people. An illuminating insight from Dewey, drawing from the *Human Conduct* book mentioned already, concerns how people define what is right for them to do. Most people get their ideas of what is morally right from listening to what others (verbally or non-verbally) tell them. Doing right "is only the abstract [expression] for the multitude of concrete demands in action which others impress upon us, and of which we are obliged, if we would live to take some account." To put this in slightly reversed terms, since Dewey is concerned with people pressured to do right things, let's say that people are also pushed to "do the wrong thing," as in an example already given where a person goes along with friends who are binging on junk foods. The same applies when an overweight child, perhaps having some self confidence, enters an environment where obesity is ridiculed. Soon enough, following the unconscious demands of others, the child is "obliged" to adopt the group opinion and look down on him or herself.

Since other peoples' first impressions of an obese person are often negative, as seen in their tendency to avoid eye contact and to be dismissive, overweight people face constant roadblocks to socializing, finding work, buying clothes, and forming healthy relationships. Employers, especially in the service industries, where personnel are waiting on or interacting with the public in some other way, will look askance at overweight individuals, being reluctant to hire them because they do not fit into the public's expectations of what a vibrant and energetic individual should look like. Even public accommodations, such as the standard-sized airplane seat, movie theatre seat, and park bench, seem to reject them.

This is particularly bad for young people, for, as my example of kids' name calling makes clear, among young people and kids, summary condemnation of obesity is fairly common. When this happens, children and teens become marginalized. Being kept out of many social gathering and friendship circles, these young people suffer from feelings of loneliness.

The social ostracism that often comes with obesity is one of a number of negative accompanying factors. People who are over-weight tend to suffer from fatigue, which affects mental alertness, stamina, and the ability to participate in everyday activities. An obese person may not be able to face such run-of-the-mill hurdles as standing in a long checkout line, climbing stairs or walking across a parking lot. Sleep apnea, in which rest is interrupted by extended pauses in taking a breath, which wake the sleeper up, is also common with the overweight. The added weight will lead to back problems and osteoarthritis in that there is excess pressure on the joints.

To sum up some other health disabilities, compared to non-obese individuals, those who are obese are:

- four times more likely to have high blood pressure
- eight times more likely to develop diabetes
- ten times more likely to suffer from hyperlipidemia (a high amount of lipids in the blood, which is associated with con-tracting heart disease)
- two and a half times more likely to have liver problems

In addition, common diseases and conditions associated with obesity include:

- Skin diseases
- Blood circulation disorders
- Joint disorders
- Menstrual problems

- Infertility
- Breast cancer
- Endometrial cancer
- A decrease in libido
- Mental and emotional stress

Youth Today: Overweight, Sugar Coated, Highly Processed, and Stressed Out

In discussing the stigma attached to obesity in the last part, I paid special attention to children, who often have a harder time than adults coping with the rejection and loneliness that are an overweight condition's usual companions. In this section, I want to look at over-weightness as it is found in young people and children, highlighting what is in store for them if they continue to be obese as well as noting how parents and counselors can work with them to turn the situation around.

We saw how type II diabetes, once nearly unknown among youth, has been growing by leaps and bounds in the younger age groups. We also saw childhood obesity is ascending in the same way. In the last thirty years, the number of overweight children in the US has more than doubled.

And being overweight, keep in mind, will often prefigure later life-threatening conditions. The higher a child's BMI from ages seven to thirteen, the greater the risk of heart disease to the overweight individual. More specifically, in females who are overweight at a young age, the likelihood of developing the disease in adulthood is 24 percent greater than it would be for non-overweight children, and in boys there is a 33 percent increased risk of developing coronary heart disease compared to the risk of their slimmer peers.

One particularly troubling fact is that where it might be thought that a parent would try to inform his or her kids about the dangers of weight gain, new research has revealed that parents often do not recognize or simply deny that their own children are at risk. This is particularly the case where the mothers and fathers themselves are overweight. Since parents are one of the primary role models for youth, the disconnect here is very troubling.

Researchers Jessica Doolen, MSN, FNP, Patricia T. Alpert, and Sally K. Miller came to these chilling conclusions after examining parental perceptions of childhood obesity in the United States, the United Kingdom, Australia, and Italy:

- Black women were more content with their extreme weight as compared to white women who were large in size.
- Children of more highly educated parents were less likely to be overweight or at risk of being overweight.
- If parents were overweight, the children's risk was very pronounced.

As the authors emphasized, if parents cannot come to grips with these health problems and help themselves and their children to overcome the risks associated with obesity, then the health problems in our country will continue to grow and diabetes will only get worse.

Let me end this subsection by again emphasizing that obesity and diabetes go hand in hand in youth, which can best be shown by citing some of the statistics summarized in a fine paper done by researchers led by Dr. Lenna Liu from the Center for Child Health, Behavior, and Development at the Seattle Children's Hospital. It begins with some interesting facts about the differences between males and females.

- Non-Hispanic white males aged from three to eleven with type I diabetes were more likely to be overweight/obese than females (34 percent versus 27 percent) while females were more likely to be overweight/obese when they were twelve to nineteen years of age (37 percent versus 29 percent).

- African-American females were significantly more likely to be overweight/obese in both age groups than males (54/55 percent versus 36/36 percent), but there were no significant differences between Hispanic males and females.
- Approximately one in eight children and youths with type I diabetes (13 percent) were obese, less than the 79 percent of subjects with type II diabetes and the 17 percent without diabetes.
- The figures for children and youths with type II diabetes showed that 91 percent of African Americans were obese, as were 88 percent of American Indians and 75 percent of Hispanics.

So, having looked at the dangers of diabetes and other diseases that weigh over the heads of obese youth and having seen the increasing prevalence of childhood and youthful obesity, one might well ask: how did things get so far out of hand?

How Did Things Get Out of Hand?

One reason the rise of obesity has been so unexpected is that the conditions that characteristically precede the disease have changed, making it emerge in unexpected precincts. Now, obesity is typically found among the children of the affluent, children who have the money and leisure to gobble junk food while sitting transfixed by their electronic devices.

This is a relatively new phenomenon. Historically, the socio-economic profile of the obese was quite different. In the old days, even until quite recently, most situations of obesity, including having diabetes or being overweight, were associated with the inadequate living conditions of being poor.

This association is backed up, for example, in a study by Dr. Siobhon Maty, an epidemiologist in Oregon at the Portland State University School of Community Health. She evaluated data from a study of adults ages seventeen to ninety-four from 1965 to 1999. Thus, her findings are based on people who largely grew up before the changed patterns of eating and of adopting sedentary lifestyles set in. Of 5,913 individuals in the study, 307 developed diabetes during the 34 years. Sixty-five percent of those getting the disease were from low-income households, and, in particular, had grown up in poverty. Fifty-four percent of those who developed diabetes were women.

Maty concludes from these findings, "Diabetes strikes harder at those who were poor as children. Participants who were disadvantaged in youth were more likely to develop diabetes than their better off peers." I'm arguing that such findings may not be transferrable to the present where the children of the affluent are getting diabetes and showing the weight gain associated with it in record numbers. What I want to take away from this study, which is not its main point, but readily gained from reading it, is that since the reality has been that diabetes and obesity were once found particularly in the lower classes (and they still are found there), their sudden expansion across class lines so that they are now a major problem for the middle class and those from even higher brackets has caught many unaware.

By the way, these last reflections shouldn't be taken to indicate that now that obesity and diabetes have become widespread in the middle and upper classes, it has abated in the lower class. Would that it were true.

Having a lower income is still correlated with high rates of childhood obesity. Another professor of epidemiology, Dr. Adam Drewnowski, director of the University of Washington's Center of Obesity Research, has put this connection clearly in these remarks. "The fight against obesity and the eradication of poverty are in fact one in the same. . . . Childhood poverty is on the rise. Does it mean that we [are in the process of] becoming an obese nation? I am afraid that it does." So while obesity spreads upward from the poor, it also continues among the lowest financial sectors.

However, there is another reason for this inattention to the phenomenal increase of obesity, beyond socioeconomic factors. Obesity has been ignored as a precursor marking disease to come. In America, many healthcare professionals appear to buy into the idea that if their patients do not have a defined illness, clearly indicated through obvious symptoms, then they are well. Let's say a male patient came to see the doctor. He was short, 300 pounds and tired all the time. If his doctor couldn't diagnose a classic disease, he would write him a clean bill of health. That was a mistake, a health-threatening mistake. Let me put it plainly. *It is not possible to be healthy and overweight.*

Remember when President Clinton, an overweight individual, got his annual checkup as all presidents are required to do and was pronounced fit as a fiddle? Shortly thereafter, he was rushed to a New York hospital for quadruple bypass surgery to save his life.

(As an aside, let me say that if we really had a preventive medicine model in mind—something much discussed by politicians and healthcare providers, but seldom followed through on—anyone who is overweight, diabetic or has any form of heart condition would get blood chemistry tests such as C-reactive protein, homeocysteine, fibrinogen, triglycerides or thyroid exams. Such a person would also be examined for his or her level of free testosterone, cytokines, and other pro-inflammatory blood markers. Testing all these people would be expensive, but hardly so when contrasted to the money saved that would have to be spent on care for the diseases that these tests would help diagnose so the concerned practitioner could nip them in the bud.)

To continue with my point about the havoc caused by physicians and other health workers' refusal to consider obesity as a disease indicator, let me just bring up something said loud and clear by a number of the experts who gave their insights in an earlier chapter. A disease is a process. It's not so much like a noun, which defines a given, static state, as like a verb, which describes movement and transition. An illness takes time to reach a full-blown state. The more negative stressors and less visible symptoms that accumulate, the greater likelihood that at some point an individual will have a biological, hormonal, physiological tipping, the emergence of an endangering physical crisis. Only when the crisis time comes, will he or she be given a classification by a health worker. "You are diabetic" the person suddenly learns.

In fact, according to Dr. Maty, it could take anywhere from ten to fifteen years "for type II diabetes to develop to the point where the individual is aware of the signs and symptoms and seeks clinical care. Being overweight or obese as an adult further increases the risk of diabetes."

An additional voice on this issue is University of Michigan C. S. Mott Children's Hospital pediatric endocrinologist Joyce Lee, M. D, MPH. She weighs in on the danger of ignoring obesity now, thus ensuring large health costs for the overweight individuals in the future, by stressing the time lag between first signs and eventual emergence of sickness. In her words, the "full impact of the child-hood obesity epidemic has yet to be seen because it can take up to ten years or longer for obese individuals to develop type II diabetes." And, this means, as we've seen, since children are becoming obese at a younger age, the typical onset age of type II diabetes is drift-ing lower. Lee comments, "Children who are obese today are more likely to develop type II diabetes as young adults. . . . Recent studies suggest that there have been dramatic increases in type II diabetes among individuals in their 20s and 30s whereas it used to be that individuals developed type II diabetes in their 50s or 60s."

Wouldn't the individual, the one mentioned earlier who suddenly learns he or she had diabetes have been better off if fifteen years before he or she, who, let us say, was obese at the time, had been told, "You are pre-diabetic, and you'd better take some steps to address the situation"? Certainly, not only the individual but our whole society would benefit from such early intervention.

Causes and Consequences, Genetic Predisposition and Low Birth Rate

In opening this chapter, I was able to give some attention to the causes of obesity, where I made a few remarks about youth, but now I want to put the focus on early life issues, ones that have not yet been discussed, but which may be influential on later developments of obesity. These factors include a low birth rate and a possibly genetic predisposition to weight gain.

Researchers at the Center for Applied Genomics at the Children's Hospital of Philadelphia, in a study led by Struan F. A. Grant, have noted the one gene variant that has been associated with type II diabetes is also found in obese children.

It is important to keep in mind, however, that while some genes have been linked to obesity and overweight risk, eating habits are the primary mediating factor, the one that turns potential for obesity into actual weight gain.

Recent (2009) research reported in the *American Journal of Clinical Nutrition* and conducted by the Marju Orho-Melander research group at Lund University Diabetes Center in Sweden has stressed the role played by food. Speaking for the group, Emily Sonestedt MSc and PhD said, "This is the first study where the effect of the gene has been studied in relation to food habits."

The pre-dispositional gene studied has been dubbed the FTO gene (fat mass and obesity associated), and is one that is widespread. Seventeen percent of the population has double copies, meaning the people received it from both parents, and another 40 percent has a single copy. In sum, the FTO gene is possessed by 57 percent of the population studied. However, thankfully, 57 percent of this population is not overweight. The Lund study suggests why.

Sonestedt provides this clarification, "When the eating habits of the carriers of the double risk variant for obesity were analyzed . . . [we saw that] the risk of obesity was dramatically increased only in the case of high fat consumption." Without poor eating habits, a person would not become fat even though he or she had a gene that was associated with obesity. In fact, this is true even when one had that gene in double force. According to Sonestedt, "For those who had a diet where less than 41 percent of the energy consumed came from fat, obesity was not more common than in the population group that was minus the gene."

While this research brings the good news that this genetic predisposition does not predetermine that one will be obese, another troubling link to something out of a person's control, low birth weight, has also been made with diabetes. First off, let's move somewhat off the focal topic and look at low birth weight and inflammation. Then we will see how these two factors mesh with obesity.

Dr. Dexter Canoy of the University of Manchester has noted, "Lower weight at birth may increase inflammatory processes in adulthood, which are associated with chronic diseases such as those of the heart and diabetes." We've seen already that obese people often have inflammation. Also noted earlier was the fact that inflammation is a normal physiologic response in the body when it is engaged in a protective response to infection or tissue injury. However, if the infection or injury is not healed by the immune system and the inflammation is long term, this may promote the development of heart disease or diabetes.

So what is the connection Canoy is finding? He wanted to look into the already established link between being born small, which typically entails having a weak immune system, and the later development of a tendency to inflammation. This link had been remarked in studies that, for example, found excessive white blood cells in six-year-olds who had a low birth size. White blood cells in excess are markers of inflammation.

Canoy's work duplicated these earlier studies, using a different population group of 5,619 children born in 1966. His results tallied with the previous work. He explained, "Our findings suggest that the link between poorer growth early in life and these adult chronic diseases may involve inflammation as a common underlying factor."

So far, this work is not directly related to obesity, but other, slightly different research has established a link. As *The Science Daily* reports, "Another group of researchers . . . has found evidence suggesting that small size at birth and excessive weight gain during adolescence and young adulthood may lead to low grade inflammation, which, in turn, is associated with an increased risk of developing heart disease." Here obesity has been brought into the mix.

It may seem counterintuitive that low birth weight would lead to obesity in childhood and adolescence, but such a pattern is frequently underlined in the research. Whether there is any causal influence (i.e., whether low birth weight predisposes a person to become obese) is not yet known. However, we do know that both states are highly correlated with abnormally high instances of inflammation in the body.

For instance, one study looked at the amount of CRP (C-reactive protein) in the body, with the understanding that this protein is seen in elevated levels at times of inflammation. The findings were that "people who were amongst the smallest at birth, but who then put on the most weight up to the age of thirty-one, had the highest average CRP levels." You see that the authors are finding ties between low birth weight, later obesity, and inflammation. As it turns out, the obesity/inflammation connection is the most noticeable one. As they go on to say, "Every extra kg/m2 (BMI) gained from the age of fourteen to thirty-one was associated with a 16 percent rise in CRP levels; this association was greatest for people who had the highest BMI at fourteen."

Paul Elliott, professor of epidemiology and public health medicine and head of the Department of Epidemiology and Public Health at Imperial College, London, remarks about the treatment implications of these findings, which link obesity to chronic inflammation, "It is essential that suitable advice is given to children, teenagers and young adults about the effect that excessive weight gain may have on their future cardiovascular health."

I might add that such advice should include suggestions on dietary changes. A study that looked simply at reduction of inflammation in overweight people turned around the level of C-reactive proteins. According to a report of the study, "Women who completed a 12-week restricted calorie diet lost an average of 17.4 pounds and reduced their C-reactive protein levels by 26 percent."

To sum up, in both cases, that of genetic predisposition and low birth weight, the adverse situation of having the gene or low weight does not by itself predetermine an outcome. Having either or both of these givens does not mean you will be overweight. It is still within your power to avoid gaining weight and to opt for a healthy, natural life.

What Is the Key Factor in Convincing a Person to Opt for Health?

Now that exhaustive consideration has been given to the multi-factorial causes of obesity, its prevalence in our society and spread across the world, it is time to turn to solutions.

Let me say at the get-go, that while flexibility is generally a good trait, sometimes it's not feasible in health matters. As those who have worked in healing groups with me have learned, I believe in some areas I have to lay down the law. One doesn't go from three juicy hamburgers a week, to two, to one, to none. With such foods, it is better to jump directly from three to none. You see, I do not start with a protocol designed to accommodate people at their level of comfort. The idea that doing a little is better than doing nothing is not productive in terms of certain parameters, such as hamburger eating.

However, going a little further, let me say that the danger of taking compromised half steps in trying to regain one's health and a better weight is perhaps more psychological than physical for, as I will show in a moment, if obesity is not "all in your mind," that's still where a lot of the force to overcome unhealthy conditions arrive from, that is, from a proactive and knowledgeable mindset.

I was convinced of this point by a study I made twenty years ago. To qualify, participants had to be obese or morbidly overweight for at least the past twelve months. (As it turns out, the average time they have been overweight was seven years.) The subjects had a myriad of other health conditions, with diabetes and heart disease being high on that list.

I wanted to try something different. I divided the participants into five 100-person support groups. The study lasted six months. There was one primary emphasis for each group, in addition to caloric restriction.

- For the first group, the focus was on exercise. Showing them each type of aerobic and resistance exercise as well as the significance of each for improving health was the primary goal. They were given personal instructions, taken to a local gym, and made frequent visits to Central Park in New York City.

- A second group put the spotlight on stress management. There were comprehensive lectures on the effects of distress as well as discussions of the inappropriate sublimation people make when they are distressed, such as overeating or choosing comforting junk foods. Each week, a different expert in the field would give a three-hour workshop and address individual questions and issues.

- A third group received, through talks and workshops, a comprehensive understanding of nutrients, including proteins, fats, carbs, vitamins, minerals, enzymes and water, as well as instructions in which ones were right for them.

- A fourth group was given a comprehensive review of all diets, including the most popular, ones running the gamut from high-protein and macrobiotic to raw and vegan. Again, this came with suggestions on which would be most appropriate for the individual.

- The fifth group was given lectures and workshops on ideas about the meaning and purpose of life, on ways of understanding and resolving conflict, and on our subconscious conditioned reactions, and how to change them so they do not debilitate us. We called this fifth group's emphasis "Overcoming the Dark Side."

Here's the finding, which I confess was something of a shock to me at the time. At the end of six months, the first four groups made very little positive progress. Failure rates in getting off the pounds were between 86 and 96 percent.

But the last group, which dealt with fundamental issues, had an over 94 percent success rate. They lost the most weight and kept it off. Equally exciting, they reported having resolved many social and psychological issues, and this resulted in high ratings in a survey we did of happiness and self-confidence. This was the group that was able to surrender unhealthy lifestyle choices or modes, giving up junk food, binge eating, comfort eating, laziness, and depression. They quickly registered improvements in blood sugar, weight, blood pressure, cholesterol, and inflammatory markers. These results were cathartic for me and the supervising physicians, including Dr. Martin Feldman and Dr. Christopher Calapi.

I also said the results were a bit shocking to me in that I had thought at the outset of the study that the other four support groups would have shown more good results. Perhaps, I had thought, some will do better than others, but I didn't fully anticipate that group five would so outdistance everyone else.

The best way to deal with shock is to examine your own assumptions. If I was shocked, I thought, it must be because while I knew one's philosophical outlook on living was essential, I didn't know it was *this* essential.

As I questioned myself, I wondered whether just giving a list of low glycemic foods and beverages, a protocol of the needed supplements, and a basic exercise program would really do much to assist a person in getting healthy? My answer, given a bit reluctantly considering my now abandoned assumptions, had to be an unequivocal "No."

I now saw the foundation upon which everything rests must be how a person deals with his or her own reality philosophically and psychologically. That is why I advise you to read very carefully the chapter "No More Excuses," which focuses on a person's emotional well being and outlook on life.

Perception Matters

What was just said about the overriding importance of perspective may be brought home to you from another angle, by looking at how people perceive themselves. Studies have shown that more than one in ten obese individuals say they are satisfied with their body weight and do not see a need to lose pounds, believing they are healthy.

A significant examination of this misperception was conducted by University of Texas's Tiffany Powell, M.D who worked with almost six thousand obese individuals in a Dallas Heart Study. The participants were of mixed background, 54 percent women, 50 percent black, 20 percent Hispanic, and 30 percent white.

Over 2,056 were obese yet said they were satisfied with their body weight because they were healthy. Yet 35 percent of this group had high blood pressure. In addition, "15 percent had high cholesterol, and 14 percent had diabetes."

Powell made these points about her findings:

- Those who misperceived their body size were less likely to go to a physician. Forty-four percent reported that they did not visit a physician during the past year, compared with 26 percent of obese participants who acknowledged that they needed to lose weight.

- There was no difference in the two groups when it came to socioeconomic status or access to healthcare insurance.
- Individuals who did not feel the need to lose weight often reported that their physicians had not told them to lose weight.
- Obese people who were satisfied with their body size didn't exercise, while obese individuals who recognized they had a weight problem exercised regularly.

We can translate this last bullet point into the following formula: an obese person's denial of being overweight = refusal to take steps to lose weight.

In the study I reported in the last section, where I split weight losers into different groups, it was found that people tended not to stay on their reduction plan if they didn't orient themselves with a thoughtful understanding of their life goals. Still, we see that even those who couldn't stay with the program were worlds closer to losing weight than those in Powell's study who won't admit they need to lose weight, even when they have life-threatening health conditions brought on by their extra pounds.

When to Eat and How Much—Three Good Meals or Many Smaller Meals?

What was just brought up about how overweight people should make revamping their mindsets a big priority, especially as dietary changes made little difference unless accompanied by a change in perspective, was in no way meant to disparage the value of proper eating habits. The point is that, without a renewed way of looking at things, dietary changes didn't work simply because the patients didn't keep to them. The value of the new outlook was that it was with it that an individual can see the value of and carefully adhere to consuming a healthy set of foods.

So, for the next few sections, let's take on the subject of the proper foods to bring with one (and eat) when walking the road to weight reduction and health.

Earlier in the book, Dr. Feldman mentioned that many carried around food and ate many mini-snacks rather than three big meals a day. I want to come back to that point, both because whether such a practice is feasible has been a subject of ongoing medical debate for the past thirty years—with researchers arguing for and against the proposition that, for overweight people as well as for those with diabetes, insulin resistance or the metabolic syndrome conditions, it is better to have many small meals per day rather than three primary, high-quality ones—but also because, having brought up already some of the hormonal mechanisms that are behind eating regulation, we can now better understand some recent research on the topic that makes a decisive contribution to the controversy.

This research was published at the end of December 2009 and was done in Zurich by a group of scientists headed by Dr. Markus Stoffel, Professor at the Institute of Molecular Systems Biology at ETH Zurich. The solid finding of the study, based on an analysis of physiological processes, is that eating three high quality meals with "no snacks, nothing in between, no sweets, is better because the body needs to fast between meals."

The center of the research depends on looking at the career of the transcription factor FOXA2. To quote from a summary of the paper, "Transcription factors are proteins that make sure that other genes are activated and converted into other proteins. The control element for FOXA2 is insulin in both the liver and hypothalamus. If a person or animal ingests food, the beta cells in the pancreas release insulin, which block FOXA2. When fasting, there is a lack of insulin and FOXA2 is active."

So what is FOXA2 doing when it is active in the bloodstream? For one thing, it moves into the brain where it assists in the formation of proteins that sharpen awareness. As the summary points out, "If mammals are hungry [which means FOXA2 is being produced], they are more alert and physically active."

However, if one is constantly snacking, there is little downtime in which FOXA2 can course through the body. Insulin is released with every snack, thus suppressing FOXA2, which in turn means that we do not feel the need for activity, such as exercise."

The findings were backed up by a discovery of a disorder in obese mice. These rodents had overactive FOXA2, which was present at all times, whether the animals are full or fasting. While this may seem to go against the early conclusions, which were based on very inactive FOXA2 production, the finding was that any disruption of the FOXA2 cycle caused problems to the energy/lack of energy balance in the animals.

Professor Stoffel concludes, considering the danger of a deficiency in FOXA2 brought on by too much insulin in the body, that "the body needs fasting periods to stay healthy." Therefore, he challenges the multiple-small-meals-a-day dogma. In effect, he believes it is healthy to get hungry between meals.

To add an important proviso to these findings, let's not forget that to regain health it is not only important to be concerned with limiting the number of times one eats a day, but also with the quality of the calories being consumed. That's where my recommendation for meals comes in.

As I touched on earlier, the optimal diet is based on whole grains and whole legumes, pulses and beans, starchy and root vegetables, green leafy vegetables and salad greens, low sugar fruits, nuts and seeds, and high quality unsweetened protein powders from rice, soy, hemp, split pea, spirulina, and chlorella. These foods can be cooked in or anointed with unprocessed organic oils, including coconut, olive, flax seed, walnut, and avocado. Creating a meal (one of three to four a day) from a balanced selection of these foods also provides healing energy that rises up like a vital living force.

It Matters What We Eat and Drink—Carbohydrates and Fats

Now that we know how often during the day it is good to eat, we can take a look at what foods are best for you. I will begin by assaying the carbohydrates, then move on to fat intake, and related matters, such as the value of foods labeled "low fat."

In considering what carbohydrates to put in your diet, it is worthwhile to pay attention to the Glycemic Index (GI). This ranks eatables based on how quickly the carbohydrates in the food raise our blood glucose. A high GI number indicates the carbs break down quickly into blood sugar, something which, as we've seen, causes difficulty by overtaxing the body's ability to produce insulin. It ultimately leads to perturbation in and damage to the insulin regulatory system. In general, the higher the fat and fiber content, the lower the GI of the food. By contrast, the more cooked or processed the food, the higher the GI will tend to be.

The Glycemic Index of what one is eating is not the only thing to consider in weighing what to consume. It is important to keep in mind that while GI value tells you the type of carbohydrate in a food, it does not say anything about portion control. Portion size is crucial for managing blood glucose and for losing weight.

Moreover, a simple GI value doesn't tell the whole story since many foods break down more quickly or slowly when they have been eaten in combination with certain other foods as opposed to how they release glucose when they are consumed by themselves alone.

Since both the amount and type of carbohydrates in food affect blood glucose, the total amount of carbohydrates is also a strong predictor of blood glucose, even without taking into account the GI value. Knowing GI, however, does help individuals fine-tune blood glucose management.

Watching your carbs in terms of their GI value will not only help you lose weight, but will curtail the blood sugar surges that commonly occur after meals packed with high GI foods. Chronic insulin overload caused by such a diet leads to further weight gain and is associated with all types of age-related diseases.

This is a sample of GI values for some common food items:

Low Gi Foods	Medium Gi Foods	High Gi Foods
Gi Value = 55 or Less	Gi Value = 56–69	Gi Value = 70+
• steel cut oats; muesli; 100 percent stone ground whole grain bread • barley; bulgur • most fruits and nonstarchy vegetables • peas, legumes, • beans, yams, sweet potato, corn, lentils	• brown, wild and basmati rice; couscous • whole wheat, rye, and pita bread • quick oats • banana	• white bread; bagels • cornflakes; puffed rice; bran cereal; pretzels; rice cakes • short grain white rice • russet potatoes • pumpkin, melons, pineapple

If high GI index foods are consumed and insulin spikes are a common occurrence in the blood, constant hunger results. Rather than gaining food energy over an extended period as happens when the glucose enters the blood at a moderate pace, the energy pours in and then sharply falls away as all the food's glucose is quickly put in the blood. So, as medical researcher S. M. Haffner has noted, this will lead to a vicious cycle of overeating, leading to even greater amounts of unwanted insulin to be secreted from the pancreas.

In discussing the danger of inrushing blood sugar, let me tag the way food producers have played on Americans' proclivities to sell them a bill of goods, in liquid form. Americans always have an eye out for a bargain. So when they hear or see one of the billboard or TV ads saying, for instance, "Drink Super Fizz Apple Juice, made of 100 percent juice," they rush to buy it. Why? For one, they think they are getting a bargain, since instead of buying, say, five apples, they are getting five apples in one glass. Moreover—and this is the insidious part—they want to be healthy and have been told, by the commercials, that these fruit juices and concentrates are good for you because they contain the nutrients found in fruits.

In fact, the very idea that the fruit is coming to you concentrated should warn you of what's wrong with this message. When you eat a whole apple or other fruit, the sugar in the food enters the bloodstream gradually as the stomach breaks down the item. If, however, a number of pieces of fruit are concentrated, the natural sugar in them is also concentrated, and put in liquid form so that there is a quick release of the fructose that can spike serum insulin. So, these juices, as the Beatles would say, are "a must to avoid."

While these advertised juices are unhealthy, fruit itself is filled with attractive qualities. There are adequate amounts of folic acid, vitamin C, fiber, carotene, and nutrients in whole fruits as well as in frozen fruit, both of which are crucial to a healthy diet.

I might add that while these juice concentrates are of little value, there are other extracted forms of fruits and vegetables that can do great good for the body. To give a single instance, I recently learned the value of mulberry leaf powder, which decreases fasting glucose levels and raises the levels of good cholesterol in the body. In studies conducted in both India and Japan, researchers found that in patients who took mulberry leaf powder daily with their meals there was a reduction in harmful lipids (which boost cholesterol) as well as a diminution of free radicals, whose perverse effects we profiled previously.

Having mentioned the *misleading* advertising used to sell fruit juice—I find food commercials are more often misleading than downright false—let me *advert* to the blandishments that are put forth in relation to another product line. Food companies plaster certain products with the labels "fat free" and "low fat," representing such commodities as always beneficial. Not so. Look at the labels. Many of them are loaded with insulin-spiking sugar calories in the form of high fructose corn syrup, sucrose and cheap, fortified processed ingredients. Whatever value might have been in the sold food in its untouched form is undermined or cancelled out completely by this raft of additives and sweeteners. A good example is green tea, which is a strong health promoter. Or it would be outside of the form it is marketed in, where the tea is sweetened with sucrose. Salad dressings also see their natural ingredients sabotaged when they are combined with high fructose corn syrup.

On the topic of fats, let me mention that here again a distinction has to be made. Recognizing and monitoring the quality and type of fat consumed is essential to maintaining a healthy weight and preventing diabetes. Most people have heard about the dangers of eating trans-fatty acids. While some of these can be found in beef, the majority are created by food processing, so that they are highly present in junk foods, baked goods and fried food, such as French fries or Kentucky Fried Chicken.

How dangerous are such trans fat? In a recent study, scientists found that "a miniscule 2 percent increase in calories from trans-fatty acids raised the risk of diabetes in women by 39 percent; conversely, a 5 percent increase in calories from polyunsaturated (good) fats reduced the risk of diabetes by 37 percent."

So, to quote another old ditty, if you have trans fats in your diet, it's time to say "move over, Rover" and let the polyunsaturated or monosaturated fats come over. You can have a rich and healthy diet by replacing these trans fats with flax oil, extra virgin olive oil, sesame oil, hemp oil, avocados, almond oil, coconut oil, and pumpkin oil.

Let me summarize what I have said so far by putting my advice into capsule form. Today, too many of us are asking our bodies to run on the wrong fuel: refined carbohydrates. Surrounding ourselves with wholesome choices that consist mostly of fruits, vegetables, grains, and legumes is the key to staying healthy and fit.

A person taking this dietary route will arrange his or her day in something like this fashion. In the morning, that person chooses a cereal that contains whole grain ingredients and no artificial sweeteners.

Later in the day, the individual may supplement lunch with a green smoothie, made from blending and juicing leafy green non-starchy vegetables. (I emphasize non-starchy for there are a few starchy vegetables, such as potatoes and corn, which should be classified with breads, grains, and other starches.) This green smoothie is a healthy, delicious alternative to soft drinks and sugared-up juices.

Recall the virtues of vegetables. They usually contain fewer carbs than fruits; many contain fiber; and they are naturally low in fat and sodium (unless they come in a can).

For dinner, our health-conscious person enjoys fresh vegetables by lightly steaming or sautéing them. He or she adds shredded cabbage or coleslaw to salad; and includes beans and legumes in a soup or salad to meet daily protein requirements.

It Matters What We Eat and Drink—Highly Processed Food

We looked at some of the dangers of advertising blandishments, which will often fool the thoughtless into expecting health benefits from attractively named foods and beverages, such as "100 percent apple juice" or "low-fat buttermilk biscuits." These advertised products frequently have few if any health benefits.

However, many refined foods, the ones I want to look at now, don't even bother with such false advertising. They are loaded with unhealthy additives and sugar, and they make no bones about it.

These items are being marketed at a much greater rate than ever before, and it is not uncommon to see foods that have at least 50 percent fructose overall.

We know that fructose is a sugar that causes glucose in the blood to unhealthily spike upward when it is consumed in any quantity. Only recently, however, have some of the devastating effects of fructose been seen. In 2008, Alexandra Shapiro and other researchers published an article pointing out sucrose's effect on leptin.

Earlier, I described how leptin acts as a signaler, telling the brain that the stomach was full and eating should cease. According to Dr. Shapiro and her colleagues, "Eating too much fructose can induce leptin resistance, a condition that can easily lead to becoming overweight when combined with a high-fat, high-calorie diet." A report on the research describes: "The research team performed a study with two groups of rats. They fed both groups the same diet, with one important exception: one group consumed a lot of fructose while the other received no fructose." After six months on the diet, the animals were tested for response to injected leptin. Normally, such an injection would lower an animal's food intake. "The researchers discovered that the rats on the high-fructose diet were leptin resistant, that is, they did not lower their food intake when given leptin. The no-fructose animals responded normally by eating less."

To summarize the study's findings, which the researchers believe can be extrapolated to humans, leptin resistance can:

- develop from eating a lot of fructose
- develop silently, that is, with very little indication it is happening
- result in weight gain when paired with a high fat, calorie dense diet

The researchers also remark that "other studies have shown that elevated triglycerides [fatty acids] impair the transport of leptin across the blood brain barrier." It could be hypothesized that since fructose increases the amount of triglycerides in the body, these fatty acids then block leptin from reaching the brain, so there is no warning that it is time to stop eating.

These findings give useful pointers that would help explain the rising rates of obesity in children, according to Richard Johnson, the former J. Robert Cade professor of nephrology at the University of Florida (UF) College of Medicine and current professor in the Department of Medicine at University of Colorado Denver. As he puts it, unlike water and low-fat milk, fruit juices and sodas, which are imbibed by many children and young people, are laden with fructose.

By suppressing the signaling capacity of leptin, Johnson notes, sucrose will cause the switching off of the "fullness" feeling that should happen after food and drinks are consumed. He explains that among kids today soda and high sugary fruit juices are common, but, unfortunately, after consuming all that artificial sugar, the body does not know that the sugar is turning into energy since the signals to the brain are blocked. So children continue to eat, and obesity is just around the corner.

His advice to parents is "limit a child's intake of fruit juice to about six ounces per day." He also noted that parents shouldn't bend their rules about how much sugary beverage a child should consume just because it is warm outside. As he explains, "We should not be increasing our [juice and] soft drink ingestion during the summer just because we're hot and thirsty. Water, sports drinks, low-fat dairy such as milk, these are all better ways to keep hydrated."

Dr. Havel, another researcher into the fructose question, remarked that juice labels can be misleading. Some juices have more sugar than soda, for example, apple juice; and many parents and children are not informed on how to read these labels. When a container is posted "100 percent juice," many purchasers don't realize that, even if it's all juice, fructose is still found in these drinks in large quantities.

Then Havel pointed to another threat of high-fructose content. "Fructose and high-fructose corn syrup, a sweetener used in most soft drinks, also cause the body to produce more uric acid." Rat experiments have shown that when rodents were fed a high-fructose diet, it "raised uric acid levels, leading to insulin resistance" and obesity. So, along with blocking leptin's signaling capacity, this indicates that, by upping uric acid, fructose also interferes with glucose control in the blood.

Some of the responsibility for our children overloading on fructose has to rest with the parents, especially those who have myriad excuses for why they allow their children to fill up on this sugar. I've heard parents defend buying juices for their kids because they think that by diluting the juice with water it will make the sugar content okay. Just reading the label to see the fructose content shoots down this rationalization. Others give their kids sports or exercise drinks to keep them hydrated, claiming that there is less fructose in those beverages than in soda or juice. But, I tell them there is even less fructose in water (i.e., zero).

It is this type of thinking—that sports drinks only have a "little" fructose, so that's all right—that has created this epidemic in the first place. All the little pieces add up to a big problem: an overweight, unhealthy society in which the children will not outlive their parents, due to the fact that at a young age, they are overweight, have rotting teeth, terrible sleeping habits, heart conditions, and diabetes, just to name a few ailments.

Moreover, when a kid's eating habits are adapted to rich sugary eatables, he or she is no longer able to appreciate the natural sugar and the good sweetness found in raw organic food. It cuts him or her off from the natural world.

If we don't reverse course and fight to save our children, they will die too soon. Then there will be no time for regrets.

Eating Your Way to Reduced Weight

The diets discussed above are ideal for any fit person looking to maintain good health but now let's look at a diet that will reduce weight.

If we want to think of this in terms of calories, then cutting calories by 300 to 500 per day should lead to a loss of between one and two pounds per week. Some may say such a cut in calories is difficult to achieve for an overeater. In my experience, though, this is a realistic target. Others may say the one to two-pound-per-week reduction is too slow. It may seem that way, but it would add up to a weight loss of more than fifty pounds in a year, of which one can be proud.

To achieve this calorie reduction, switch off the fats, which contain more calories per serving than what is found in carbohydrates and proteins. For nutrition, lean heavy on the whole grains, beans, fruits and vegetables.

Here are some rules of thumb that will help you achieve the weight-loss goal:

- Eliminate alcohol from the diet
- Replace sugary treats in between meals with whole grain snacks, fruit or green juices
- Learn to eat smaller portions mindfully
- Do nothing else during the meal. Stop multi-tasking and eating on the go
- Eliminate coffee and all caffeinated drinks
- Replace milk products with soy or rice-based diary foods
- Enjoy ice water with lemon, lime or orange rather than drinking your calories by consuming fruit cordials

Finally, don't be tempted to skip breakfast or any meal to lose weight. While skipping a meal will reduce your calorie intake for that moment in time, it will leave you much hungrier later on. When it comes time to eat, you will be tempted to overeat to compensate. Irregular eating habits also disrupt your body's metabolism, which makes it harder to lose weight in the long run.

On this diet, it will take a week or two before you notice any changes, but they will steadily appear. After about thirty days, you will notice your clothes are looser, your energy is greater, and your self-esteem is increasing.

Keeping your motivation up is one of the most difficult aspects of dieting. There will be days when you backslide. Perhaps, you go to a party and see a table overflowing with junk food. Everyone else is eating it. The host offers you a platter and without thinking you chow down. It happens. Healthy eating has gone out the window for that one night, only to be continued the next day. There may be weeks when due to such lapses you may not lose much or any weight. But remember at such times that weight loss is a process that will be slow but sure with this change in eating habits. Even if you only lose one pound in a single month, it's much preferable to having that one pound put on.

Celebrate the new you as you achieve weight loss goals. What pleasure can top that of stepping on the scale and seeing the weight drop? Your only regret will be you have to restock your wardrobe as you drop in pants or dress size.

Parents and Children—Making the Right Food and Lifestyle Choices

A parent who is overweight and decides to alter his or her diet to lose weight, may momentarily cringe in facing the the new weight-loss regimen because her or his kids—kids very often being both hyper-critical of their parents and super-vigilant in watching the parent's behavior—will note and frown over any lapses the parent makes in keeping to the plan.

However, there is a much more positive perspective one can take, from a parent's point of view. Look at it this way, the parent can say to him or herself, "I have the opportunity to help my children at the same time as I'm helping myself."

Household meals will be prepared that are chockfull of healthy grains, vegetables and fruits. Sugary drinks will be replaced with green juices and unsweetened teas. While only the one parent is making this shift to lose weight, every member of the house is reaping the benefits.

The importance of getting your kids on a good diet young has been underlined by Dr. Kelly Brownell, director of the Rudd Institute for Food Policy and Obesity at Yale University. She said, "If you are trying to prevent the [obesity] problem, then you want to establish good food habits early. You want to keep children away from the food industry messages to eat unhealthy food." She emphasizes the parents' role. "The key is prevention and the effort cannot be left up to the individual. Parents ought to be the first to take responsibility. Dismissing childhood obesity as baby fat or relying on a kid's will power is simply not a solution. We cannot consider it to be a cosmetic problem. It's a health risk problem. We can no long sit back and wait and think a child may grow out of it."

All of which makes me think of a further note. Even if a parent doesn't need to diet, he or she should be eating the type of healthy diet I have outlined if not for his or her own sake then for the children's good.

Diets Don't Make It

I occasionally use the word diet to describe the change in eating patterns I'm advocating, but that's really not the right word, at least with the connotations that word now has. Think about it: going on a diet usually suggests taking a temporary detour away from normal eating patterns. For the time being, while on a diet, the person eats foods that are healthy but generally not liked. As soon as the weight is off, provided the diet is a success (which, in fact, is not that likely), the person can rush back to eating junk food again.

You can see that is not what I envision for weight losers. My "diet" is not a temporary aberration from one's normal eating. Instead, it is a lifestyle change. What I am prescribing are the eating habits you should stay on for your whole life, provided you want that to be a long and healthy one.

Lifestyle changes will make the difference when diets don't make the grade. But the lifestyle changes laid out in this book do not stop at eating (as you've seen). Eating is part of an integrated, multi-layered program. The typical diet (profiled a few paragraphs back) is food only. It has no other components, such as advice on how to cope with emotional crises. As explained before, people often eat as a way to face emotional difficulties, rather than because they're hungry. For example, after a bad day at work or after a row with a loved one or as an end to a long week, the person will "allow" him or herself a junk food meltdown, as it were, in which the individual overeats on chips or ice cream or another guilty pleasure.

Dieting does nothing to cope with the possible emotional roots of eating. If anything, it makes people more depressed because it becomes one of the issues that cause overeating. When a person "falls off the wagon," and breaks his or her diet plan, this may engineer later meltdowns, in which, unable to deal with the self blame for the violation of the plan, the person binges once again.

The only people who lose weight and keep it off are those who make permanent changes to their (and to their family's) eating and exercise habits. They, to borrow a phrase from Leonard Cohen, are the "beautiful losers."

Exercise Is a Must

Another component of a well-thought-out, successful weight-loss program is exercise. Truth to tell, even if someone didn't change their diet one iota, if that individual increased the amount of time spent exercising, he or she would certainly lose weight.

You may hate gyms. Fine, avoid them. Exercise can be done at home or by doing a light exercise outside, such as a short 40-minute power walk. Each time you do that exercise, you burn calories and fat.

I was not saying avoid gyms by my earlier remark. I was saying follow your preference. There are lots of pleasant ways to increase the amount of activity you do. Team sports, racket sports, aerobics classes, running, walking, swimming and cycling are all beneficial. Your aim should be to find something you enjoy, something that's easy for you to do in terms of location and cost. If it's not only healthy but fun to do, you are more likely to build it into your routine and continue to exercise, despite missing the odd session through such occasions as holidays and family commitments.

A few pages ago I laid out some rules of thumb for good eating. Now let me complement that list with a few pointers on exercise.

- Get out and about on the weekend. Leave your car behind and walk to the shops. Try to incorporate longer walks into outings to the park, coast or countryside, and take a picnic so you can control what you are eating that day.
- Know that every extra step you take helps. Always use the stairs instead of the lift or get off the bus a stop before the usual one and walk the rest of the way.
- If you are watching TV, hopefully a program of value, use commercial breaks between shows to stand and do exercise. Or consider using an exercise bicycle in the living room so you can pedal a few miles while watching your favorite program.

Through exercise, the body will shed the extra pounds. I might add, although you probably know this already, that exercise is effective in treating insulin resistance and reducing the risk of diabetes. What you might not know is that one reason for this is that the muscles become more conditioned with exercise, and there is an increase in the number of insulin receptors on the muscle cell, which allow for a greater uptake of glucose so that blood sugar is balanced effectively.

Having worked with thousands of individuals over the years, I have found that my protocols, which call for regular exercise along with a healthy diet, can perform wonders in promoting weight loss. And exercise, like good eating, pays off not only in reinvigorated health but in the joy found in the moments of working out or eating delicious food.

Case Study—Natalie

Having summarized the healing strategies I believe are de rigueur for weight loss, I think this might be a good place to look at an actual case, that of a woman who I saw go from poor health and obsessive behavior to a state of renewed vigor and well being. She was not grossly overweight but had various fixations and phobias about food that made for a very unhealthy life.

Natalie (not her real name), a long-time employee at my health food stores and restaurants and also a dancer, is now a forty-five-year-old tall brunette. Looking at her—she exudes a healthy glow—you wouldn't realize what a hard struggle she fought to achieve her current plateau of health and liveliness.

Growing up, Natalie was very sensitive to the risks of developing an illness since there was a lot of sickness in her family. Her father had battled cancer throughout Natalie's youth, and her mother was bipolar and an obsessive compulsive.

Although she was neither a full-blown obsessive compulsive person nor an anorexic, she did become fixated on staying in shape, exercising constantly, doing hundreds of crunches several times a day. She also cut her calories intake way down, drinking coffee as one way to repress her appetite.

She was afraid to eat too much because, occasionally, she would lose control and binge. Such behavior arose from overindulgence in her childhood. She recalls, "My mother, on her good days, would carefully craft thick loaves of ten-grain bread from my grandmother's recipe. They were irresistible to me. Straight out of the oven, they seemed to practically glow with warmth, safety, and love. I would eat until much of the loaf was gone. I literally couldn't stop until I felt sick."

Her reasons for eating such a large quantity were tangled up with love for her mother, but also fear that mom would have another mood swing and withdraw from the family space. We can call it anxiety eating.

Throughout her twenties and thirties, Natalie says, she was not only apprehensive that she might resort to bingeing but also because she had seen other members of her family abuse food. "I was so frightened of being addicted to eating like other members of my family had been that I cut out all grains and all sugars entirely." This was done without a good eating plan to back her up and without supplementation, but haphazardly. Later, when she dropped sugar from her new eating regimen, it was as part of a wholesome plan of positive eating and supplementation.

Meanwhile, along with her food phobias, she was scared, partly in reaction to all the illness in her family, that she would get sick. This turned her into a "germaphobe." As she explained in an interview, "I would clean and scrub down my room, and then the bathrooms for hours. I took several showers a day. In my mind, this was all positive. I was the cleanest person I knew."

The constant exercising, restricted eating and paranoia about germs ended up sapping her. By thirty-seven, Natalie had zero energy, her menstrual periods stopped, and tests revealed that in addition to low thyroid function, she was vitamin-deficient. Moreover, there were health troubles. She described, "I had developed recurrent sinus problems, severe eczema on my hands, and I was constantly fighting off yet another viral or bacterial infection."

In 2001, Natalie called, seeking my advice on how she could rebalance her life. I set up an informal team of holistic nutritionists, chiropractors, and other healthcare professionals, and we all pitched in to help her turn things around. Listening to our advice, and also drawing some hints from my books *The Ultimate Lifetime Diet* and *For Women Only,* Natalie isolated her nutritional needs and shifted to a healthier diet.

Following my protocol, she began eating a variety of fats, proteins, and carbohydrates; adding juices, fiber, and supplements to her diet; and exercising moderately. She eliminated milk, egg, meat, and wheat products, as these were all affecting her functioning.

As she began to live according to this healthier regimen, Natalie's menstrual periods returned, her mood swings disappeared, and the quality of her sleep improved. She had begun listening to her body's signals. As she reported, "I noticed that my body felt tired and weak when I ate dairy products, so I cut them out." She added. "And when I ate lean red meat, it made me sluggish, so I've shifted to a completely meat-free diet."

She cooks organically and takes a variety of supplements on a daily basis, including a spectrum of digestive enzymes. Also among the health boosters, she consumes a full arsenal of antioxidant supplements, along with multi-vitamins, multi-minerals, and brain-specific nutrients, such as ginkgo biloba and phosphatidylserine. She mentions, "I'm also big on anti-inflammatory supplements, such as omega-3 fatty acids."

Her supplement list can be extended to vitamins A, C, and E, as well as quercetin, CoQ10, flax seed oil, selenium, alpha-lipoic acid, carnitine, carnosine, and resveratrol. You'll note most of these items are contained on the protocol given earlier in the book.

When it comes to nutritional supplements, Natalie proceeds by trial and error. Here is her explanation: "Just as there is no magic diet for everyone, each individual has to experiment with the supplements that are right for him or her." She added, "As holistic healthcare professionals will tell you, your supplement intake may vary according to the weather and the circumstances of your lifestyle. Your body requires different support when the seasons change or when you are under extra stress."

In addition to eating an organic diet, Natalie has started meditating and practicing calming and rejuvenating breathing exercises. On a spiritual note, Natalie observes that, "The greatest health supplement of all is love. Without it we are incomplete." A committed family woman, Natalie has two daughters with her husband of twenty years. However, in her darker days, before she committed herself to change, she feels she did not appreciate all the love her family had to give her.

Natalie has been able to sort out her priorities and streamline her lifestyle. Instead of obsessively cleaning or exercising, she is living in a mindful way, keeping in touch with her feelings, and extending these positive emotions to her family and circle of friends.

Breathe and Meditate

Like Natalie, you can learn how to eat, breathe, exercise, and relax in a whole new way if you stay focused and disciplined. And the choices you make in one area will support the choices you make in another without your having to think about it. They will naturally integrate.

One little exercise that will have multiple ramifications is a great destresser. When you feel unsettled or sick and out of sorts, try a two-minute breathing exercise. This yogic breath technique helps to balance the right and left hemispheres of the brain. You can try this anywhere and at any time:

1. Raise your right hand to your face, and place your pinky and ring finger lightly on your left nostril. Hold your right nostril closed, and inhale slowly up your left nostril.

2. Pause and while your lungs are full of air, press the left nostril closed while lightening the pressure on the right one. Exhale slowly from your right nostril, then inhale up your right nostril. Pause, and while your lungs are full of air, switch your fingers so that your right nostril is closed again. Exhale.

Do ten cycles of this breathing exercise, increasing length as you get comfortable. Try this in the early morning before meditating, during your lunch hour to regroup your energies, perhaps in the bathtub or before bed to wind down a busy mind.

Building a balanced lifestyle rests on mind/body self-awareness and proactive self-care. Along with breathing, meditation can be very beneficial. Meditation involves listening to yourself and cultivating calm and emotional resilience regardless of life's turbulence. I find meditation inspiring and energizing, and it is also a time to reflect on all the people, animals, and things in my life that I appreciate.

Done in the middle of a busy day, it can be a time to step back and hear your body's messages. During meditation, you can query your body's actual state, a state probably covered over as you were immersed in the day's business. Once this inner state comes to consciousness, you may take self-nurturing action in response to its needs. For example, letting your body talk to you and then responding to it might play out like this. "I feel like I'm getting a cold again. I'd better take some immune-enhancing supplements." Or, "I feel so sluggish. I'd better get some exercise and get my energy flowing before I go back to work." I will outline various meditation techniques a little later.

Both the breathing exercise and the meditation involve an interruption. Break the smooth rhythm of the day, a rhythm that can often hide the fact that you are being heedless and insensitive to your body's experiences. A constant sensitivity to your inner state is one of the hallmarks of a healthy lifestyle.

Detoxification: Eliminating Toxins, Rejuvenating Organs, Restoring Your Being

Detoxification, as the name indicates, is a process of flushing poisons out of the system. The body already has its own detoxification center in the liver. Chemicals, drugs, medications, caffeine, alcohol, nicotine, and anything else foreign that comes into the body and needs to be expelled is filtered out by the liver.

One difficulty arises when the liver has so many toxins to wash out that it has to stop or limit everything else it is doing—besides detoxifying the body, the liver has 400-plus other functions—such as balancing hormones and making the cholesterol that every cell needs for normal production.

In a detoxification, the liver is given a rest because the food eaten and other activities eliminate the toxins that have accumulated, lowering the poison overload.

Modifying the diet is the first move that will help you clean the liver. Adding a variety of quality fiber to your foodstuffs is important in that fiber binds to some of the toxins that have been eliminated in the gut, carrying them out of the system. On the herbal front, dandelion and milk-thistle encourage detoxification

The skin is the largest organ of elimination, and in a detoxification program individuals can take advantage of all the surface area. One way to do so is by dry skin brushing. In this technique, using a natural fiber brush or loofah pad, one brushes the extremities and works towards the heart. Some of the benefits of this practice are that it gets rid of dead skin, aids circulation, and opens pores that may have been clogged with dead cells.

Saunas also promote skin detoxification by slowly heating the skin at about 120 to 140 degrees Fahrenheit. At this temperature the oil glands close and only the sweat glands remain open. In this way, varied toxins, including urea, are "sweated out."

Other ways to reduce toxins include washing yourself with a sugar or salt scrub and taking an Epsom salt bath. Mixing up a bath of sea salts and pure essential oils, and then relaxing in the tub is a pleasurable way to draw some toxins out of the body through the skin.

Also a helpful way to expel toxins is flushing out the intestinal tract by drinking a lot of water. One can initiate a short fast, eliminating foods and replacing them with water for a controlled period of time, as a way to push out fecal matter faster and more thoroughly.

The occasional use of enemas and colonics, perhaps one a year, can be useful in eliminating accumulated waste. Enemas can be administered from the comfort of home or you can visit a colon hydro-therapist.

For maximum results, abstain from solid foods during a colon cleanse and supplement with nutrient-dense vitamins and minerals, green juices that contain spirulina and algae, fresh wheatgrass juice, and fresh vegetable juices. These supplements and drinks will help dampen hunger and are packed with vitamins and minerals.

Any and all of these are ways to help take the load off your liver and allow the body to function more ably, being freed from the interference of toxins.

Live Mindfully

A number of the doctors we met earlier were quite enlightening in discussing how contemporary life can disturb the stress/de-stress system in the body, one set up to deal with intermittent, short-lived situations of threat that are followed by longer times of calming down. Nowadays, though, many people find themselves in a constant "state of emergency," in which their bodies don't have time to recover from one intense bout of stress before plummeting into another.

The doctors and therapists who spoke of this outlined some of the havoc this out-of-whack stress/de-stress configuration causes to the body, which don't need to be repeated, and they also offered their own opinions on healing strategies that would break one out of this overstressed pattern. They had different specific methodologies, but all shared the opinion that the individual seeking to escape the constant stress treadmill had to cultivate the ability to relax.

I heartily concur. The relaxation response brings your system back into balance by deepening your breathing, reducing stress hormones, slowing down your heart rate and blood pressure, and relaxing your muscles. One has to become adept at evoking the relaxation response, which will bring on a state of deep rest that is the polar opposite of the stress response. Once one practices a deep relaxation technique on a regular and daily basis, these benefits will flow from relaxation:

- Produces calming physical effects
- Increases energy and focus
- Combats illness
- Relieves aches and pains
- Heightens problem-solving abilities
- Boosts motivation and productivity

A number of disciplines, often originally created as a set of spiritual practices, contain relaxation techniques that were once used to get the adherents into a proper state of mind to approach religious ground. I will turn to detailing some of these techniques in a minute. First, let me lay out some general parameters on how to bring them into your life.

I recommend you leave time each day for at least twenty minutes of stress-relieving relaxation. In order not to forget this essential if brief time for pausing, taking stock, and de-stressing, incorporate it in your daily routine. Schedule a set time either once or twice a day for your practice.

You may want to do your relaxing early in your day. Such a suggestion may seem surprising. It would appear that right after one gets up, hopefully from a refreshing sleep, is the time one *least* needs to relax. However, there are two points in favor of doing the relaxing at that time. Some of us are involved in a draining and nerve-wracking occupation or project. Individuals in these situations normally "switch on" the moment they waken, immediately thinking of all the things they have to do in the day ahead, mentally gritting their teeth and girding their loins. Those people will benefit by entering their days relaxed. But even if one doesn't fit into this profile, a busy day may make it hard to find time to relax as one is pressed by many chores. In this case, it may be best to do your relaxing first thing in the morning, before other tasks and responsibilities get in the way.

Don't practice when you're sleepy. These techniques can relax you so much that they can make you nod off. The center of this practice is to be relaxed *and* awake, acclimatizing yourself to a state of aware, tension-free consciousness, which is the opposite of a lazy stupor one might adopt in front of a TV.

Choose a relaxation technique that appeals to you, considering your needs, preferences, and fitness level. If you crave solitude, solo relaxation techniques, such as meditation or progressive muscle relaxation, will give you the quiet mind, which will allow you to recharge your batteries. If you crave social interaction, a class setting will give you the stimulation and support you're looking for. Practicing with others may also help you stay motivated.

You may recall (if you've read) Ralph Nader's recent novel, *Only the Super-Rich Can Save Us*, highlights the use of deep relaxation techniques in a group setting.

The book, as the title might hint, is the story of how Warren Buffet, a super-rich investor, gathers a number of his wealthy peers, including Bill Cosby, Ted Turner, and Yoko Ono, at a secret retreat and propose they dedicate parts of their fortunes to a project of turning the US around with an agenda that includes shifting the nation to clean energy and expunging the influence of money from politics. This is not an unexpected storyline from the pen of Nader, a celebrated, indefatigable reformer, but how Buffet ends the first round table meeting with his fellow millionaires may well be. As the session winds up:

> Warren consulted his watch. "I was so absorbed in our discussion that I lost track of the hour. We've put a lot on the table tonight for thought, response, and decision. If you'll indulge me just a little longer, I'd like to ask that we remain here for another hour in total silence, thinking about what we've heard and said and jotting down any additional reflections and ideas. It's a technique I've learned from some of my business partners in Asia and, like the prospect of hanging, it concentrates the mind wonderfully. I've used it with my executives to great effect, so give it a try, my friends, and then we'll retire for the evening."

His fellow movers and shakers are a bit surprised at this time for deep relaxation, but as the book progresses, they all find that such intermissions are key to helping them find new ideas as well as allowing them to re-energize for the continuing struggle.

What can I say? If millionaires and billionaires see the value in this practice (at least in an imagined scenario), perhaps it's something that should be part of your daily routine.

Here are some useful relaxation techniques to consider.

Meditation

This has to be carried out in a quiet environment, anything from a secluded place in your home, office or garden, place of worship or in the great outdoors. Get comfortable, but avoid lying down and drifting off to sleep. Sit up with your spine straight, either in a chair or on the floor. You can also try a cross-legged or lotus position. The object of meditation is to find a center and stay there, without undue forcing of consciousness. It is not the time to daydream but fix the mind, perhaps on a meaningful word or phrase, perhaps on an object in your surroundings. This is not done because the phrase or object will reveal new sides to you as you give it attention (although this may happen), but because such practices have proven best at emptying your mind of stray or obsessive thoughts. In the religious traditions from which this technique is drawn, the empty mind was considered most fit to receive god-given (literally) insights, but used for relaxation, the empty mind has been found to be the one that most brings you to a state of calm and tension-less fluidity. Don't think, though, that the emphasis on focus means you have to unmercifully police your thoughts. Keep an observant, noncritical attitude, and don't worry about distracting thoughts. If they intrude, don't fight them. Instead, gently turn your attention back to your point of focus. This action itself, of trying to keep a focus without forcing things, is an exercise in gentle, but firm self control that will have ramifications in other actions in your life. It may seem difficult at first, but with regular practice, it comes naturally. And mindfulness meditation actually changes the brain, strengthening the areas associated with joy and relaxation.

As said, there are different points of focus one can choose for a meditation's center and there are also different types of mindfulness meditation techniques, a few are:

- *Body scanning*—This involves focusing your attention on various parts of your body. As is done in progressive muscle relaxation, you start by focusing on your feet, then work your way up. However, instead of tensing and relaxing your muscles, you simply non-judgmentally focus on the way each part of your body feels.
- *Walking meditation*—You don't have to be seated or still to meditate. In walking meditation, mindfulness involves focusing on the physicality of each step: the sense of your feet

hitting the ground, the rhythm of your breath, and the touch of the wind on your face.

- *Mindful eating*—Instead of snapping up a snack when you're under stress or gulping a meal in a rush, try eating mindfully instead. Sit down at the table and focus your full attention on the meal. Eat slowly, really taste and savor each bite.

Visualization

This technique might be considered a special type of meditation in which, instead of emptying the mind, the engaged participant imagines a restful scene in which he or she feels at peace. If you choose this technique, find in your mind a place of tranquility, such as a place from your childhood of which you have fond memories, like a playground or park, or a vacation spot, a beach, mountain or forest glade, or even a place you have never visited, such as a lush jungle or desert oasis. The main thing is that the mind's picture is one of maximum quiet and calm. Some people get started on this type of meditation with a therapist's help or use an audio recording, for example, one of waves rolling in to stimulate thoughts of a beach. Picture the scene as vividly as you can, noting everything you can see, hear, smell, and feel. For example, if you are thinking about a dock on a quiet lake:

- *See* the sun setting over the water
- *Hear* the birds singing
- *Smell* the pine trees
- *Feel* the cool water on your bare feet
- *Taste* the fresh air

Progressive Muscle Relaxation

A moment ago I mentioned, in the context of body scanning meditation, progressive muscle relaxation, which scanning resembles. At the time of that reference I did not fully elucidate the muscle relaxation process. It takes place in two steps, during which the participant systematically tenses and relaxes different muscle groups. As with meditation, it takes a little practice for you to find your rhythm, but once you have made a number of trial runs, you begin to get an intimate sense of how muscles feel in a relaxed or tensed state. This growing awareness has the spillover effect of heightening your perception of sudden increases of muscular tension that accompany stress, helping you counteract a sudden ascent of anxiety. Further, spillover number two, as your body relaxes, so will your mind. You can combine deep breathing with progressive muscle relaxation for an additional level of relief from stress. When you are ready for a few moments of relaxation, begin by loosening your clothing, dropping your shoes, and in general getting comfortable. Take a few minutes to relax, taking slow, deep breaths. When you're ready, shift your attention to your right foot. Take a moment to focus on the way it feels. Slowly tense its muscles, squeezing as tightly as you can. Hold for a count of ten. Then relax the foot. Be aware of the tension flowing away as your foot becomes loose. Stay in this relaxed state for a moment, maintaining your slow, deep breathing. When you're ready, shift attention to your left foot, and go on with same sequence of muscle tension and release. Move slowly up through your body: legs, abdomen, back, neck, and face, contracting and relaxing the muscle groups as you go. When the exercise is completed, you will rise, put your shoes back on, straighten your clothes, and step forth rejuvenated.

Deep Breathing

A couple of the experts who pitched in earlier to offer advice on healing gave strong recommendations concerning deep breathing exercises. Following their wise discussion, let me add my own take on this topic. To me, the key is to draw your wind deeply from the abdomen, pulling as much fresh air as possible into your lungs. When you breathe from the abdomen, rather than sucking shallow breaths from the upper chest, you inhale more oxygen. That's a major plus since the more oxygen you get, the less tension you feel. As the common saying has it, when you are tense, you are "short of breath," so, in keeping with that, a good way to head off an escalation of inner tense, is via feeling "long of breath." Breathing is best done in the same comfortable setting in which you might practice meditation. Sit comfortably with your back straight. Put one hand on your chest and the other on your stomach. Breathe in through your nose. Ideally, the hand on your stomach should rise, the hand on your chest should move very little. Exhale through your mouth, pushing out as much air as you can while contracting your abdominal muscles. The hand on your stomach should move in as you exhale, but your other hand should move very little. Continue to breathe in through your nose and out through your mouth. You might refer back to Dr. Richard Brown, who spoke earlier, for more details on the optimal number of breaths per minute and for some further pointers. This relaxation technique is both the easiest and most stress-reducing of them all.

Yoga

There is a vast literature on yoga as a stress relief technique. For further knowledge of it, you should consult this writing or, as a better alternative, take a beginner's class. Here, suffice it for me to say that a yoga session involves going through a series of both moving and stationary poses, combined with deep breathing. Yoga that emphasizes slow and steady movement, along with some preliminary stretching, offers the best stress relief.

Tai Chi

On occasion I make my way down to New York City's Chinatown where, if I'm early enough, I see collections of twenty to thirty people, usually middle-aged, but with a few younger individuals sprinkled in, going through a non-competitive series of slow, flowing body movements. They are practicing tai chi, an Asian technique that emphasizes concentration, relaxation, and the conscious circulation of vital energy ("chi" in Cantonese) throughout the body. Though tai chi has its roots in martial arts, today it is primarily practiced as a way of calming the mind, conditioning the body, and reducing stress. As in meditation, tai chi practitioners focus on their breathing and keeping their attention in the present moment. Tai chi is a safe, low-impact option for people of all ages and levels of fitness, including older adults (such as those you see in Chinatown's parks) and those recovering from injuries. Once you've learned the moves, you can practice it anywhere, at any time, by yourself or with others. And if you have occasion to go to China and visit a large city, such as Guangzhou, on a Sunday morning you will see groups of 100 to 150 people quietly going through their relaxing tai chi moves.

Massage Therapy

Massage generally takes place when a therapist gently or with a harder pressure rubs a person's body, an activity which soothes and relaxes the muscles. The most common type of massage is Swedish, a soothing technique that relies mainly on long, flowing strokes. Not only does it relax, but can reduce pain and relieve joint stiffness. Another common type of massage is Shiatsu, also known as acupressure. In Shiatsu massage, therapists use their fingers to manipulate the body's pressure points. The same points that are pierced with ultrathin needles in acupuncture. If you cannot afford to go to a spa or health center to work with a therapist, there are many simple techniques of self massage or ones that can be done with a close friend or partner. Not only does the latter relax you and release stress but it also deepens your bonds with the massage giver/getter. Let me describe a few self-massage methods.

- "Scalp Soother"—Place your thumbs behind your ears while spreading your fingers on top of your head. Move your scalp back and forth slightly by making circles with your finger-tips for 15 to 20 seconds.

- "Easy on the Eyes"—Close your eyes and place your ring fingers directly under your eyebrows, near the bridge of your nose. Slowly increase the pressure for five to ten seconds, then gently release. Repeat two or three times.

- "Sinus Pressure Relief "—Place your fingertips at the bridge of your nose. Slowly slide your fingers down your nose and across the top of your cheekbones to the outside of your eyes.

- "Shoulder Tension Relief"—Reach one arm across the front of your body to your opposite shoulder. Using a circular motion, press firmly on the muscle above your shoulder blade. Repeat on the other side.

These last few pages have suggested a large number of alternatives that can aid you in relaxing. With our stressed-out lifestyles and with the way too much tension plays havoc with the hormones and other bodily systems, these methods are invaluable. But remember that many of them also increase awareness, something on which I need to say a few more words.

Dewey: on Education as Mindfulness

Anyone with even the slightest familiarity with Dewey may have felt my mentions of his work thus far are off base. Dewey is primarily known as a theorist of education (though he wore many hats), indeed many label him the greatest thinker on education of the 20th century. Yet all I have spoken of is his psychology.

Still, if we go back to my initial treatment where I discussed his conception of choice, it will be seen in a moment that I did allude to his educational ideas.

I noted that for Dewey good choice involves an integrated bundling of varied desires and options. Secondly, I noted that one wasn't able to accomplish such choice-making unless *one knew oneself and knew the world* well enough to have a range of desires and options to integrate.

So far, so good. Now if we look into Dewey's *Democracy and Education* to find a central formulation of his notion of what education is, we find, in words that may at first seem off-putting, "We thus reach a technical definition of education: It is that reconstruction or reorganization of experience which adds to the meaning of experience, and which increases ability to direct the course of subsequent experience." Put more simply, in real education a person expands his or her views, seeing both more inside (as to personal feelings and capabilities) and outside (in the world). Dewey develops this thought: "The increment of meaning [mentioned] corresponds to the increased perception of the connections and continuities of the activities in which we are engaged."

To explore this in terms of the type of situations faced in this book, a person, a man, say, who is overweight and pre-diabetic, if he is truly being educated in this area, starts seeing new connections (new to him) between such things as sucrose consumption and weight gain or between lack of exercise and lack of energy.

But there's something more to this definition. Recall, he said this expanded mindset "increases ability to direct the course of subsequent experience." Dewy elaborates, "The other side of an educative experience is an added power of subsequent direction or control. To say that one knows what he is about is to say that he can better anticipate what is going to happen; that he can prepare in advance so as to secure beneficial consequences and avert undesirable ones."

One is only learning if the newly revealed connections and continuities are helping an individual to act more consciously. To use our previous example, if the man is truly being educated, after he finds out the impact of sugary soda, he drinks them no longer. We could say he stops dead (before he is dead). Now if he gets thirsty, he drinks water or a tea flavored with a natural sweetener.

In this way, Dewey ties together two strands I have been stressing in this book. True learning comes when you see more connections between things in your world, making you more aware, and this new understanding leads you to make affirmative life changes. To slightly alter a famous quote from early scientist Francis Bacon, "Education is power."

Thyroid Breakdown: Recognizing and Reversing It

Having gone through my suggested healing strategies for dealing with obesity and overweight conditions, and having also looked at a case study, I want to move to another feature of the book, in-depth examinations of some of the health problems, such as depression, which commonly accompany obesity. After looking at these ailments and saying something about their etiologies, I will suggest recuperative methods. First up is the thyroid.

Our bodies are constantly being bombarded by environmental toxins from lead, cadmium, mercury and silver amalgam fillings in teeth; the chlorine and fluoride from our water system, and from viruses and bacteria. This plays havoc with our hormones. Hormones are the messengers in our body, switching on and off metabolic processes. If they are interfered with the body's signaling system is awry. This can make it difficult to lose weight. It is crucial to have a thorough check of your hormonal functioning before you begin a weight-loss program and make dietary changes since a hormonal imbalance can scotch your effort to lose pounds.

One part of the hormone system that is frequently wounded by all these toxins is the thyroid. This is a butterfly-shaped gland located at the base of your neck, just below your Adam's apple. Although it weighs less than an ounce, it is a heavy-duty regulator, playing a part in every aspect of your metabolism.

The thyroid produces two major hormones, thyroxine and triiodothyronine, that have significant responsibilities for body functioning. They maintain the rate at which your body uses fats and carbohydrates, help control body temperature, influence your heart rate, and aid in regulating the production of protein. Your thyroid also produces calcitonin, a hormone involved with controlling the amount of calcium in your blood.

Hyperthyroidism is characterized by too much thyroxine. Scientists have suggested several additional reasons for this abundance, beyond the fact that the thyroid may have been damaged by the intrusion of toxins in the body. In some cases, antibodies mistakenly attack the thyroid. This happens in a condition called Grave's disease. Furthermore, if the gland becomes inflamed, this state will cause excess thyroid hormone stored in the gland to leak into the bloodstream.

If this gland is not working in tiptop shape, a number of health problems are sure to follow, including, especially weight gain. Its dysfunction also results in fatigue, intolerance to cold, infertility, swelling of the neck, face or abdomen, constipation, fibromyalgia (chronic pain and sensitivity), allergies, and arthritis. It will also have repercussions that affect the brain, such as depression, slowed thinking processes, difficulties with concentrating, and poor memory. If hyperthyroidism, a state in which the gland's imbalance is exhibited by the overproduction of its hormones, results and continues, it is likely to become an underlying factor in diabetes, elevated cholesterol levels, heart disease, stroke, and kidney failure.

Dr. Alan Cohen, a leading nutritionist, feels that many of the health problems associated with thyroid dysfunction arise from the fact that the gland helps regulate body temperature. He says, "We have enzymes that control every function that occurs in the body, and they are all temperature sensitive. When your body temperature is low because of a low thyroid, then everything begins to slow down and many cells can begin to malfunction."

He also warns that many doctors misdiagnose the condition as simple depression, because the outer signs of thyroid breakdown are similar to those of the mental state. He says, "I classify people with hypothyroidism as the walking wounded. They just do not feel well; they're tired; they cannot concentrate, and they can't lose weight. They're able to function, but not at their optimal level of health." This dispirited condition may mislead a doctor. As Cohen suggests, "When these patients go to their doctor, their blood tests are normal, and they're put on medication for depression. But that doesn't get to the underlying cause of the problem."

While there are a number of thyroid diseases, including hypothyroidism, in which not enough hormones are produced, the most common, the one Dr. Cohen was concerned with, is hyperthyroidism. Its common symptoms and signs include:

- Heart palpitations
- Heat intolerance
- Nervousness
- Insomnia
- Breathlessness
- Increased bowel movements
- Light or absent menstrual periods
- Fatigue
- Fast heart rate
- Trembling hands
- Weight loss
- Muscle weakness
- Warm moist skin
- Hair loss
- Staring gaze

Alternative therapies have often proved effective at minimizing symptoms of mild thyroid dysfunction. These concentrate on eating and supplementation.

The first thing is to look out for possible allergies that are tampering with the body's smooth functioning. It may be helpful before beginning any dietary change to have your healthcare provider test you for food allergies. In the meantime, eliminate suspected food allergens, such as dairy (milk, cheese, and ice cream), wheat (gluten), soy, corn, preservatives, and chemical food additives. Also be careful about foods that can interfere with thyroid function. Some of these are broccoli, cabbage, Brussels sprouts, cauliflower, kale, spinach, turnips, soybeans, peanuts, linseed, pine nuts, millet, cassava, and mustard greens. Also things to watch out for are refined foods, such as white breads, pastas, and sugar, along with meat and anything containing trans-fatty acids. Avoid alcohol and tobacco.

What you should be eating are foodstuffs high in B-vitamins and iron, such as whole grains (if you have no allergy to them), fresh vegetables, and sea vegetables. Also consume antioxidant foods, including fruits (such as blueberries, cherries, and tomatoes) and vegetables (such as squash and bell pepper). Beans and grains are good sources for protein. I also suggest using healthy cooking oils, such as olive oil, sesame oil, almond oil, hazelnut oil, sunflower seed oil, and flax seed oil.

A good supplementation regime is this:

- A daily multi-vitamin, containing the antioxidant vitamins A, C, E, the B-complex vitamins, and trace minerals, such as magnesium, calcium, zinc and selenium.
- Omega-3 fatty acids, such as fish oil, 1 or 2 capsules or 1 or 2 tbs. of oil daily to decrease inflammation and boost immunity.
- Vitamin C as an antioxidant and for immune support.
- Alpha-lipoic acid for antioxidant support.
- L-carnatine for decreasing thyroid activity.
- Probiotic supplement (containing *Lactobacillus acidophilus*) for maintenance of gastrointestinal and immune health.

Along with these supplements, herbs are a safe way to strengthen the body, and many can be taken in teas. Unless otherwise indicated, teas should be made with 1 tsp. herb per cup of hot water. Steep covered for 5 to 10 minutes for leaf or flowers, and 10 to 20 minutes for roots. I advise two to four cups per day. A couple you might try:

- Green tea (*Camellia sinensis*) for antioxidant effects. Use caffeinefree versions.
- Lemon balm *(Melissa officinalis)* for thyroid support and because it helps normalize an overactive thyroid.

Not all herbs are beneficial to this condition and some should be avoided in that they may stimulate hyperthyroidism. These include ashwagandha (*Withania somnifera*) and bladderwrack *(Fucus vesiculosus)*. Stimulating herbs, such as caffeinated green tea products and Chinese or Korean ginseng (*Panax ginseng*), are also no-nos.

Let me end by saying that changes in the diet are crucial but exercising five days a week for at least forty minutes is also invaluable. If you have mild thyroid dysfunction, and take up this eating, supplementation and exercise program, you will have a good chance of beating this glandular setback and getting the thyroid back to healthy operation.

The Adrenals

Let me more briefly speak about the adrenal glands, another part of the hormonal system that can stimulate weight gain. Small and triangular, these two glands sit near the top of both kidneys. They release cortisol, a hormone called into play when the body faces stress.

If the adrenal glands are not working properly, one is faced with such symptoms as extreme fatigue, inability to sleep, decreased ability to handle stress, craving for salty and sweet food, having more energy at night instead of in the morning, confused or murky thinking, pain in the joints, poor digestion, lowered immunities, and PMS and other menstrual problems. Food cravings can lead to weight gain.

As may be recalled, Dr. Martin Feldman, whose views were canvassed earlier in the book, is very careful in his treatment of the adrenals and mentioned important tests that should be administered to check on their health. He also recommended vitamin C, pantothenic acid, and rodiolo herb for their curative power in treating this gland.

Depression Is Often Present—Don't Ignore the Signs

As Dr. Cohen noted, many doctors seeing overweight patients who have hyperthyroidism misdiagnose this as depression. This is understandable because depression has been connected to obesity. This link has recently been the subject of a number of scientific investigations.

Researchers led by Sarah M. Markowitz, MS, asked the questions whether people who are depressed are more likely to become obese, and whether people who are obese are more likely to suffer from depression than thinner people. Their answers were published in the March 2008 issue of *Clinical Psychology: Science and Practice*.

Their conclusion shows that the connection flows both ways. In the words of the article, "People who are obese may be more likely to become depressed because they [are] in poor health and are dissatisfied with their appearance. . . . People who are depressed may be more likely to become obese because of physiological changes in their hormone and immune systems that occur in depression. Also, they have more difficulty taking good care of themselves because of symptoms and consequences of depression, such as difficulty adhering to fitness regiments, overeating, and having negative thoughts."

The writers prescribe, as treatments that will address obesity and depression at the same time, exercise and stress reduction. They look askance at dieting, which can worsen mood, and antidepressants, "which can cause weight gain."

The depression/obesity tie was also examined in a paper, also published in 2008, that had as its lead author Gregory Simon, M.D a psychiatrist and researcher at Group Health Cooperative in Seattle.

The investigation focused on the middle-aged, and found that women with clinical depression were more than twice as likely to be obese than women without the psychological problem. Counterposed to this, it also revealed that obese women were more than twice as likely to be depressed.

In an interview, Simon talked about the equation, saying: "Depression and obesity likely fuel one another. When people gain weight, they're more likely to become depressed, and when they get depressed, they have more trouble losing weight." He added that the depression-obesity association held even when the researchers controlled for marital status, education, tobacco use and antidepressant use.

He said that the subjects of his study, "who were predominantly white and middle-class women," may have slightly biased the results upward in that "there is some evidence that being overweight is less stigmatized for men, for lower-income people, and for women in nonwhite ethnic groups."

The conclusions of both these studies give additional evidence to the conclusion I reached earlier (on diabetes not obesity as such) that psychological factors are key to one's state of health. These findings are also important for health care professionals, who need to consider treating depression and obesity in a more integrated way since the conditions are interrelated.

This is the same conclusion reached by Richard Rubin, a Johns Hopkins University psychologist. He remarked, "Health care providers should glean a similar message from the [Simon] study results. Providers need to monitor for depression and treat it in overweight individuals."

Treating Depression and Obesity Simultaneously

While weight gain tends to bring on depression, healthy weight loss improves mood. This is hardly a surprise, but a number of researchers have looked into this more positive connection in order to turn an intuition (that one feels better when weight is shed) to a more exact sense of, for example, how much weight loss is necessary to elevate mood.

In a 2009 University of Pennsylvania School of Medicine Study led by Lucy Faulconbridge PhD, researchers found that after a six-month, weightloss program, depressed patients not only dropped 8 percent of their initial weight, but reversed many of the symptoms of depression.

The weight-loss program included a strict meal plan and some lifestyle modifications, such as engaging in some physical activity and having the subjects spend less time in front of the TV. In it, a group of overweight and depressed individuals took part beside a group of overweight but more lighthearted people. Throughout the study, not only did the two subsectors of patients lose poundage, but glucose, insulin, and HDL cholesterol significantly improved in both groups.

This not only offers hope to depressed, overweight people who should be able to foresee the alleviation of the tandem problems, but it hits on an issue that will probably only strike a chord in health professionals who are aware of this problem. It reverses a therapeutic trend of keeping depressed people from taking part in weight trials. As Faulconbridge explains, "Clinically depressed individuals are not usually included in weight-loss trials due to concerns that weight loss could worsen their depression." However, as she goes on to say, "These concerns are not based on empirical evidence, and the practice of excluding depressed individuals from clinical weight-loss trials means that we are learning nothing about this high-risk population."

Her views are echoed by Group Health Research Institute Senior Research Associate Dr. Evette J. Ludman, who for years has been researching the link between depression and obesity. She agrees with Faulconbridge that weight-loss programs should not exclude depressed people.

Her own research comes with the development of a one-year behavioral weight-loss intervention involving twenty-six group sessions. The intervention, developed at the University of Minnesota over the past twenty years, has proven equal in success to any other currently available non-medical treatment. In her study, she mixed 190 female Group Health patients, age 40 to 65. 65 of the participants had major depressive disorder and 125 were without this difficulty.

The results were even better than hoped in relation to the depressed part of the enrolled group. "We expected women with major depression to lose less weight, attend fewer sessions, eat more calories, and get less exercise than those without depression," Dr. Ludman said. "We were surprised to find no significant differences between the women who had depression and those who did not have it." Women lost around the same amount of weight at six months (eight or nine pounds) and twelve months (seven or eight pounds), with no significant differences between the groups with and without depression.

The last point she raised in discussing her findings is highly relevant to what we have been talking about in this book. Listen to what divided those who lost weight from those who didn't. Ludman expresses it in this way, "What made a difference was just showing up." It broke down like this. "Women who attended at least 12 sessions lost more weight (14 pounds at six months, and 11 pounds at 12 months) than did those who attended fewer sessions (4 pounds at both six and 12 months), regardless of whether they had depression. Being depressed didn't lead them to attend fewer sessions or lose less weight."

In other words, if you want to lose weight, the first step is to make a commitment, then make those eating and exercising changes. The healing and personal growth will follow.

Eating Disorders

The term eating disorders does not refer to simply eating too much junk food, but to highly irregular patterns, such as anorexia, where a person starves him or herself, or bulimia, in which a person causes him or herself to vomit, as a (slightly demented) way to lose weight.

Certainly, this type of poor eating is not as widespread as obesity, but it is more common than you might think. In 2009, the Royal College of Psychiatrists estimated that eating disorders affect roughly seven young women in every 1,000, and one in every 1,000 young men.

These statistics indicate that seven out of eight people with eating disorders are female, which means that females are the largest group involved, but also indicates that the problem is not confined only to women. Recently, the men affected have been characterized in two ways. One claim is that of those men with eating disorders, 25 percent are gay and 75 percent straight. It's also claimed that the vast majority of men with such disorders had been bullied at school.

Where do we look for the origin of eating problems? Let's start with last point raised, bullying. Young people who are bullied or even just living in bossy or super-achieving households may not be able to stand up to the pressure. Let's picture the bullied individual as a male anorexic. He begins to feel others are controlling him. To counter that, he looks for a place where he can have power himself and finds it in control of his body. He rigidly governs how much food he'll allow to pass his lips. The sense of power can be very elevating—at least initially. While a bully might steal this young man's food at school, he won't be able to make him eat more. Here the bully has to yield to this beleaguered individual.

This is only one factor that may spur out-of-control non-eating. Other young people, ones suffering a deficit of self-esteem, arrive at the disorder when they become convinced that if their bodies were more perfect, they would feel better about themselves.

They may have come to this perception under the baleful influence of the mass media. This is the source of the idea that the successful are thin. Television, magazines and newspapers continually bombard us with images of extremely slim people. The ultra-thin models and movie stars are shown as rich and living enviably glamorous lives. It is not surprising then that, exposed to enough media messages, even young children will go on diets.

The influence of these media pictures of ideal body types is discussed by social worker Carol Bloom in these terms, "As long as products are being sold that have to do with image, you are going to have people transform their outer selves [to copy these ideals]."

Indeed, the globalization of this American thin imagery was seen when television reached the Fiji islands. It wasn't long before the young women there became so concerned about their figures, for the first time ever, that 15 percent of them began to induce vomiting as a means of controlling their weight. This trick was probably also learned on TV.

Eating disorders have also been linked to stress. This may come in the aftermath of a traumatic event, such as bereavement or sexual abuse, which hits a child in her or his early years. It can also be due to later anxieties, ones that occur between the ages of fourteen and twenty-five, when the sufferer is under stress at high school or college, perhaps in relation to academic achievement or from uncertainties about sexual orientation or attractiveness.

(By the way, many people overlook the fact that though the bulk of eating disorders are found in young people, there are a few cases of people well into mid-life who are having these eating difficulties.)

The problem of eating disorders is hardly a new one. It's now thirty-one years since the therapist Suzie Orbach published her classic book *Fat Is a Feminist Issue.* Here she laid bare some of the social components, such as the Barbie doll image of the ideal woman, that drive women toward becoming trapped in eating disorders.

Far from these problems slackening over the years, they are now as prevalent and shocking as they were when Orbach's volume first hit the bookstores. In 2007, though, the way the topic was nuanced was that it came up in relation to the fashion industry, and the scandal of many of its "Size Zero" models, who had or were perceived to have eating disorders.

One might consider this both a loss and gain from the days of Orbach. For one, where the earlier author concentrated, as I do, in helping everyday people in confronting and solving health problems, the new media interest is in celebrities. Yet, on the other hand, it might be said that at least critics were taking on the media, which for so long had its own, unimpeded way in foisting unobtainable images on American women.

Having given you this brief background, with some suggestion on how these problems may originate, let me now lay out some basic facts about the three main eating disorders, starting with the most well known.

Anorexia nervosa

- Anorexics restrict the amount they eat and drink, often to dangerous levels.
- The usual age range for the onset for anorexia nervosa has been reported to be from 14 to 25 years.
- Anorexics often come from families where there is not much communication but where there is considerable pressure to perform well or to "be perfect."
- In anorexia, there's a refusal to maintain weight at a normal level.
- Anorexics have an intense and growing fear of gaining weight or of becoming fat.
- As time goes by, an anorexic loses a proper perspective on his or her own weight, so the person frequently believes that he or she is much bigger than that person is in reality.
- Anorexic girls can become so seriously undernourished that their periods stop and downy hair appears on their bodies.
- Anorexics frequently have mood swings.
- Anorexics will often have dizzy or fainting spells and will usually feel cold.

Bulimia nervosa

- A bulimic has an uncontrollable urge to eat vast amounts of food. After binging, the bulimic then vomits or uses laxatives or diuretics as a means of controlling weight.

- Bulimics are frequently of normal weight.
- Bulimics often suffer from mood swings.
- Bulimics sometimes have abrasions on the back of one hand. This happens because their teeth graze that hand whenever they stick their fingers down their throats to induce vomiting. This tell-tale sign can be useful for friends, parents, or doctors in identifying the problem.
- Bulimics frequently have sore throats because of their constant vomiting. This again is a symptom that may help doctors identify the problem in their patients.
- Bulimics develop problems with tooth decay, because of the acid in their vomit constantly washing over their teeth. Dentists are often the first people to spot this problem.
- Bulimics often eat to gain emotional satisfaction but as they start to feel full they are overcome by feelings of guilt and shame.
- In severe cases, the bulimic can develop dangerously low levels of essential minerals in the body, which can adversely affect, sometimes to a fatal extent, the vital organs.
- Occasionally, severe bulimia can lead to heart attacks.

Compulsive/binge-eating

- A compulsive eater will indulge in regular episodic overeating of large amounts of food.
- A sufferer will constantly entertain thoughts about food and weight.
- A compulsive eater will have a sense of being out of control.
- A compulsive eater will indulge secretly.
- A sufferer will eat until she feels uncomfortably full.
- A compulsive eater will suffer guilt and remorse after eating.
- Some sufferers say that they never feel full and that they always have a sense of emptiness.

The one thing that all the experts agree on in the treatment of eating disorders, particularly in the case of anorexia nervosa, is that it is better to begin sooner rather than later. Treatment is likely to consist of one or more of the following:

- counseling
- family therapy
- group therapy
- support group involvement
- drama or arts therapy
- nutritional advice

You can see the emphasis here has to be psychological since the problem is beyond eating right. It doesn't make any difference what you eat if you later throw it up, or eat too little of it to sustain health. Since it originates with a person who is suffering so badly that he or she is engaging in self-destructive behavior, there is little chance to reverse it unless the person is interested in getting better.

Like an excessive smoker, drinker or drug taker, the person with an eating disorder has becomes locked into an addictive form of behavior, this one concerning food. The ill health accompanying the addiction is accepted as the price to pay for this one security blanket. To be asked to change is often as if the sufferer was being asked to cut him or herself off from the one thing that spells safety and control.

Once the person has said yes to moving to a different manner of controlling stress, feelings of rejection and other negative emotional states, treatment strategies can be put in place. With bulimics, the therapy often centers on avoidance techniques: the bulimic is encouraged to delay bingeing or to delay vomiting, perhaps for one meal, perhaps a day. However, it turns out that in many cases bulemics view treatment in the same way they do food: at first they long for it and consume it, and then they violently reject it. So with therapy, at first compliant and willing to follow the counselor's advice, then unexpectedly and suddenly, they drop out of the program and revert to their old activity.

Another approach to eating disorders is known as cognitive behavior therapy (CBT), which has been tried most successfully with bulimia nervosa and overeating. In one typical version of CBT, the person tries to simply change his or her actions. An overeater will be asked to eat regularly, perhaps keeping a diary of what foods he or she consumes each day. This is the behavior part of the therapy, which ignores how the person may be feeling and puts emphasis simply on controlling actions. The cognitive part involves the sufferer trying to undermine any part of a belief system that is sustaining the poor behavior. For instance, if a woman eats when she is feeling lonely, she will be encouraged to challenge the idea that eating makes her feel less lonely. She will also (behaviorally again) be asked to try different ways of overcoming loneliness that do not include food.

Both these therapies have had some success, but many feel that it will be hard to overcome these eating problems until the time when young people are not constantly and one might say unthinkingly exposed to so many idealized and lauded images, which are impossibly far from the average body.

Perceptions Matter 2: Eating Disorders and Interaction

Another therapy, aside from those mentioned in the last section, which has been productive in helping those with eating disorders is interpersonal therapy (IT), which focuses particularly on interpersonal interactions and an individual's mental health issues.

As we learned earlier, eating disorders may be triggered or stimulated by adverse family or peer relations. I noted, for instance, the situation of a youth in a family who made high demands that he or she felt couldn't be fulfilled. Interpersonal Therapy allows an individual to explore his/her interactions with others and how these interactions affect the person. During therapy sessions, individuals suffering from eating disorders can learn how to best cope with the tension and frustration that result from negative interpersonal interactions as well as build their self-confidence and self-esteem.

The value of this type of therapy was testified to by a study led by Dr. Marian Tanofsky Kraff at the Uniformed Services University of the Health Sciences and the National Institutes of Health. The researchers worked with overweight girls, who reported that they binged and lost control over their food consumption. Tanofsky Kraff reported the therapy classes "helped prevent these girls from gaining excess weight."

Another important study also looked at how interactions play a role in eating disorders, especially behavior that led toward anorexia. It was piloted by Dr. Eleanor Mackey from the Children's National Medical Center in Washington, DC, and her colleague Dr. Annette La Greca from the University of Miami.

These researchers found that girls from ages thirteen to eighteen were highly influenced in their eating patterns by the type of groups they hung around with or considered the norm. So, those who identified with athletic peers "were less concerned about their own weight and seemed less likely to be trying to control their weight," than outsiders who identified with fellow nonconformists, and the rebellious, who skipped school and often got into trouble. Still and all, those who were the most likely to use drastic slimming strategies were those outside of interaction altogether, "girls who did not belong to any particular peer group."

The indication here is that while interaction, which is helpfully dealt with in interpersonal therapy, can push a person toward eating disorders, lack of interaction, which occurs when a youth is isolated and friendless, is also a key stimulator of these problems.

This makes a fit ending point for this whole chapter in that throughout these pages I have emphasized how significant a role psychological factors play in the genesis of obesity.

Chapter 7

Sweet Suicide

In our discussion of obesity, we had occasion more than once to allude to the dangers of sucrose, one particularly noxious form of sugar. As we saw, while blood sugar is itself a needed element of human metabolism, if sugar that comes from food, such as a candy bar, enters the bloodstream in a big swoop, rather than in the gradual way it would if it were contained, say, in an apple, there is hell to pay in the sense of a disturbance of the distribution of insulin. Repeated stress to this system leads to diabetes.

This problem of the over consumption of sugar is the heart of the rising trajectories of both diabetes and obesity, and has so many hidden angles (such as the ads I mentioned that suggest drinking concentrated apple juice is healthy), that I want to spend some time covering the problem in depth.

The association of health problems with sugar has long been known to doctors. Indeed, going back to the beginning of the last century in England, doctors lamented the ever-increasing amount of sugar being consumed and its relationship to various illnesses. When having heard someone mention the interesting discussions that went on in the medical journals concerning these issues, I decided to flip through a few of them. I was surprised not only at the intelligence of the debate, but at the amount of concern over sugar consumption in the scientific community. The British were annually consuming approximately five pounds of sugar per person in those days. By contrast, in 1999 according to Department of Agriculture figures, Americans were consuming 158 pounds per person a year! So if the British doctors were alarmed then, our doctors should be in an uproar.

Perhaps because the profession has been concerned with this issue for so long or perhaps just because they were astute observers of society, I found many doctors in Great Britain honing in on the diabetes/sugar connection a few decades back.

I visited England circa 1972 to meet with three leading medical specialists: Dr. John Clease, Dr. John Yudkin, and Dr. Dennis Burkitt. These men opened my eyes to the epidemic of diseases that were related to our over consumption of refined carbohydrates and sugar.

I was particularly impressed by Dr. Yudkin, the first professor to hold a chair in nutrition in England. If he wasn't a scientist I would suspect he was a magician in the tradition of Merlin, because the predictions he made in '72 have all been proven true about forty years later. He forecast the rising occurrence of type II diabetes. He could foresee that as a nation becomes increasingly obese, with their traditionally healthy diets being replaced by fast or highly processed food, diabetes would emerge in alarming numbers.

He even guessed what the food industry's "house" scientists would say. They would seek to convince the public that the cause of the increase in diabetes was in the genes not the foods people chose to eat. Furthermore, he predicted, all of the medical conditions associated with diabetes (i.e., weight gain, high blood pressure, elevated cholesterol, inflammatory conditions and arthritis) would be presented by house medical specialists as genetic ailments, to which fast food, sugar, and so on, made no or insignificant contribution.

All these predictions came true—too true. He made them over forty years ago when people in the United Kingdom and the United

States were consuming approximately 100 pounds of sugar a year. I gave you the figure for 1999, over 150 pounds of sugar, and it has climbed since then.

Of course, the corporate toadies among scientists don't only point to genetic factors as behind these medical problems. If that seems unconvincing, they seek to persuade the public that the rise in diabetes is the result of the population being too sedentary. Their solution is simple. They say, "Just exercise more. And, by the way, bring a sugar-rich sports drink with you to the gym, because, after all, sugar has nothing to do with ill health." I imagine after such an "expert" finishes making a speech on the need to exercise, the "scientist" rushes off to check his or her stock in Mega Sucrose Corp.

On the other side of the diabetes debate stands a growing number of holistic dieticians, nutritionists, physicians, nurses, and other medical scientists, who will point you to the increasing number of studies, all telling the same tale: processed sugars, in even normal amounts, can disrupt the body's biochemistry in many harmful ways.

If you note the year-by-year increase of sugar consumption by the American population, you can guess which of the two sides of the debate has the media's ear and which can afford to flood Washington and state capitals with their boosters and money. Their influence is felt at many agencies, including the FDA, USDA, CDC, NIH, NIAID and the US public health service. This is in stark contrast to the muffled voices of the scientists who warn the public against the dangers of sugary food and drink, something they do because they have a very comprehensive understanding of the dangers of sugars. The media generally turns its back on these thinkers, no matter how many studies they have as evidence.

The skeptic may object, "Oh, yes, Gary, you say there are an ever growing number of studies on the subject. Surely, you are exaggerating. Maybe one or two."

The skeptic would be wrong and I am about to bring such material to public attention. In this chapter I am presenting a summary, in lay language, of the most important studies presented on the dangers of sugar and artificial sweeteners. This information comes from peer-reviewed literature and was independently verified and reviewed by Dr. Dorothy Smith. Following that, I have included a list of natural sugars and a brief description on healthier sweetener options. Replacing processed cane sugar with these recommended sweeteners will enable you to eliminate sucrose, high fructose, and aspartame from your diet without sacrificing the pleasures of taste.

It is important to note that even natural and healthier sweeteners must still be used judiciously. Hence, we have included total calories and grams of sugar per serving.

Also, in the recipe section, you will not see any sweeteners in the dishes. It is up to you to select the sweetener you prefer and add as much as you desire in the preparation. Try, however, to work with a minimal quantity of the sweetener in order to keep the total grams of carbohydrates and calories at the lowest possible threshold.

Don't worry if you can't immediately adjust to healthy natural sweeteners and feel almost magnetically drawn back to refined and processed sugar. It will take anywhere from a week to several months to break the habit. Be patient, the transition will be worth it. Not only will your health improve but you will begin to savor your food more, since its tastes won't be buried under a load of sugar.

Following this chapter, I have one on Super Foods. These are individual foods that have extraordinary amounts of antioxidants, phytonutrients, phytosterols, chlorophyll, and healthy fibers.

I can't help but offer a preview here of one super food, but in a way that will allude to some of the points about sugar, an additive that often appears in sheep's clothing.

One super food is the goji berry, whose complete profile will appear later. You can purchase bags of freeze-dried powdered goji berries, and in this powdered form it might be stirred into the health drinks served by health-food stores. But beware, the drink may also contain cane sugar, counteracting the health-giving effects of the goji.

Very few people ever eat any goji plain. Instead, it is sugar-coated, as it were. For instance, when you eat a goji bar, the goji part of the bar is miniscule and, in most cases, virtually insignificant to your health. The number one ingredient in that "health" bar is fructose. That's at the top of the list (since ingredients are listed so those that contribute the most are put first). Goji will appear near the bottom, if not being the last, on the list. The end result is that manufactures have marketed an unhealthy product in a deceptive manner. It's the equivalent of a bait and switch: focus on goji in advertising the bar—*Eat a Goji Treat*—but provide the consumer with what is largely a sugary supplement.

As an alternative, as you will see in the power foods section, you can incorporate these foods into your diet yourself. One good way is by making a protein shake in the morning. By adding rice milk, Noni powder, a teaspoon of goji powder, some fresh blackberries, and a scoop of non-genetically engineered rice powder, you will have created a drink that is low in calories and very low in sugar, but high in nutrients, with a heavy emphasis on antioxidants, phytonutrients and polyphenols.

However before turning to super foods, we have to look at super liabilities to your diet, in particular, many forms of sugar.

Sugar

Before looking at how sugar consumption has been growing by leaps and bounds (or should I say leaps and pounds) in the United States, let's clarify what sugar is since it comes in a number of sub-varieties.

In 2002 statement the American Heart Association (AHA) and the USDA provided a broad, succinct definition of what constitutes "sugar": Simple carbohydrate (sugar) refers to mono- and disaccharides; complex carbohydrate refers to polysaccharides, such as starch. Common *disaccharides* are sucrose (glucose + fructose), found in sugar cane, sugar beets, honey, and corn syrup; lactose (glucose + galactose), found in milk products; and maltose (glucose + glucose), from malt. The most common naturally occurring *monosaccharide* is fructose (found in fruits and vegetables). Intrinsic or *naturally occurring sugar* refers to the sugar that is an integral constituent of whole fruit, vegetable, and milk products; extrinsic or *added sugar* refers to sucrose or other refined sugars in soft drinks and incorporated into food, fruit drinks, and other beverages.

The sugar in that definition that is the most concern to the health conscious is added sugar, which can also be termed sweeteners, (i.e., something added to a food to make it sweeter than it already is). These are the sugars that are adding so much to American consumption.

As a recent report from the USDA notes, "per capita consumption of caloric sweeteners increased by twenty-eight pounds, or 22 percent, from 1970 through 1995, and has continued to increase since 1995."

A similar sugar explosion was detailed in a separate *USDA Report on Food Consumption, Prices and Expenditures,* during the period 1970–1997. Instead of using pounds, the report's authors broke consumption into teaspoons, pointing out that their figures, translated into such terms "amounted to more than 53 teaspoonfuls of added sugars per person per day in 1997." Meanwhile, the "USDA's Food Guide Pyramid suggests that people consuming 1,600 calories limit their intake of added sugars to 6 teaspoons per day." The guide suggested those who consume 2,200 calories a day limit themselves to 12 teaspoons while those eating 2,800 calories keep their consumption down to 18 teaspoons."

In other words, Americans are consuming close to *three times the maximum* of 18 teaspoons recommended by USDA food guidelines for even the highest calorie diets!

As I mentioned, it is the sweeteners that are really hoisting up the consumption figures, and these sweeteners are particularly found in soft drinks. The USDA report just mentioned showed that the steep rise in caloric sweetener consumption since the mid-1980s coincided with a 47 percent increase in annual *per capita* consumption of regular (non-diet) carbonated soft drinks. This soared from 28 gallons per person in 1986 to 41 gallons in 1997. Carbonated soft drinks provided more than a fifth (22 percent) of the refined and processed sugars in the 1994 American diet.

All this sugar consumption is closely related to a spectrum of increased disease. That's why I have often commented while these sodas are called soft drinks, they are certainly hard on your body.

Sugar and Health

Refined sugar only became a major part of the human diet over the last few hundred years, and only began its gallop to such over-consumption in countries like the US and England in the last few decades. Looking at its recent rise and the simultaneous increase of sugar-related diseases, most obviously diabetes, some clear-eyed scientists have suggested these two processes are related. However, on the other end, what we have called the house scientists, with ties to food makers, have taken the position that, given the recentness of the phenomenon of large sugar consumption, it is too early to draw any conclusions.

In the first camp would be found the authors of *Sugar Busters!*, who argue that it is quite logical that we should have added refined sugar to the priority list of things that are, or may be, "Hazardous To Your Health" when you see the increase in disease caused by our huge consumption of refined sugar and certain other carbohydrates. Sugar just may be the number one culprit in lowering the quality of life and in causing premature death. There is certainly enough evidence to bring us to that conclusion.

Another clear-eyed thinker is Robin Edelman MS, RD, CDE, who, in an article for *Eating Well,* explained that added sugars are found in virtually every type of prepared food we buy. She pointed out that a 30 percent increase in sugar consumption during the last two decades has led to a doubling in the number of overweight and obese children over the same time period.

Alarmed by such figures, The Center for Science in the Public Interest (CSPI) petitioned the Food and Drug Administration to require new food labels declaring just how much sugar is added to soft drinks, ice cream, and other foods. Their petition was joined by thirty-nine organizations, ranging from the American Public Health Association and former Surgeon General Koop's Shape Up America! to the YMCA and Girl Scouts.

At one time the American Medical Association (AMA) would have been seen on the side of the angels. In 1942, the organization made the statement that it would be in the interest of public health to limit the consumption of sugar in any form when it is not combined with significant proportions of foods high in nutrients.

How times have changed. While the AMA and other medical organizations stop short of endorsing high sugar consumption, they are notably silent about the problem. And this quiet can be taken as an "enabler," in that the authorities' lack of comment encourages the soft drink industry's (and other sugar-laced product makers') consistent portrayal of its products as being absolutely healthful.

And if they are as healthful as claimed, why not get kids to drink them? That's the pernicious reasoning of these food giants. Thus, in 1997, Coca-Cola spent $277 million in advertising that was targeted towards children. The advertising placed their logos and products within easy reach of kids. These pitches to children are made despite the fact that Coke is filled with caffeine, which increases the excretion of calcium in urine, which is no good for the bones. And not to be outdone by its rival, Pepsi, Dr. Pepper, and Seven Up, who have licensed their logos to the baby-bottle manufacturer Munchkin Bottling, Inc., so infants can get familiar with the soft drinks.

Earlier, in the 1960s and 1970s, the companies might not have gotten away with this marketing to tots for public outcry would have hindered their plans. But now the public is much less concerned about sugar.

Writing in 1998, Ron Lord explained this changed mood in an article in the *Agricultural Outlook Forum*. He wrote that sugar once "had a rather negative public image." Families generally viewed excessive sugar as a health risk and avoided processed sweets. "Then in the 1980s," Lord goes on, "public attention became focused on fat as something to avoid; and about the same time a rather successful advertising campaign to promote the healthy and natural aspects of sugar was conducted."

The result was predictable if tragic. There was a drastic increase in carbohydrate consumption, particularly sugar consumption. Emboldened by this changed, relatively pro-sugar stance on the part of the general public, sugar began to be placed into foods that had traditionally never been thought of as sweet, such as many fast foods and processed goods.

Consumption of sugar skyrocketed as a result, and sugar addicts, the type of people you characterize as having a "sweet tooth" or who need a "sugar fix," were on the rise. By the way, I used the term "addicts" advisedly. Dr. Anne C. Colantuoni, an obesity researcher, has shown that excessive sugar intake causes serious dependence and that the removal of sugar creates withdrawal symptoms. She and colleagues have found that withdrawal from heavy use of sugar is qualitatively similar to getting off morphine or nicotine. Other researchers have backed up Colantuoni's conclusions.

This point about addiction may be surprising to some. Even the better informed of my readers, while they will know about the connection of high sugar intake to some diseases, such as diabetes and to obesity, will not be cognizant of other ramifications of such a diet. We will look first at these known connections and then turn to lesser known aspects, such as high intake's connection to aging, cancer and appetite suppression.

Sugar and Obesity

My previous discussion of American youth today, in a section that called them "sugar-coated," suggested that obesity in American children is becoming an epidemic. No, it is an epidemic. Let's look at the children first, before getting to overweight adults.

Let me cite some figures from the December 2001 issue of *The Journal of the American Medical Association,* which presented a comprehensive national picture of weight trends among children. From 1986 to 1998 the number of overweight, non-Hispanic white children doubled, shooting from 6 to 12 percent. By the end of the same time period, roughly one in five African-American and Hispanic children were overweight, a 120 percent increase from the numbers in 1986.

A year ago Bill Cosby, in a comedy routine, talked of a childhood friend, Fat Albert, who later became a cartoon character. One point of Cosby's anecdotes, however, was that the friend was called Fat because he stood out from the other, gangly or skinny kids in the neighborhood. Now, a kid who stood out would be Thin Albert!

The relationship between increased sugar consumption and obesity in children is well documented in recent studies. In the late 1990s, The Children's Hospital of Boston and the Harvard School of Public Health conducted a long-term study to examine the impact of soda and sugar-sweetened beverages on children's body weight. The study involved 548 sixth and seventh graders over a 21-month period. Of course, they didn't give them or encourage the youth to drink soda, but simply observed their intake and compared it to their weight.

During this time, 57 percent of the children increased their daily intake of soft drinks, more than half of them by nearly a full serving. The researchers' conclusions were that the odds of becoming obese increased 1.6 times for each additional can of soft drink consumed above the daily average.

Similar work was done more recently by D. S. Ludwig, MD, and colleagues. Looking also at the correlation between consumption and adding pounds, they found that one daily soda increases the risk of obesity by 60 percent. These researchers noted that drinking soda was the norm among adolescents. About 65 percent of adolescent girls and 74 percent of adolescent boys consume soft drinks daily.

While childhood obesity is reaching new heights, adult obesity is following it up a steep incline. Shocking as it might seem, being overweight is also a new norm. Researchers at the CDC report that in 2000, most Americans were overweight (more than 56 percent), and nearly 20 percent of adults were obese. The total number of individuals who are morbidly obese (at least 100 pounds overweight) rose from 0.78 percent in 1990 to 2.2 percent in 2000.

Although adults may not drink as much soda as adolescents, they are still putting on the pounds by eating other sugar-laced foods and beverages. And, as we just saw, with this sugar goes added weight.

In *Sugar Busters!* authors Samuel S. Andrews, MD, who is an endocrinologist with the Audubon Internal Medicine Group, and Morrison C. Bethea, MD, who is in private practice, point out a new facet in the progress from high sugar intake to obesity. We've already covered how sugar from food that enters the blood quickly can draw a disruptively high amount of insulin into the system. The authors point out that such an insulin uptick does not only "lower our blood sugar, but in the process, insulin causes the storage of fat and also increases cholesterol levels. Insulin also inhibits the mobilization [that is, loss] of previously stored fat."

Add this to the strong possibility mentioned later, that sucrose blocks the stomach's signal to the brain that it is full, and we have a recipe for creating obesity.

It is not necessary to do anything but recall the association of obesity and disease discussed earlier in these pages. We've seen there are links between being overweight and encountering such health problems as heart disease, osteoarthritis, diabetes, high blood pressure and certain types of cancer. Also implicated in this circle are hypertension, gall bladder problems, and sleep disturbances.

While, as we've seen, many medical associations had sat back or looked the other way when it came to identifying the link between sugar and disease, there have been outstanding exceptions, such as

Surgeon General David Satcher, who served from February 1998 to January 2001.

In a December 2001 *Washington Post* article, Sally Squires reported on Satcher's views. Squires said, "He called for sweeping changes in schools, restaurants, workplaces, and communities to help combat the growing epidemic of Americans who are overweight or obese."

These weren't just words, because he, for one, acknowledges the direct link between sugar consumption and obesity. So the changes he envisioned included that schools make their lunch programs "less fattening, restrict students' access to vending machines that sell calorie dense foods and soft drinks, and resume daily physical exercise classes for all children and adolescents, as well as recess for elementary school students."

Such a far-seeing program, like the one suggested by the Surgeon General, which would promote a healthy, lowered-sugar lifestyle for our children, is the type of direction we need to move in to reduce obesity.

Sugar and Diabetes

We've seen that diabetes is a disease rooted in problems with insulin, and also that high sugar intake throws the insulin system out of whack, so it's a no brainer to connect diabetes with heavy use of sugar.

This link has been demonstrated scientifically by a host of studies. For instance, J. Salmerón and colleagues from the Harvard School of Public Health examined the relationship between glycemic (i.e., sugar oriented) diets, low fiber intake and the risk of type II diabetes. They found that this type of diet increased risk of diabetes in women. This is one among many studies that have brought out such evidence as how sucrose added to the diet of laboratory animals or increased in the diet of healthy volunteers is associated with impaired glucose tolerance, retinopathy (eye disease) and nephropathy (nerve damage), and reduced insulin sensitivity of the tissues, all major factors of diabetes.

I've already commented on the epidemic growth of type II diabetes, which is now not only adult onset, but is being found in youth in unprecedented numbers. One fact I haven't yet mentioned is that with the rising number of adults with the disease, there is also a rising number of birth defects in children born from mothers with the illness. Researchers studied 23,000 pregnant women and found that obese women with type II diabetes are three times more likely than non-obese, non-diabetic women to have a baby with a birth defect, and seven times more likely to give birth to a child with a craniofacial defect such as cleft palate or abnormal limb development. Nearly 6 percent of all women with type II diabetes had babies with major defects, compared with 1.34 percent of women without diabetes.

Sugar and Aging

Of particular concern to those reaching the middle stages of life should be sugar's effect in promoting premature aging. I've already talked about glycation, using the metaphor of a turkey baked in an oven as an example of this process's effect. I also gave some of the more physiological background earlier on. At this point, let me simply point out that sugar consumption promotes glycation, whose baleful effects include thickened arteries, stiff joints, pain, feeble muscles, and failing organs.

The link I am getting at was assessed by Dr. L. Joseph Melton, who notes that diabetics suffer a very high incidence of nerve, artery, and kidney damage, because high blood sugar levels in their bodies markedly accelerate the chemical reactions that form advanced glycation products. As Melton pithily puts it, "After years of [eating] bread, noodles, and cakes, human tissues inevitably become rigid and yellow with pigmented glycation deposits." As we know, it is the breakdown of such foods as overly processed cakes and bread that flood the blood with sugar and spur the development or furthering of diabetes.

Sugar and Cancer

Above I talked of links between diabetes and cancer. This discussion only noted connections via correlation, that is, I noted studies recording that diabetics were more prone to contracting certain cancers than the general population. The researchers did not suggest any physiological mechanism that linked the two.

In the case of sugar and cancer, by contrast, Dr. Otto Warburg, PhD, a Nobel Laureate in medicine, discovered in the 1930s that cancer cells have a fundamentally different energy metabolism than healthy cells. He found upped sugar intake could increase cancer cell production.

The reason for cancer cells' proclivity for sugar was simply that, because of the more primitive nature of cancer cells, they required a direct supply of glucose, not being able to master the more complex synthesis of glucose from larger molecules. This indicates a direct relationship between sugar ingestion and the risk of cancer.

A vast, four-year epidemiological study conducted in the Netherlands by the National Institute of Public Health and Environmental Protection examined people in twenty-one industrialized countries and found that sugar intake is a strong risk factor that contributes to higher breast cancer rates, particularly in older women.

These findings are mirrored in the studies of D. S. Michaud and fellow researchers at the National Cancer Institute, who followed up on two large studies conducted over the past twenty years on approximately 50,000 men and 120,000 women. They were looking at pancreatic cancer and didn't stop at mere correlation but kept looking deeper into the causal nexus. Their first conclusion was that obesity significantly increased the risk of coming down with this disease. However, more relevant for our point in this section, they went further and found evidence from both animal and human studies that abnormal glucose metabolism plays an important role in pancreatic carcinogenesis. Then, they examined whether diets high in sugar were to blame for this abnormal metabolism and learned that a diet high in sugar may significantly increase the risk of pancreatic cancer.

More evidence, if more is needed, that eating sugar is a risky business.

Sugar and Cardiovascular Disease

As I noted, many health organizations have been shy at condemning sugar use and doctors groups have also often been wary at blasting such panderers of sugar as the deep-pocketed fast-food and soft-drink industries. One notable exception to this faintheartedness is the American Heart Association, which on July 23, 2002 released a report on "Sugar and Cardiovascular Disease." The report cited scientific data that indicated sugar consumption is detrimental to human health, and added that no data indicates that sugar consumption is advantageous, and that high sugar intake should be avoided. The report also stated that obesity is a definite cause of cardiovascular disease and death.

It's hard to top that as far as "telling it like it is," but I also might mention a recent study that delved into the way sugar acts in the body to promote cardiovascular disease. This work was done at the State University of New York at Buffalo, headed up by Dr. Paresh Dandona, and looked at the production of free radicals, whose adverse effects on the body have already been seen. As we know, the effects include damaging the arteries.

In the study, healthy adults were given a drink containing 75 grams of pure glucose, the equivalent of two cans of cola. They experienced a significant rise of free radicals in the blood one hour after the drink, and a doubling of free radicals after two hours. Dandona and his colleagues concluded, "We believe that in obese people, this [free radical production stimulated by high sugar consumption] cumulatively leads to damage and may cause hardening of the arteries."

The way drinking the soda-like beverage leads to free radical increase should give pause to anyone who is contemplating quaffing a sugary soft drink.

Sugar and Dental Caries

I don't have to tell you that sugar causes dental caries, a disease in which bacteria damage the teeth with decay and cavities. This, at least, is something the public gets: that eating sugar ruins your teeth.

If we look deeper into the problem, we might point to a study by Aubrey Sheiham, a professor of epidemiology and public health at University College, London, which found that both frequency of consumption and the total amount of sugar one eats are important factors in determining whether one gets caries. According to Sheiham, the intake of sugar beyond four times a day leads to an increased risk of dental caries.

Looking more narrowly at soft drinks, research that studied over 6,000 fourteen-year-olds concluded that consumption of sugary and carbonated drinks was associated with significantly higher levels of dental caries.

Just as it's common knowledge that sugar damages teeth, which these studies only confirm, so it should also be well known that as we age, our teeth often become weak from a lifetime of sugar damage, calcium depletion and wear. Cavities may be ignored and, as a result, become worse. The best way to avoid this is to remove excess sugar from the diet and focus your meals on nutrient-rich foods.

Sugar and the Immune System

The immune system, the part of the body that takes action when the body is threatened by, for example, hunting down and eliminating viruses, is one of the most important layers of our body's interconnected structure. It could be said that the better our immune system, the better our other systems.

That's why, though it's not always been explicitly pointed out, so much of the advice in this book is aimed at bringing optimal health to the immune system, something to be done by, among other things, keeping away from hormone-treated meats, pesticides, and other toxins. One of the other things that should be high on your list for putting your immunity in top shape is strict regulation of sugar intake.

We've seen how sugar promotes different illnesses, such as different varieties of cancer, now let me say a few words about how it disrupts the actions of a number of the body's immune-system agents.

In one careful study, similar to the one we just looked at in which drinking a soda-like beverage increased free radicals, ten healthy people were first assessed for blood-glucose levels and for the presence of neutrophils, immune system cells that target invaders such as cancer. Then the ten's glucose and neutrophil levels were examined after they had eaten 100 grams (24 teaspoons) of carbohydrates, variously from glucose, sucrose, honey and orange juice. In all ten, the ability of the neutrophils to engulf bacteria was significantly decreased, indeed, the neutrophils became "paralyzed," after this consumption.

Another study, this one by N. Yabunaka, turned its attention to macrophages, white blood cells that defend the body against invaders, such as bacteria and viruses. The work learned that sugar caused an increase in a protein that inhibits macrophage activity. This weakens the immune system's ability to function.

Overall, excessive sugar intake has been shown on many levels to deplete and weaken the immune system. This is one part of the body that must be kept in good working order since it is the first line of defense against the outriders of any invading infectious disease.

With all these marks against it in terms of diseases, it is fostering, you might say sucrose has a lot to answer for, but we are the ones who are paying the price and must take steps to end the offensive reign of sugar in our diets.

Sugar and Appetite Suppression

Another noxious effect of high sugar intake at first might not seem particularly unhealthy, at least in comparison to some of the other threats we have been surveying. This is that a high sugar use can suppress the appetite.

J. W. Anderson and fellow researchers have shown that sugar intake, by dampening appetite, can lower your intake of necessary nutrients. As we've seen, when refined sugars and simple carbohydrates enter the blood, they quickly become glucose. Anderson and his group learned that with the consumption of sugary food or drink, your body may not be getting any of the nutrients it needs, but it is being tricked into thinking it has ingested the proper amount of energy. That's why candy bars can be recommended by advertisers as a way to tide over your appetite till you get a full meal.

In this way the "empty" calories of many sugary treats can give you a paradoxical feeling of "empty fullness," the sense you are full when you haven't eaten a balanced diet with proper nutrients.

Sugar and Children's Behavior

Let's get back to common knowledge. As mentioned a few sections back, it's explicitly understood that sugar and good teeth don't mix. Something also well known is that if children "overdose" on sugar, they often get out of hand, overexcited and overactive in distressed, not productive ways. This is acknowledged by parents who often joke about their children being on "a sugar high" when they are rowdy.

Like the tooth decay idea, this one about too much sugar adversely affecting young people's behavior is based firmly in reality. Between 1973 and 1977, Dr. William Crook did extensive work laying out the truth that a majority of children could have their behavior affected by the removal of particular foods. He wasn't centrally concerned with sugar consumption, but the behavioral effects of junk (or should we call them junky) foods and sugary treats were highlighted by Dr. Stephen Schoenthaler, who conducted diet research on children for almost thirty years. It was his original, seminal studies that led to the introduction of sugarless and junk food-less lunch programs for one million school children in over eight hundred New York schools during a seven-year period (1976–1983).

In a study accompanying and following through on this dietary shift, it was found that as high sucrose foods were gradually eliminated or reduced in schools, there was a 15.7 percent gain (from 39.2 to 55 percent) in learning ability in comparison to schools in which the lunch programs were left as is.

In other words, removing sugary foods made children smarter! However, the increase in learning ability probably wasn't because kids' IQs suddenly jumped, but because of their changed behavior in the classroom and during their studies when they were less antsy and distracted once they removed the excess sugar in their diet. (It should be noted that today, sugar intake in children and teens is much higher than it used to be. A corresponding spike in behavioral problems and dropout rates should trouble concerned parents who see the importance of diet in their children's future.)

Schoenthaler went on with his work by studying thousands of juvenile delinquents on junk-food-free diets. The removal of these sugary foods always produced the same result: an observed dramatic improvement in mood and behavior.

Setting up the Los Angeles Probation Department Diet-Behavior Program, he and those working with him observed 1,382 incarcerated delinquents at three juvenile detention halls. When put on a low-sucrose diet, these young delinquents showed an averaged 44 percent drop in antisocial behavior.

These results were replicated in other studies he conducted in Alabama and California. Schoenthaler's work with juvenile delinquents and sugar intake presents cold, hard evidence of the effect a sugary diet has on children's behavior. As we often think about the effects of taking drugs on teen delinquency, it may be time we begin to consider what our kids are snacking on, as well.

To try to counter this massive evidence and act as if sugar does no harm to our children, the sugar industry usually cites four very small scale studies that claim there is no link between the consumption of sugar by children and hyperactivity. Although there were many flaws in their studies, the conclusions are used, nonetheless, to quash any objections to the increasing amount of sugar in children's diets.

Among the problems with the sugar industry's studies is that they used an insufficient amount of sugar to warrant a reaction. In one of the four studies, an average of only 65 grams (13 teaspoons) of sugar were given daily to a trial group of twenty-one persons. This is the average amount of sugar in a single ten-ounce can of soft drink. A milkshake alone has 30 teaspoons of sugar, and a sugar-loaded birthday party can net a child as much as 100 teaspoons of sugar within several hours.

If one were going to measure the overall effect of too much sugar on children, you would think a researcher would start at a higher rate, which represents the reality of the amount of sugar the children actually consume in daily life.

Some researchers have calculated that a growing pre-teen may consume, on average, as much as 50 teaspoons of sugar a day, far more than the meager 13 teaspoons that were used in the study. A clinical study based on giving children only 13 teaspoons of sugar, or about 25 percent of their normal daily consumption of sugar, should not have produced any appreciable results. Once the study was finished, it hadn't. Yet, by giving the children less sugar than they usually absorb per day, the conclusions, which said the mothers of these children were wrong in saying their children were hyperactive because of the sugar they consumed, were hardly justified.

Let's look at a second problem, trial size. The pro-sugar scientists, in the four favorable studies, studied from ten to thirty children. In contrast, in one of Schoenthaler's studies, 800,000 schoolchildren were studied. In six of his other studies, 5,000 juvenile delinquents were studied. Alexander Schauss, a colleague of Schoenthaler's, who worked with him on some studies, did two studies that examined over 2,000 juvenile delinquents. Both of his studies concluded sugar has detrimental behavioral effects. As anyone who has followed political polling or any other type of statistics knows, you get closer to the facts when you survey the greatest number.

Third, the sugar lobbyists' studies only followed the children they were studying for a few hours. Compare that to the work performed by Schoenthaler and Schauss, who in looking into how diets high in sugar can lead to juvenile delinquency and behavioral problems in children, were conducted over a period of several years, not just a few hours. Compare this to the "pro-sugar" studies. For example, Behar's gave twenty-one males their 13-teaspoon sugar drink and observed them for only five hours on three mornings. Even more outrageously, Wolraich observed his thirty-two hyperactive school-age boys for only three hours! That was enough evidence for him to conclude the consumption of sugar has no effect on human behavior.

Fourth, in some of the pro-sugar work, the sugar replaced rather than, as it would in normal life, supplemented the child's diet. So, in the studies, the children were told not to eat any breakfast in the morning. They would then go to school where they would be given a sugared drink was equivalent to their missing breakfast, and would therefore not necessarily cause any changes in behavior.

Here are the camps on the question. On one side, studies championed by the sugar industry, which, by way of suspiciously unscientific studies, find children's behavior is unaffected by sugar. On the other, work from researchers not associated with the sugar industry and its lobby, who hold that sugar does have an effect on children, causing behavioral problems that range from hyperactivity to delinquency.

I, for one, put my money on this second group, and hold with them that the best choice is a diet that removes unnecessary sugar and processed foods, doesn't have a negative effect on children's behavior, and creates a positive effect of lifetime health.

Socioeconomic Impact

Though it does not directly affect health, it is always good to know the facts behind the products we take for granted. Often when we consider a product we may be ready to do without, finding out the moral costs of that product helps to solidify our decision. As with the moral problems raised by meat consumption, sugar has its own moral complications. The sugar industry has a long and sordid history of using both slave labor and child labor to harvest sugar, refine it, and bring it to market. In an October 17, 2001 article for *Creative Loafing,* senior editor John F. Sugg reported the current exploitation of child labor by the sugar industry:

> While we're talking sweet, take a hard look at your sugar bowl. Much of the sugar on American tables comes from the Dominican Republic. The Reverend Kirton recalls seeing cane-cutters, *braceros,* as young as six, labor dawn-to-dusk shifts. And it's not a Dominican company that works the children. "Those plantations were owned by Gulf & Western, the same people who make movies at Paramount studios," Kirton says. (In 1985, Gulf & Western sold its 240,000 acres of plantations—along with a posh resort— to the politically powerful Fanjul family of Palm Beach. That clan is often accused of widespread abuses of labor in its fields in the Everglades, so it is unlikely to have improved conditions in the Dominican Republic.)

The sugar industry was also one of the largest exploiters of slave labor. The University of Calgary, in its applied history tutorial *The Sugar and Slave Trades,* provides a concise review of sugar production's historical origins:

Sugar cane cultivation had its origins in Southwest Asia. From there it was carried to Persia and then to the eastern Mediterranean by Arab conquerors in the twelfth and thirteenth centuries. Shortly after sugar cane's introduction to the Mediterranean, it was being grown on estates similar to the later plantations of the Americas. By the fourteenth century, Cyprus became a major producer using the labor of Syrian and Arab slaves. Eventually sugar made its way to Sicily where a familiar pattern of enslaved or coerced labor, relatively large land units, and well-developed long-range commerce was established. The Portuguese and the Spanish both looked to Sicily as a model to be followed in their own colonies in the Atlantic, and in 1420 Prince Henry sent to Sicily for cane plantings and experienced sugar technicians.

An innovation in sugar production, the roller mill, was introduced to the Mediterranean in the fifteenth century. The roller mill reduced the time and labor needed to prepare the sugar cane. It was this technology, which was transplanted and expanded to the Atlantic Islands. The final component necessary for the industry's growth was satisfying its requirement of a large labor force. The solution was the incorporation of African slaves.

Herbert Klein, in his book *African Slavery in Latin America and the Caribbean* (1990), traces the history of the sugar industry and compares it to other exploiters of African and indigenous Indian slavery:

> Once we enter the more familiar history of the "Atlantic Islands," sugar and slavery become the economic foundation for European imperialism, even more so than the cotton and tobacco industries. Before the cotton and tobacco plantations, there was the sugar industry in Brazil. When the Dutch became the direct competitors of their former Brazilian partners in 1630, their first step was to deny pivotal component of the sugar industry.

According to Klein, by the 1650s, with the decline in Brazilian production, the Dutch were forced to bring their slaves and sugar milling equipment to the French and British settlers in the Caribbean. When the Dutch themselves migrated to the Caribbean, the sugar plantation system took hold on the islands, and by the 1670s sugar became a larger commercial operation than tobacco and indigo. The accompanying slave trade led to a declining population of indentured whites and soon blacks outnumbered whites on Barbados for the first time. By 1700 every year saw the arrival of at least 1,300 black slaves, and Barbados, with 50,000 slaves, became the most densely populated region in the Americas.

Norman Kretchmer and Claire Hollenbeck, authors of *Sugars and Sweeteners* (1991) estimate that in the four centuries prior to the abolishment of slavery, the transport of slaves involved 22 million people, 12 million of whom were utilized in the Americas. The remainder died onboard ship or shortly after arrival. Further, "a number of historians state that sugar was responsible for 70 percent of the traffic of slavery."

Kevin Bales noted in his book *Disposable People: New Slavery in the Global Economy* (2001), that even today, large amounts of slave labor exist in Africa, Asia, Pakistan, Brazil, and the Caribbean, among other places. As a result of globalization and the international commodities markets, products tainted with slavery are being broadly distributed throughout the world.

According to Bales, "Maybe 40 percent of the world's chocolate is tainted with slavery. The same is true of steel, sugar, tobacco products, jewelry—the list goes on and on. Thanks to the global economy, these slave-produced products move smoothly around" the world.

Bales points out that the global market in commodities, such as cocoa and sugar, functions as a money-laundering machine. Cocoa, for instance, coming out of West Africa and entering the world market almost immediately loses its "label." If you're a buyer for a candy maker, you don't say, "I'd like to buy six tons of Ghanaian cocoa." You just say you want six tons of cocoa. When the cocoa is delivered to your factory, you can't tell where it's from, so you may be passing on a slave-tainted product without knowing, and consumers will buy it without knowing. The same is true of sugar and other commodities, where the source is not easily identifiable.

Peter Cox in the *New Internationalist* (November, 1998) asked the question, "Slavery on sugar plantations is a thing of the past. Or is it?" Cox's investigation revealed the following:

"We suffered all kinds of punishment," one witness told the Brazilian Justice Ministry. "We were hit with rifle butts, kicked and punched. I tried to escape, so did my uncle. He was shot and killed by farm gunslingers."

The word is *peonage*—a vicious system of forced labor, common in many parts of Latin America, Asia and even in the southern US. A recruiter entices the poor and the homeless with promises of employment, good wages, food and shelter. Then they are trucked long distances to toil on remote plantations where they are held prisoner and compelled to work at gunpoint. The victims aren't paid cash—they receive notional "credits," which are offset by extortionate charges for the tools they use and the hammocks they sleep in.

"Life for these people is worse now than it was under slavery," says Wilson Furtado, of the agriculture federation in Bahia state in Brazil. "Then the owners had some capital tied up in their slaves so it cost them if one died, but now they lose nothing." No matter how hard the victim's work—cutting sugar cane or felling trees—they can never break even. A loaded rifle keeps them in line, but it's debt that keeps them working.

However, Cox points out an irony for those countries relying on sugar as a cash crop while the sugar industry focuses on more research and development into artificial sweeteners. According to Cox, the plight of non-Western nations whose economies are dependent on cash crops such as sugar is identical to the position of the victims of *peonage*. Both are held to economic ransom by a system that ensures they can never free themselves of debt—no matter how hard they try. The more they produce, the more indebted they become. In 1981, the Dominican Republic earned $513 million from its sugar exports, yet by 1993 its income had dropped almost by half—to $263 million, despite increasing its production by 84,000 tons. This disastrous decline in income saw the Dominican Republic's debt swell from $600 million in 1973 to a staggering $2,400 million in l983. And not only sugar producers are crippled: plummeting prices for commodities in general have impoverished many Third World economies, leading to widespread starvation.

Cox also investigated how one of the richest islands of the Philippines could become the setting for another Ethiopia-type famine, where an estimated 85,000 Philippine children under six were suffering from moderate or severe malnutrition. This was partly, according to Cox, because the corrupt Marcos regime mismanaged the industry. Also, the US market for Philippine sugar had disappeared (being replaced by corn syrup), throwing a quarter of a million sugar workers out of their jobs. And the land, rich and fertile, was exclusively used for sugar cane, which prevented self-sufficiency in food production. Cox concludes that a disaster was waiting to happen. Quite a few other authors have documented the exploitations of modern slavery, and its variants, by the sugar industry.

Enough has been said, I think, to make one wonder if sugar with such a foul history, and which even now to be farmed is drawing labor from people working in outright or slightly disguised slavery in many countries, should be permanently boycotted for moral as much as health reasons.

Sugar and the Environment

Sugar production also causes stress on our natural environment. As nation's cash-crop economies vainly struggle to repay the debts, which we saw in the last section, are growing rather than being paid off, environmental devastation becomes another consequence of the modern sugar industry. In 1997, the American University in Washington, DC, issued a special-case study on the effects of the sugar industry on the environment of the Philippines:

> The relationship between sugar production and environmental damage is found in deforestation, soil erosion, and consequent bio-diversity loss caused by forest conversion to sugar cane fields. Forest clearing caused widespread soil erosion and had a devastating effect on the ecology, wiping out a third to a half of the known species of snails and birds in the Philippines.
>
> In the overall Philippines, cultivated upland areas increased from 582,000 hectares in 1960 to over 3.9 million hectares in 1987. Soil erosion was estimated at about 122 to 210 tons per hectare annually for newly established pasture, compared to less than 2 tons per hectare for land under forest cover. Forest cover declined from 50 percent of the national territory in 1970 to less than 21 percent in 1987.

The deforestation rate of the Philippines, driven in large part by the sugar industry, is now pegged at 25 hectares an hour or 219,000 hectares a year. Experts say the country can expect its forests to be gone in less than forty years.

This is not the only country where sugar production is tearing up the ecosystem, and those who want to look into it can usually find books describing similar devastation in Africa, the Caribbean, and other places where sugar is grown. However, from this one example, you can see why the ecologically sensitive tend to forego the use of sugar.

The Multinational Corporations

As my previous remarks on the involvement of Gulf & Western in the sugar cane industry in the Dominican Republic (DR) should suggest, quite a few large multinational companies are invested in the sugar industry. For example, to continue with Gulf & Western's involvement in DR, Daniel Hellinger and Dennis Brooks in their book *The Democratic Façade* (1991), write:

> Gulf & Western came to the Dominican Republic in 1966, two years after an invasion by US Marines. Aided by major tax concessions granted by President Balaguer to foreign investors, economic penetration of the country quickly followed US military and political intervention. With loans from Chase Manhattan Bank, Gulf Western gained a foothold in the island's economy with its purchase of the South Puerto Rico Sugar Company. By 1976, its investment had grown to $300 million in sugar, meat, citrus, tourism, and tobacco. Other transnational corporations also operated in the Dominican Republic, but Gulf Western dominated the economy as the country's largest landowner, employer, and exporter. Because the yearly revenues of Gulf Western were greater than the Dominican Republic's Gross National Product, it could accurately be called "a state within a state."
>
> Immediately on entering the country, Gulf Western broke the sugarcane workers' union, Sindicato Unido. Denouncing the union as communist controlled, the corporation fired the entire union leadership, annulled its contracts, and sent in police to occupy the plant while the American Institute for Free Labor Development (an agency financed in part by the CIA) formed a new union that obtained immediate acceptance from the Dominican president. The possibility of free unions on Gulf 's sugar plantations disappeared (along with dozens of labor leaders), with the result that of the country's 20,000 cane cutters, only one out of ten is Dominican. Most of the cane

> workers are Haitian immigrants paid $1.50 to $3.00 a
> day to do what Dominicans call "slave work."

Hellinger and Brooks also describe how Gulf Western set up the first of the industrial free zones that thrive in the Dominican Republic. Often called "runaway shops" (because businesses relocate there from US communities) or "export platforms," such zones offer a low-wage labor force, government subsidies and freedom from taxes and environmental regulations. Unions are not permitted in these zones. So, in the mid-1980s, in these zones, 22,000 workers earned an average of 65 cents per hour working in factories that were surrounded by barbed wire and security guards.

Rather than saying more, let me just comment that the criminal misbehavior of Gulf Western is not unexpected as making a buck is its bottom line for this, as for very many business enterprises. While there have been and are responsible corporations, the last place you seem to find them is in the food production business.

Conclusion

Whereas there are many health foods, sugar might be dubbed a *stealth food* in that it is often hard to know, even if you consult the label, how much sugar is in what you eat. Moreover, the sweetener's grim effects on health are being downplayed by the industry that sells it and by its myriad shills and spokespeople. In that way, too, it tries to get in under the awareness radar.

Because of the public's unconsciousness of the dangers of high sugar diets, excess sugar ingestion is rampant in today's society. And this excess sugar has saddled us with alarming health risks like obesity and diabetes. The sugar industry, with its carelessness for workers and the environment, cannot be trusted to tell us the facts about its stealth food. Instead, it uses misleading tactics, such as having athletes guzzling its wares in commercials as if their sports success were connected to drinking these sugary brews.

The truth is that, just as athletes don't really drink these beverages, this massive amount of sugar doesn't have to be a part of our everyday life. We can dump sugary products and adopt a diet based on nutrient rich, natural foods. Diets centered on vegetables, legumes, and whole grains provide everything a body needs for optimal health. Young people who transfer to this type of lifestyle have a zestful, hearty, rich, enriched life, while those who are older can pick up these healthy alternatives to ensure a long and happy life.

Sugar Alternatives and Natural Sweeteners

Let me say a few words to people who are pre-diabetic or diabetic, though what I will talk about, sugar alternatives, also merit studies by all readers who want to get away from sugar without giving up sweetness.

Just because you are diabetic does not mean you are relegated to a diet that includes no desserts or food with a trace of sweetness. Diabetics need only switch over to sugar alternatives and natural sweeteners. Although we charge you to act responsibly, being conservative and judicious with any type of sweetener, these alternatives will prove a wonderful way to enhance a healthy cuisine.

When thinking of eating something sweet, you should first educate yourself on the source of the sweetener you want to try and check out its glycemic index (GI) rating. Recall, this index charts how quickly a given food breaks down into sugar in the bloodstream. The higher the GI, the quicker the food breaks down and the more risk it poses to the balance of the insulin regulation system. Using the chart, you can evaluate possible sweeteners and chose ones that are low on the glycemic index chart. Most of the sweeteners in the list that follows are low in sugar, calories and carbohydrates and have low glycemic activity.

When a recipe calls for sugar, honey or maple syrup, replace these items with a sugar alternative from this list. Not everything on the list may be equally appealing to your palate, so test them out to find which is most pleasant to your taste buds, appropriate for your recipe, and healthiest for your body.

Remember, be responsible and conservative, and enjoy the tasty alternative sweeteners of the world! They can be found at almost any health food store and are also available at many retailers online. Here they come.

Agave nectar is a natural liquid sweetener that comes from a mature agave plant, which is grown, harvested, and cultivated in Mexico. It is a sweet, sticky, syrupy sugar located in the center of the plant. It is great for cooking, baking, and sweetening beverages, such as iced tea. Any recipe that calls for sugar can be replaced with agave.

Agave is low on the glycemic index while it is about one and half times sweeter than refined sugar. However, cooking agave can increase the amount of fructose, so it is important to check with the manufacturer for ideal usage. As with most sweeteners, agave is best in its organic and raw form.

Agave nectar comes in three grades: light, medium and amber. Light agave is sweet but flavorless, making it great for recipes where the stronger flavor of maple or honey may interfere. The two darker grades possess a more intense agave flavor, so they are more fitting for use with a richer meal or beverage.

The glycemic index of agave is 11, so it's good for diabetics as long as they monitor their carbohydrate intake.

Nutrition Facts:
  21 grams = 60 calories
            16g carbohydrates
            15g sugars

Barley Malt: Dark, sticky, with a strong and distinctive flavor, barley malt sugar is a mix between honey and molasses in taste and texture. This malt is composed primarily of maltose, a natural sugar, and enters the bloodstream slowly. It contains trace amounts of eight vitamins and several minerals.

Nutrition Facts:
    100 grams = 316 calories
                76g carbohydrates
                62g sugar

Birch sugar, also known as xylitol, is a derivative of birch bark. This one is a great replacement for brown and white sugar. It is excellent for baking, dissolves quickly, looks and tastes like sugar, and, as another key attraction, has only half the calories of sugar. It is a pure carbohydrate that metabolizes very slowly.

Unlike refined sugars, it does not further gum decay or dental caries, and for this reason birch sugar can often be found in tooth-pastes and mouthwashes.

However, one has to be careful with how much is used since xylitol taken in high dosages can cause gas and diarrhea.

Nutrition Facts:
    1 teaspoon = 4 grams
                 9.6 calories
    1 cup = 200 grams
            480 calories

Brown rice syrup is made from a variety of enzymes and, as the name indicates, brown rice. It is amber in color, mild butterscotch in flavor, and less sweet than sugar. It can be used well in some baking, but note, baked goods made with rice syrup often end up with a brittle, coarse texture. So, this works well when making crunchy, baked items such as granolas and hard cookies. On the other hand, it is not recommended for cakes, breads or soft baked goods.

For sugar substitution recommendations, please consult the product label or manufacturer.

Nutrition Facts:
    1 tablespoon = 50 calories
                    42g carbohydrate

Coconut palm sugar is made from the nectar of the coconut palm blossom. In earlier times, it was taken from the sap of the palmyra palm or date palm, but now it is obtained from sago and coconut palms, and sometimes sold as palm sugar or coconut sugar. It has a slight coconut taste with overtones of caramel. It benefits from a low glycemic index of 35, and so is absorbed into your bloodstream slowly. It can be used in a 1:1 ratio against white/cane sugar, so that for every teaspoon of sugar called for by a recipe, substitute one of coconut palm sugar.

Nutrition Facts:
    1 teaspoon = 10 calories
                  2.5g carbohydrate
                  2.5g sugar

Date sugar is made from ground, dehydrated dates, and is a mix of sucrose, glucose, fructose, and complex carbohydrates, with a little folic acid. A dark, mahogany color, date sugar is comprised of moist, coarse granules. Dates are high in fiber, and rich in a wide variety of vitamins and minerals. As with coconut palm sugar, date sugar can be exchanged measure for measure for sugar in baking cakes, muffins and breads. Also it's good for crumb toppings for pies and fruit crisps in place of brown sugar. It shouldn't be used as a beverage sweetener because the tiny granules do not dissolve.

Nutrition Facts:
    1 teaspoon = 12 calories

Maple sugar is the yellowish brown sugar produced by boiling down maple syrup. Once called sinzibukwud, it was a sugar frequently used by the Native Americans because it is long lasting. You can usually buy it in small blocks or as a translucent candy. By composition, this sugar is about 90 percent sucrose, with the remainder consisting of glucose and fructose. It is quite a bit sweeter than cane sugar, but it should be used more sparingly than most of the other sweeteners we have mentioned because it does not have a low glycemic number.

Nutrition Facts:
   1 teaspoon = 11 calories
                      3g carbohydrate
                      3g sugar

Mesquite pod meal is an aromatic powder ground from the bean pods of the mesquite tree. It tastes like molasses, but it has more nutritional value. The entire mesquite pod is rich in protein, and the meal is also high in the amino acid lysine, and in calcium, magnesium, potassium, iron, and zinc. Mesquite pod meal is high in fiber, so it's a good sweetener for baking when it is mixed with flour. It also can be a useful adjunct in cooking, and for including in soups and sauces. It can also be put in salads and fruit smoothies. This sweetener is particularly helpful to diabetics because it is a very slow-to-digest protein.

Nutrition Facts:
   15 grams = 30 calories
                      2 calories from fat
                      0 sodium
                      6g carbohydrates
                      3g dietary fiber
                      1g sucrose
                      2g protein

Rapadura, also known as panela, comes from evaporated cane juice. It is commonly used in Latin American countries where it is most often sold in the form of a brick. It is an unbleached, unrefined sweetener to use in place of refined sugars. Rapadura has a mild, caramel flavor, which makes it a great sweetener for baking and drinks. Because it is not heated during its processing, it retains its original vitamins and minerals, including silica and iron. It also has a natural balance of sucrose, glucose, and fructose.

Being metabolized more slowly than white sugar, rapadura is a good choice for diabetics, who can avoid that white sugar rush.

Nutrition Facts:
   1 cup rapadura = 1 cup sugar
   1 teaspoon = 15 calories
              = 4g carbohydrates

Stevia is a South American herb that's been used as a sweetener for hundreds of years. It's actually thirty times sweeter than sugar. The leaves of the small, green *Stevia rebaudiana* plant have a delicious and refreshing taste. As a sweetener, Stevia has many excellent properties:

- The body does not break down the glycosides (organic plant compounds that contain sugar) from stevia, so rather than being low calorie, it is a natural *no* calorie option!
- Stevia is ideal for diabetics because it has been found to enhance insulin secretion, and it doesn't adversely affect blood glucose levels. It possesses anti-hyperglycemic properties, making it one of the best options for individuals suffering from type II diabetes.

A perennial shrub of the aster family, stevia can be purchased as whole or broken leaves. It also appears on the market in powder form and as a liquid extract. Dried stevia keeps its flavor for months. Use one teaspoon in place of one cup of sugar. To make your own liquid solution, dissolve 1 teaspoon of white stevia powder in 3 tablespoons pure water and refrigerate.

Nutrition Facts:
  0 calories = 0 carbohydrates
  0 on glycemic index, and no chemicals

Sweet Fiber is a fiber-based all natural sweetener. Its ingredients include inulin, also known as chicory root fiber, with low glycemic fruit extract. It has no artificial ingredients. Each spoonful has about the "sweetness" of one teaspoon of sugar.

Nutrition Facts:
  ½ teaspoon = 0 calories
                1 gram carbohydrate

Yacon syrup, a natural sweetener derived from the yacon root, has been used in South America for centuries. It is similar to molasses, and can be used as a healthy honey or maple syrup substitute. Yacon syrup is naturally low in calories and low in mono- and disaccharides, making it a great option for a diabetic.

Nutrition Facts:
  1 tablespoon = 30 calories
                  0 fat
                  0 protein
                  7g carbohydrates

Zsweet® is a sweetener made of erythritol, a fermented sugar, which is infused with natural botanical extracts and then crystallized. All the ingredients are gluten free and contain no known allergens. In a recent study conducted by Glycemic Index Laboratories, Zsweet® was shown to affect 0 percent increase in blood sugar levels.

Nutrition Facts:

1 teaspoon = 0 calories

4g carbohydrate

Glycemic Index of Popular Food

Let me repeat myself here, just to remind you of what I said about the Glycemic Index earlier in the book. This index charts how quickly a given food breaks down into sugar in the bloodstream. The higher the GI, the quicker the food breaks down and the more risk it poses to the balance of the insulin regulation system.

The following tables provide the glycemic index of popular food. Eating food that is low on the Glycemic Index can help reduce your risk factor for heart disease, cancer, Alzheimer's disease, and diabetes.

Grains and Pasta

Low Glycemic Index (< 45)		Medium Glycemic Index (46–60)		High Glycemic Index (> 60)	
Barley Chapati	43	Brown Rice	55	Bagels	72
Barley Kernel Bread	39	Buckwheat	55	Cheerios	74
Chickpea Flour Chapati	27	Bulgur	47	Corn Chips	83
Fettucini	32	Corn	55	Corn Flakes	83
Pearl Barley	25	Cracked Barley	50	Cornmeal	69
Rice Bran	27	Linguini	46	Couscous	65
Soy Lin Bread	19	Linseed Rye Bread	55	Crackers	67
Spaghetti	36	Macaroni	46	Cream of Wheat	70
Vermicelli	35	Muesli	56	English Muffins	71
Wheat Bran	42	Oat Bran	55	Gnocchi	67

Whole Rye	37	Oatmeal	60	Melba Toast	70
		Pita Bread	57	Millet	71
		Popcorn	55	Puffed Wheat	74
		Pumpernickel Bread	50	Rice Cakes	74
		Rice Vermicelli	58	Rice Krispies	82
		Special K	54	Rice Pasta	92
		White rice	58	Rolled Barley	66
		Wild rice	57	Rye Bread	64
				Semolina Bread	64
				Shredded Wheat	71
				Taco Shells	68
				White Bread	95
				White Flour Products	71

Beans

Low Glycemic Index (< 45)		Medium Glycemic Index (46–60)		High Glycemic Index (> 60)	
Black Beans	31	Baked Beans	48	Fava Beans	79
Black-Eyed Peas	41	Romano Beans	46		
Butter Beans	30				
Chana Daal	8				
Chickpeas	33				
Green Lentils	29				
Kidney Beans	29				
Mung Beans	38				
Navy Beans	38				
Pinto Beans	38				
Red Lentils	25				
Soybeans	17				

Dairy

Low Glycemic index (< 45)		Medium Glycemic Index (46—60)		High Glycemic Index (> 60)	
Plain Yogurt	14			Ice Cream	61
Skim Milk	32				

Fruits and Nuts

Low Glycemic Index (< 45)		Medium Glycemic Index (46–60)		High Glycemic Index (> 60)	
Apple	38	Banana	54	Pineapple	66
Cherries	22	Blueberry	57	Raisins	64
Dried Apricots	31	Canned Peaches	47	Other Dried Fruit	70
Grapefruit	25	Kiwi	53	Watermelon	72
Nuts	15	Mango	56		
Orange	44	Orange juice	52		
Peach	42				
Pear	37				
Plum	38				

Vegetables

Low Glycemic Index (< 45)		Medium Glycemic Index (46–60)		High Glycemic Index (> 60)	
Brassica Family	<15	Raw Carrots	49	Beets	64
Green Beans	<15	Sweet Potatoes	54	Cooked Carrots	85
Green Vegetables	<15	White Potatoes (boiled)	56	French Fries	75

Herbs	<15	Yams	51	Mashed Potatoes	70
Peas	<15			Parsnips	98
Powdered Greens	<15			Pumpkin	75
Tomato	<15			Rutabaga	72

Charts from *The GI Factor: The Glycemic Index Solution* by Dr. Jennie Brand-Miller, Kaye Foster-Powell, and Dr. Stephen Colagiuri.

Chapter 8

Super Foods

What does it mean when we say a food is super? No, it's not that the foodstuff is so powerful that, as might happen in a Hollywood movie, a few bites will cure cancer or diabetes. Nature's products don't work that way, but move gradually to improve health where it is weak or to maintain it where it is strong.

Rather a super food is one that *simply does better what all natural, healthy foods do*. All natural foods have nutrients and work to boost different bodily processes. Super foods are those that perform these offices in a big way. Native traditions throughout the world have long known that certain vegetables, fruits, and grains are especially powerful purveyors of protective, preventative, and therapeutic health benefits. However, it was not until there were studies of these natural products by modern biochemistry, botanical science, molecular biology, and medical clinical research that many of these foods' extraordinary properties were more widely known.

This section briefly introduces these super foods, which all should be a permanent part of your diet. The benefits I ascribe to them are those I have culled from reading the medical literature. An appendix, "Super Foods: Supporting Scientific Evidence," has been included, and it contains some of the more conclusive evidence supporting the specific preventative and curative properties of these foods, which you may want to look into for yourself if you are interested in learning more about the enhancing properties of the different organic substances.

Apples

For thousands of years, apples (malus sylvestrsis) have been used for a wide variety of medical complications and diseases, including diabetes, fevers, inflammatory conditions, and heart ailments. In addition to having confirmed many of the healthful properties of apples, modern research has identified invaluable phytochemicals contained by the fruits. Phytochemicals are chemical compounds that are found in plants and which have been used to treat illnesses. One of these found in apples is phloretin, a natural antibiotic. The fruits also contain pectin and pectic acids that provide essential bulk to a diet. The apple's tannins, quercetin, alpha-farnesene, shikimic acid, and chlorogenic acid also promote health benefits, such as increasing production of the neurotransmitter acetylcholine, so helping offset cognitive decline due to oxidative damage. With high levels of phenols, polyphenols, and other anti-oxidant, chemoprotective properties, apples have been shown to help guard against a variety of cancers, including leukemia and those that target the colon, lung, breast, liver, and skin. These apple's chemicals also provide essential nutrients to improve cardiovascular health, reduce the risk of coronary heart disease and stroke, and prevent atherosclerosis.

Apricots

This fruit had a long and rich history in the medical practices of China and India. In traditional Chinese medicine, apricots and their kernels are prescribed for treating asthma, cough, and constipation. The fruit is a stronghold of vitamins C and K, beta-carotene, thiamine, niacin, and iron. Japanese scientists have called attention to the apricot's ability to inhibit the pathogenic bacteria frequent in ulcers and acute gastritis.

Bananas

Bananas are low in calories while providing essential nutrients, among them vitamin B6, vitamin C, potassium, and manganese. They also stimulate probiotic activity, which sustains healthy gut flora. Bacteria in our gastrointestinal system are critical for proper digestion and absorption of nutrients. Bananas help keep this system on track. Recent findings have indicated that bananas may offer protection against kidney cancer, particularly in women, and aid renal function.

Blueberries

Many berries have health-boosting properties. Berries that are black, blue, and red are especially known for their possession of antioxidant nutrients. Blueberries specifically contain the antioxidant groups of flavonoids, phenolic and polyphenol compounds, all of which have shown some ability to reverse cellular aging of the cognitive and motor functions. The fruit's power was brought home in a recent study that compared the antioxidant levels of 100 different foods. Blueberries scored highest! Other examination have shown blueberries acting to protect brain health, improve memory, and sustain coordination by, for one, enhancing communication between nerve cells. This activity provides protection from serious neurodegenerative diseases, such as dementia and Alzheimer's. On top of this, blueberries have anti-inflammatory properties that protect the skin, joints, and the cardiovascular and neurological systems. Eating of the fruit has proven beneficial to those suffering from diabetes. It consumption prevents bone loss and inhibits cancer cell proliferation, particularly in the cases of prostate and colon cancer. With all these life-giving properties, blueberries have certainly earned the soubriquet "super food."

Broccoli

What makes broccoli a super food is its high concentration of the phytochemicals diindolymethane and isothiocyanate, which are powerful immunomodulators, that is, substances that have strong effects on the immune system. Because it fosters immune system strength, broccoli empowers that system in the fight against cancer (breast and prostate cancer, in particular) and provides protection from bacterial and viral infections. Along with the two aforementioned phytochemicals, broccoli also contains other anticancer agents, such as glucoraphanin. Due to these observed properties, right now a substantial amount of research is being conducted on broccoli's mutagenic qualities.

This vegetable is rich in vitamins A, B5, B6, B9 (folate), C and K, and provides plenty of dietary fiber. It will also give anyone who eats it moderate amounts of calcium, iron, phosphorus, and potassium. As with other leafy green vegetables, it contains lutein and zeaxanthin, which foster eye health. Since it has more calcium than even most dairy products, it can protect bones and increase bone mass. Thus, it's another plant well deserving of its super food classification.

Carrots

Carrots can be looked to as chief provider of carotenoids, a family of antioxidants proven to block DNA and cellular membrane damage caused by free radical activity. This vegetable is rich in the phytochemicals alpha-carotene and lycopene, both shown to have anti-carcinogenic properties, fighting against cancer especially in the colon, lung, prostate, and stomach. The less-known black and purple carrots have high levels of anthocyanin, a powerful anti-cancer biochemical that studies have found slowing cancer cell proliferation by as much as 80 percent. Other work indicates the commonplace belief that carrots improve memory is far from mythical since the vegetable has shown capacity in boosting brain function. Add to that cardiovascular benefits, such as decreasing cholesterol.

Another adage has it that carrots improve vision. This has been backed by the fact that carrots are high in retinoids that benefit ocular health. Since carrots are a good source of vitamin A, they should be kept in the diet of diabetics, given that A lowers blood sugar and aids in the development of insulin-producing cells in the pancreas. One cup of raw carrots can provide almost 700 percent of the daily recommended consumption of vitamin A and 220 percent of vitamin K, a substance critical for bone health. Thus, we have to dub carrots another superhero among edible plants.

Garlic

While garlic contains phytonutrients similar to those found in onions, it also possesses selenium, a substance that, according to some studies, offers protection against various cancers and against the deterioration of the body caused by free radicals. Different studies have looked at and remarked on its ability to both guard against heart disease and arterial calcification (hardening of the arteries), and to reduce cholesterol and blood pressure. Since it is a source of the flavonoid quercetin, it contains antibiotic properties that empower it to fight colds, stomach viruses, and yeast infections.

Ginger

Ginger is already widely employed throughout the world by anyone who wants to cure dyspepsia (stomach upsets), reduce gastrointestinal gases, and to relieve nausea that arises from pregnancy, seasickness, and even from chemo drugs used in cancer and other medical therapies. Ginger is largely composed of fragrant essential oils, which give it a distinctive aromatic flavor. One of these oils, gingerol, makes it a natural sedative for calming the gastrointestinal tract. This oil also provides some protection from pathogenic bacteria that upset the stomach. All in all, ginger is rich in antibiotic properties that combat the GI infections that bring on diarrhea and dehydration. Beyond this, new evidence suggests ginger helps lower cholesterol, a boon that provides protection from cardiovascular disease.

Folk medicine has long honored ginger. Bear in mind, by the way, that while some scientists look down on folk medicine, numerous modern pharmaceuticals have been derived from folk remedies, suitably renamed and price-tagged. This folk science, now supported by modern science, has seen ginger as a mild immune booster, which wards off colds and flus, sinus congestions, and coughs. There have also been some preliminary findings in animal studies suggesting that ginger may help to treat diabetes. This is an exciting new perspective.

Goji Berry

In the "Sweet Suicide" chapter, I touched on the way the goji berry, a fruit with many health-giving properties, has sometimes been traduced by more unscrupulous food companies by being sold in such things as (to imagine a name) "Goji Power Plus Bars," which are actually low on goji as an ingredient and high on unrefined sugar. Now let's look at the value of goji, which has caused such companies to try to trade on its good name.

Also known as wolfberry in its native Europe, the plant is found through much of Asia, where it appears in exotic (to Westerners) Tibetan and Himalayan descriptions. The word goji is actually a Westernization of the Chinese word for the berry, which can be transliterated as "gouqi." The berry is a common ingredient in traditional Chinese medicine, dating back thousands of years in its use.

The oblong red goji berry has no problem fulfilling the requirements to be designated a super food. It has a high concentration of phytochemicals, amino acids, vitamins B and C, and beta-carotene. Additionally, it contains eleven essential and twenty-two trace dietary minerals, is moderately high in alpha-linolenic acid, and an outstanding source of the antioxidant lycopene. One can look to the goji berry for extra protein, dietary fibers, calcium, zinc, and selenium. With all these nutrients found in it, the goji will obviously have many health-lifting effects, and these include protection from cardiovascular and inflammatory diseases as well as from age-related vision disorders (such as glaucoma and macular degeneration). Studies have pointed to its neuro-protection, positive immunomodulatory, and anti-cancer properties. This last benefit has been underscored by a study published in the *Chinese Journal of Oncology*, which indicated cancer patients responded better to treatment while on a diet that included goji. However, the study recommended that individuals on blood-thinning medications avoid eating goji berries, which may interfere with the drugs.

Last but far from least, it offers liver protection and can improve sexual function.

Green Tea

The ingredient in tea—in green tea particularly—that has stirred the most scientific interest is catechin. Approximately 25 percent of a dry tea leaf is catechin. Although traces of catechin are also found in chocolate, wine, and other fruits and vegetables, it is tea that offers the greatest amount of this super nutrient.

The multi-tasking catechin not only has been shown to reduce the plaque buildup that is part of atherosclerosis, but it gives protection against infectious bacteria, and reduces oxidative stress. In our polluted world, tea catechins are especially needed due to another of its curative features, which is that it can improve DNA replication and protect against genetic damage from environmental toxins. Studies in recent years have noted its inflammatory properties and suggested it can play a role battling against cancer. Other scientific examinations note that green tea can improve bone density and cognitive function, reduce the risk of developing kidney stones, and strengthen heart function. There is also some evidence showing that green tea's polyphenols protect against the brain cell death that is associated with Parkinson's and Alzheimer's diseases.

I remember reading about the traditional Chinese dental hygiene procedure of brushing with tea. At the time, years ago, I thought it was humorous, but I realize now, that like many folk practices, it is rooted in real insight. Even if brushing with tea doesn't prevent cavities, it is full of other health enhancers.

Legumes

The modern Western diet, especially in America, ignores most legumes at its detriment. Sometimes I think the only way that Americans would take to legumes would be if they came in a hamburger bun and were sloshed with catsup and mustard. But, to be more serious, when I mention legumes, most people think of beans, peas and lentils. However, alfalfa, clover, peanuts, and cashews are also legumes.

These vegetables and grains are excellent sources of cholesterol-lowering fiber. When you consume a legume, its fiber content helps you manage blood sugar levels. One cup of lentils can provide upwards to 65 percent of the minimum, daily necessary dietary fiber. With this high fiber content in a serving, when legumes are frequently included in meals, we are assured to have better gastrointestinal and colon health.

Legumes in general contain energy-boosting protein and iron. Looking at specific entities in this group, black beans are rich in the potent antioxidant anthocyanidins, which promotes heart and vascular health. Green beans are excellent sources of vitamins C and K. Garbanzo beans, commonly known as chickpeas, are a superb source of molybdenum, which strengthens teeth and preserves tooth enamel.

Another important legume that is not as familiar in the US as some of those just mentioned is adzuki beans. Originally from the Himalayas and standard in East Asian cooking, it is a rich source of magnesium, potassium, iron, zinc, and B vitamins. Very high in soluble fiber, the adzuki helps eliminate bad cholesterol from the body. In Japan, it is treasured for its kidney and bladder health-promoting function, and used in weight-loss programs.

To maximize the benefits of legumes in the diet, combine them with whole grains. The reason for this recommendation is that legumes are very low in methionine, an essential amino acid that supports cellular life, while whole grains are replete with this amino acid, but low in lysine, which is abundant in legumes. A wholesome, integrated vegetarian diet will contain a balance of legumes and grains.

Leafy Vegetables

Another "league of superheroes" among foods is found in the dark green leafy vegetables. This band includes spinach, kale, arugula, Swiss chard, cabbage, collard greens, and watercress. While they should be united in your diet, each eaten in turn, they all have individualized, singular health benefits. One thing they hold in common, however, is that they are high in carotenoids and other antioxidants that guard against heart disease, cancer, and problems in blood sugar regulation.

To choose one example from among them, one cup of cooked kale provides over 1,300 percent of the daily requirement of vitamin K needed for maximum bone health. It is also rich in calcium and manganese, other nurturers of bone density. As does broccoli, kale contains the anti-cancer phytochemical sulforaphane.

To note the value of a few more of the green leafy vegetables, look at cabbage, which contains manifold glutamine, an amino acid that contributes to the anti-inflammatory activities in the body. This acid also protects from infectious complications due to human papilloma virus (HPV). The juice from cabbage will quicken the healing of peptic ulcers.

Now, turn to spinach. It is one of the best sources for iron. Per gram, it generally contains over 30 percent more iron than a hamburger. (Any diet heavy in spinach should include sufficient vitamin C to help assimilate the iron.) Spinach is also an excellent source of folic acid, calcium, copper, zinc, selenium, and omega-3 fatty acids.

Although I can't give details on every green leafy vegetable, let me end with two more. Watercress is a superb source of phytochemicals. It has been shown to be a diuretic and digestive aid as well as an aid in protecting against lung cancer and strengthening the thyroid. Collard greens supply ample quantities of immune response modulator diindolylmethane.

Mushrooms

My friends who have travelled to the Yunnan province in China, mention how there some of the most prized eatables are the wide varieties of mushrooms. Where an average, un-health conscious American would find his or her greatest culinary delight in choosing between cuts of steak, the Yunnan citizen is delicately discriminating between different mushrooms.

A wealth of growing peer-reviewed science, which would recommend the Yunnan culinary emphasis, shows that many edible mushrooms are among the more important immune builders in the plant kingdom. In particular, medicinal mushrooms inhibit tumor growth, have anti-pathogenic and blood-sugar-lowering activities, and strengthen immunity.

Among approximately two hundred different varieties whose health-enhancing skills have been noted are the chaga, cordyceps, maitake, oyster, portobello, reishi, shiitake, and turkey tail mushrooms. Although it is possible to find all of these in fresh or dried form, at the moment in the US the shiitake mushrooms are the easiest to obtain.

A list of the benefits obtained from mushrooms would have to mention their antiviral and antibacterial properties, which in different mushrooms have shown some effectiveness against a wide spread of pathogens, including those from polio, hepatitis B, influenza, candida, Epstein-Barr virus, streptococcus, and tuberculosis. The mutagenic benefits of mushrooms that one can read about in the scientific literature note how mushrooms can be enlisted in the fight against leukemia, sarcoma, and the bladder, breast, colon, liver, lung, prostate, and stomach cancers, even in advanced stages.

Onions

A rule of thumb is that the more pungent the onion, the greater its health benefits. It's as if you could smell its disease-thwarting power.

Onions are particularly important to include in diets for diabetics, for one, because they are rich in chromium, a trace mineral that helps cells respond to insulin. Moreover, refined sugar depletes the body's chromium levels, so for anyone that has this sugar in his or her diet, onions are an excellent source of replacement. Onions are also rich in vitamin B6, vitamin C, manganese, molybdenum (essential in preserving tooth enamel), potassium, phosphorous, and copper. They are also just about the best source of quercetin, which works hand-in-hand with vitamin C in help the body eliminate bacteria and strengthen immunity.

The onion's health benefits don't stop there. Inclusion of onions in the diet help individuals lower blood pressure and cholesterol, and strengthen bone health. Onions also have anti-inflammatory benefits, reducing symptoms related to inflammatory conditions, such as asthma, arthritis, and respiratory congestion. Some studies have noted that they lessen the adverse effects from colds and flus.

Oranges

The orange is a vitamin and mineral-packed treasure chest of a fruit, rich in vitamins A, B and C, potassium, and calcium, as well as being an excellent source of fiber. One phytonutrient in oranges that boosts it into the super food category is the flavonoid hesperidin. This biochemical works to support healthy blood vessels and reduces cholesterol.

What has been established so far overlooks what the public considers the orange's defining health trait, its being stocked with vitamin C, an important antioxidant that limits free radicals while also building the immune system. Vitamin C's healing properties are well known and have been repeatedly scientifically validated. These include the lessening of arterial plaque as well as protecting from Alzheimer's, Parkinson's and Crohn's diseases, arthritis, and diabetes.

Peppers (capsicum)

Native American folk medicine, which has so many features we can still learn from, gave a prominent place in its pharmacology to peppers of the capsicum family, which includes bell and chili peppers. Recent work suggests that the nutrient capsaicin, found in these peppers, is a natural analgesic and a neuro-inflammatory blocker that relieves aches and pains to joints and muscles. This is one reason why Native American medicine prescribed a topical application of pepper to painful areas of the body.

Capsaicin is particularly deserving of mention in this book because recent, promising research in Canada has explored the uses of capsaicin in the treatment of type I diabetes. Other work has noted it can benefit sufferers from prostate cancer and leukemia. Some scientists have noted that this much studied nutrient found in peppers helps with weight loss, stimulation of insulin-producing cells, and prevention of LDL cholesterol oxidation. Another benefit recently uncovered is that the nutrient protects from stomach ulcerations and induces apoptosis (cancer cell death) in lung cancer.

Setting aside the value of capsaicin, peppers can also be prized because they are rich in the antioxidant vitamins A as well as in vitamins B1, B6, E, and K. They are also high in potassium, magnesium, and iron. Yellow peppers are rich in lutein and zeaxanthin, which protect from eye disease and blindness.

Soy

Comparative studies that have considered dietary reasons for the lower cancer rates in the East as compared to the West always point to soy as one of the major foods that distinguish these global eating patterns and so may have something to do with lower cancer rates. Scientists have taken this suggestion and done a number of studies that give evidence that the phytochemicals in soy protect against the genesis of cancer. Isoflavones, including genistein and daidzein, that are major constituents in soy, seem to be some of the active ingredients that provide natural protection against various cancers: breast, colon, endometrial and prostate. One important Japanese study involving over twenty-four thousand women found those who had the highest soy content in their diet were best protected against breast cancer. A later Japanese study noted the soy isoflavones could reduce breast cancer risk by up to 54 percent.

Along with this exciting attribute, soy has given evidence of an ability to lower blood LDL cholesterol and promote good HDL cholesterol, improve cardiac function, strengthen bone mass, and stabilize blood sugar.

In vegetarian diets, soy-based foods are an excellent replacement for animal protein. Soybeans are also high in iron, omega-3 fatty acids, phosphorus, riboflavin, magnesium, and potassium.

Tomatoes

You have probably gotten the idea by now that one thing that distinguishes super foods from other eatables is that they contain very potent organic compounds, such a phytochemicals, that boost their health giving propensities. Tomatoes are no exception. They are the best source for lycopene, a carotenoid biochemical that gives tomatoes their red color, and is packed with positive properties. It has been estimated that approximately 80 percent of the lycopene consumed in the US derives from tomatoes and tomato-based foods. There is a vast body of scientific literature confirming lycopene's antioxidant and anti-mutagenic properties. This chemical is noteworthy for its protection against and treatment of various cancers, running the gamut from bladder, breast, cervix, lungs, and mouth to ovarian, prostate, and stomach cancer. Because diabetics often have low levels of lycopene in their blood, tomatoes should become a regular part of their diets.

Tomatoes have been shown to prevent cholesterol oxidation, lower blood pressure, and decrease the risk of atherosclerosis. Among other benefits that may accrue to the eater of these plants is improved renal function. Tomatoes also have anti-viral and anti-bacterial qualities. In particular, lycopene can protect against human papilloma virus, one pathogen that has been associated with cancer.

Tomatoes are also rich in most of the B complex vitamins as well as in potassium, manganese, chromium, folate, and iron. You can look to the tomato as an excellent source of the amino acid trypto-phan, which is important for neurological health and can improve sleep.

Whole Grains

By now most Americans are aware that whole grain breads and pas-tas are healthier than those made from white flour, and brown rice is higher in nutrients and health benefits than white rice. However, once a person has changed over to brown rice and whole grain breads, he or she still has a rich world of whole grains to explore, each of which offers unique health benefits and phyto-nutrients.

As with legumes, whole grains are rich in fiber. Take spelt, which is being used in breads and pastas and will provide 75 percent of the recommended daily requirement for vitamin B2. Spelt is highly water soluble, which means its nutrients are easily absorbed. There is evidence that spelt is a good choice for diabetics. Another grain, barley, is distinguished by being an excellent source of selenium, a substance that reduces the risk of colon disorders and colorectal cancer. Because barley is high in tryptophan, it will aid in sleep regu-lation. A third important grain, millet, is high in manganese, magne-sium, and phosphorous, all of which support cardiovascular health.

You are probably familiar with the grains I've just mentioned, but two that you may not have been alerted to are kamut and quinoa. The Glycemic Research Institute in Washington, DC, has trumpeted the value of kamut for its low-glycemic properties, which makes it an ideal super food for diabetics, athletes, and people suffering from obesity. It is also an excellent substitute for those with wheat allergies, giving them the benefit of its possessing 65 percent more amino acids than wheat.

Quinoa has been identified as a super food among grains for its ability to balance blood sugar and provide high quality fiber and protein to the diet. It is higher in calcium, phosphorus, iron, and zinc than are wheat, barley and corn. In addition to balancing insulin resistance, quinoa is one of the most complete foods in nature, earning its super food status not only by the aforementioned traits but because it protects against atherosclerosis and breast cancer, and acts as a probiotic to foster the good micro-flora in the gut.

The last few pages have shown you some of the amazing properties and multiple actions of the super food family. However, simply reading about foods may not prompt you to rush out to buy them, because, after all, although many can and should be eaten raw, they are probably more appealing combined in salads or other recipes. To really be enthused you have to imagine them in delectable recipes. That's why I recommend you turn quickly to the next section of this book, which is filled with mouth-watering recipes, ones which will get you stopping as soon as possible at the health food grocery where you can stock up on super food in preparation for trying them out using the recipes provided.

Chapter 9

Your Recipe Repertoire

All of the recipes in this book are vegan and gluten free. However, I realize that most people cannot make recipes that they would consider to be a radical transition from what they are normally used to eating. Transitional foods are an option. Another approach is to lessen the amount of meat, dairy, and refined products before you are able to wean yourself completely.

So, if you wish to use the protein source you are used to within any of the recipes until such time that you are able or willing to give them up completely, that is an option.

Since I've allowed you this ability to move gradually, I don't want to hear readers saying (or writing me), "I am not used to any of these foods" or "I don't like the way they taste" or "The average person doesn't eat them." Instead of balking at eating these delicious but unfamiliar foods, modify the recipes on your journey to making the full transition.

My hope is that you will realize the variety of flavors and tastes in these unique combinations and recipes.

BREAKFAST CEREALS AND OTHER EARLY DAY DELIGHTS

Tips

Rather than provide a quantity of any one sweetener for any given recipe, I have decided to give you all of the different, natural, and healthy sweeteners from which you can select, which can be found listed at the end of the "Sweet Suicide" chapter.

- Always begin with a low amount of sweetener and choose sweeteners that are low calorie and of low glycemic content.
- Each single serving of protein suggested is equivalent to 15–20 grams of protein.
- Grains cooked in advance may be reheated by steaming.
- Grains are more flavorful when cooked with ½ teaspoon sea salt per cup of dry grain.
- Although unhulled barley is most desirable because it is the whole grain, it has a longer cooking time than "pearled" barley. I suggest you look for the darker varieties of pearled barley, found in health food stores, as they are minimally processed.
- Rice milk or soy milk may be used interchangeably, with slight taste variation; however, soy milk adds a protein complement to grains.

NUTTY CINNAMON CEREAL
½ cup cooked pearled barley
3 oz. almonds, chopped
1 serving of protein
¼ teaspoon of cinnamon
Sweeten to taste

Combine barley in a medium-size saucepan with water. When water comes to a boil, lower heat and cook until water is absorbed,

stirring occasionally. Add remaining ingredients and mix well. Serve immediately. When cereal is ready to eat, add sweetener to taste.
Serves 1

AMISH COUNTRY
½ cup amaranth
1 ¼ cup (approx.) water for amaranth
3 tablespoons carob powder
½ cup blackberries
⅛ teaspoon fennel seeds
1 serving protein powder
Sweeten to taste

Bring amaranth and 1 ¼ cups water to a boil and cook covered over low heat for 25 minutes or until tender.

In a saucepan, stir carob powder into 3 tablespoons of filtered water. Add berries. Let simmer for 5 minutes

Pour carob sauce over amaranth. Sprinkle protein powder over sauce. Add sweetener to taste. Serve immediately.
Serves 1

OLD WORLD CEREAL
½ cup teff
1 ¼ cup water
¼ teaspoon sea salt
½ cup pomegranate seeds
1 serving protein powder

Bring teff and salted water to a boil. Lower heat, cover, and cook until tender, about 25 minutes. Then let stand 5 minutes.

Sprinkle protein powder over cereal. Add the pomegranate seeds. Serve immediately.
Serves 1

BANANA-COCONUT WALNUT CEREAL
½ cup millet
1 ½ cups water
1 cup mashed banana
¼ cup coconut flakes
4 tablespoons chopped walnuts
½ cup rice or soy milk

Combine millet and water in a medium-size saucepan. Bring to a boil over medium heat. Lower heat and cook 3 to 7 minutes, or until tender.

Add the remaining ingredients (except milk). Wait 1 to 2 minutes.

Serve with rice or soy milk on top.
Serves 2

BARLEY IN THE MORNING
4 tablespoons carob powder
3 tablespoons water
½ cup raspberries or dried cherries
1 cup cooked pearled barley
1 serving protein powder
Handful of almonds
Vanilla rice milk or vanilla soy milk
1 serving of friendly fiber

In a small saucepan, stir carob powder into water. Add raspberries. Let simmer 5 minutes.

Pour raspberry carob sauce over cooked barley. Sprinkle protein powder and slivered almonds over sauce and serve immediately with vanilla soy or rice milk on the side.
Serves 1

BLUEBERRY BLAST

1 cup cooked brown rice (at room temperature)
½ cup blueberries, cut in half
3 tablespoons sunflower seeds
1 serving protein powder
1 oz. flax seed oil
Sprinkle of unsweetened, flaked coconut

Combine all ingredients. Mix well.
Serves 1

BREAKFAST FROM THE ANDES

½ cup quinoa
1 ½ cups water
1 ripe pear, quartered and sliced
Dash sea salt
Handful of chopped cashews
1 serving protein powder
Dash of cinnamon
Dash of fennel
Sweetener (to taste)

Cook quinoa in 1 ¼ cups of water with the sea salt.

Cook pears with sweetener and the remaining water over low heat until tender, about 3 to 5 minutes.

Spoon pear mixture with cinnamon and fennel over cooked quinoa.

Sprinkle protein powder and cashews on top and serve immediately.
Serves 1

RICE 'N' NUTS

1 cup rice milk
Sweetener (to taste)

¼ cup pure vanilla extract

½ cup raw macadamia nuts

Pinch sea salt

½ cup sliced strawberries

1 cup cooked brown rice, hot

In a blender, combine rice milk, vanilla extract, sweetener, nuts, and salt.

Sprinkle strawberries over hot rice. Pour macadamia sauce over all. Serve immediately.

Serves 1

CAROB OATS DELIGHT

1 cup oats

¾ cup water

3 tablespoons carob powder

½ cup raspberries

1 serving protein powder

Sweeten to taste

¼ cup ground or handful raw sunflower seeds

Bring oats and ¾ cup water to a boil, cover, lower heat and cook until tender, about 15 minutes.

In a small saucepan, stir carob powder into 3 tablespoons filtered water. Add raspberries and sweetener. Let simmer 5 minutes.

Pour carob sauce over oats. Sprinkle protein powder and sunflower seeds over sauce and serve immediately.

Serves 1

AMARANTH SMOOTH

½ cup amaranth

1 ½ cups water

¼ teaspoon sea salt
½ cup tofu
½ cup macadamia nuts
1 cup raspberries
1 serving protein powder

Mix amaranth and salted water and bring to a boil. Lower heat and cook covered until tender, about 25 minutes. Let stand 5 minutes.

Mix in the rest of the ingredients until creamy.

Sprinkle protein powder on top and serve immediately.

Serves 1

BARLEY FOR BREAKFAST

½ cup cooked pearled barley
½ cup tofu
2 tablespoons chopped almonds
1 banana, mashed
1 serving protein powder

In a saucepan, combine all of the ingredients except barley and protein powder over low heat until creamy.

Add barley, stirring until hot.

Sprinkle protein powder on top and serve immediately.

Serves 1

IRISH OATMEAL

½ cup steel cut oats
¾ cup water
¼ teaspoon salt
½ cup soft tofu
2 tablespoons walnuts
1 peach, diced
1 serving protein powder

Bring oats and salted water to a boil. Lower heat and cook covered until tender, about 15 minutes.

Mix the rest of the ingredients, except protein powder, stirring until creamy.

Sprinkle protein powder on top and serve immediately.

Serves 1

RED QUINOA

½ cup red quinoa

1 cup water

¼ teaspoon sea salt

2 tablespoons walnuts

1 cup blueberries

1 serving protein powder

Bring red quinoa and salted water to a boil. Cover and cook over low heat until tender, about 15 minutes.

Mix in the rest of the ingredients, except protein powder, stirring until creamy.

Sprinkle protein powder on top and serve immediately.

Serves 1

SWEET RICE

½ cup short grain brown rice

1 cup water

¼ teaspoon sea salt

½ cup soft tofu

3 tablespoons of raw macadamia nuts

½ cup blackberries

1 serving protein powder

Bring rice and salted water to a boil. Cook, covered, over low heat until tender, about 40 minutes.

Mix in the rest of the ingredients, except protein powder, stirring until creamy.

Sprinkle protein powder on top and serve immediately.

Serves 1

HOT SPELT CEREAL

½ cup spelt

1 ¼ cups of water

¼ teaspoon sea salt

3 tablespoons Brazil nuts

½ cup pomegranate seeds

1 serving protein powder

Bring spelt and salted water to a boil. Cover and cook over low heat until tender, about 1 ¼ hours.

Mix in the rest of the ingredients, except protein powder, stirring until creamy.

Sprinkle protein powder on top and serve immediately.

Serves 1

FLUFFY RAISIN AMARANTH

1 cup cooked amaranth (at room temperature)

Handful of raisins

1 tablespoon honey

Pinch cinnamon

Combine all ingredients.

Mix well.

Serves 1

CINAMMON AMARANTH

½ cup amaranth

1 ¼ cup water

½ teaspoon cinnamon

¼ teaspoon ground nutmeg

1 serving protein powder

1 banana, sliced

6 strawberries, sliced

Bring amaranth and salted water with maple syrup to a boil. Cover and cook over low heat until tender, about 25 minutes. Let stand 5 minutes.

Sprinkle with spices and protein powder. Add fresh fruit and serve immediately.

Serves 1

MANGO QUINOA

1 cup cooked quinoa (at room temperature)

¾ cup unsweetened mango, chopped

¼ cup pecans, chopped

½ teaspoon cinnamon

Pinch of allspice

Combine all ingredients.

Mix well and serve immediately.

Serves 1

RASPBERRY BANANA PANCAKES

2 tablespoons egg substitute

2 tablespoons vanilla extract

1 banana, mashed

¼ cup unsweetened rice milk

¼ cup whole spelt flour

1 cup oat flour

½ cup soy flour

1 teaspoon baking powder

1 teaspoon baking soda

2 tablespoons unsweetened flaked coconut (optional)

½ cup raspberries
1 tablespoon coconut oil
Sweeten to taste

In a medium-size mixing bowl, combine egg replacer, vanilla, banana, and rice milk. Mix with fork until well blended.

In a separate bowl, combine flour, baking powder, and baking soda. Mix well. Add flour mixture to banana and milk mixture, blending well with a spoon. Stir in coconut if desired, and raspberries.

Heat oil in large skillet over medium heat. Pour in 2 to 3 tablespoons of batter at a time. Cook each pancake for 3 to 5 minutes on each side until light brown. Re-oil skillet as necessary to prevent sticking.

Yields 14 pancakes

POWER OATS BREAKFAST
¾ cup rolled oats
¼ teaspoon sea salt
1 cup filtered water
4 dates
Sweetener (to taste)
1 serving protein powder

Cook oats in salted water for 10 to 15 minutes over medium heat, stirring occasionally until tender.

Dice dates. Add sweetener to cooked oats and mix well. Sprinkle with protein powder and serve immediately.
Serves 1

QUINOA BROWN
½ cup quinoa
1 cup plus 3 tablespoons water
¼ teaspoon sea salt

3 tablespoons carob powder
½ cup raspberries
Sweetener (to taste)
1 serving protein powder

Bring quinoa to boil in 1 cup of salted water. Lower heat and cook, covered, 10 to 15 minutes until tender.

In a small saucepan, stir carob powder into 3 tablespoons water. Add raspberries and sweetener. Let simmer for 5 minutes.

Pour carob sauce over quinoa. Sprinkle protein powder over sauce and serve immediately.
Serves 1

SPELT VITALITY
½ cup spelt
1 ¼ cup water
Sweetener (to taste)
¼ teaspoon sea salt
½ teaspoon cinnamon
¼ teaspoon ground nutmeg
1 serving protein powder
1 banana, sliced
4 strawberries, sliced

Bring spelt, sweetener, and salt to a boil in a medium saucepan. Lower heat and cook, covered, about 1 ½ hours or until tender. Add more water if necessary.

Sprinkle with spices and protein powder. Add fresh fruit and serve immediately.
Serves 1

VERMONT PUMPKIN
1 small whole pumpkin
Water

2 tablespoons almond butter
1 serving protein powder
Pinch of allspice

Preheat oven to 400 degrees F. Cut pumpkin in half, remove the seeds, and discard them.

Place pumpkin halves in baking dish cut side down. Add enough water to measure ⅓ inch. Bake for 40 minutes.

When cooled, spoon out pumpkin and place in bowl. Add remaining ingredients. Mix well.
Serves 2

AMARANTH PEACH DELIGHT
1 ½ oz. pecans, chopped
Pinch of clove
Pinch of allspice
6 oz. amaranth, cooked (room temperature)
3 oz. dried peaches, chopped

Combine all ingredients.
Mix well.
Serves 2

FLUFFY RAISIN COUSCOUS
6 oz. couscous, cooked
1 tablespoon stevia
Pinch of cinnamon
3 oz. raisins

Combine all ingredients.
Mix well.
Serves 2

HAWAIIAN RICE CEREAL

1 ½ cups coconut milk or tropical fruit juice

1 banana, sliced

½ cup pitted fresh or frozen cherries

½ cup chopped pineapple

¼ cup shredded unsweetened coconut

2 cups cooked basmati rice

½ cup chopped macadamia nuts, toasted (see note below)

In a medium size saucepan, combine the milk, banana, cherries, and pineapple.

Cook over medium-low heat for 2 to 3 minutes.

Add the remaining ingredients, mix well, and cook an additional 2 to 3 minutes.

Serve hot. Serves 2

Note: To toast nuts, preheat oven to 375 degrees and place nuts on ungreased cookie sheet for 10 to 15 minutes or until light brown.

JUICES AND SHAKES

Tips

As you know, I recommend using juices and shakes as liquid breakfasts. However, if these are not sufficient for your appetite, you may have a piece of fruit not less than one hour after your drink.

WATERMELON SHAKE

1 cup watermelon chunks, peeled with seeds

1 banana

¼ cup plain rice milk

1 serving protein powder

½ teaspoon pure almond extract

½ teaspoon cinnamon

1 cup ice

Juice watermelon.

In a blender or food processor, combine 1 cup watermelon juice with remaining ingredients. Blend for 2 minutes or until smooth.

Serve immediately.

Yields 1 cup

APPLE CHERRY JUICE
Fresh apples (juiced to yield 1 cup)
1 plum (¼ cup juice)
1 lemon (2 tablespoons juice)
¼ cup pitted cherries, frozen
1 serving protein powder
1 cup ice

Separately juice apples, plums, and lemon. Set aside.

In a blender or food processor, combine 1 cup apple juice, ¼ cup plum juice, and 2 tablespoons lemon juice with the remaining ingredients. Blend for 2 minutes or until smooth.

Serve immediately.

Yields 1 cup

AVOCADO AND STRAWBERRY SHAKE
Note: May have 6 whole strawberries one hour after this breakfast shake if necessary.
1 apple (¼ cup juiced)
¼ cup avocado
¼ banana
½ cup strawberries, fresh or frozen
½ cup plain rice milk
½ teaspoon pure almond extract

1 serving protein powder

1 cup ice

In a blender, combine all the ingredients.

   Yields 3 cups

BLUEBERRY AND PAPAYA MACADAMIA NUT SHAKE

1 papaya (¼ cup juice)

½ cup blueberries

½ cup ground or whole macadamia nuts, unsalted

1 banana, mashed

¾ cup unsweetened rice milk

1 serving protein powder

½ teaspoon pure lemon extract

1 cup ice

Juice papaya.

In a blender or food processor, combine papaya juice with the remaining ingredients. Blend for 2 minutes or until smooth.

   Serve immediately.

   Yields 1 ½ cups

CAROB NUT MILK SHAKE

Fresh apples (to yield 1 cup juiced)

1 banana

4 tablespoons of ground walnuts or walnut butter, unsalted

1 cup plain rice milk

1 ½ tablespoons pure unsweetened carob powder (pure
   unsweetened cocoa powder may be used as a substitute)

1 teaspoon almond extract

1 serving protein powder

1 cup ice

Juice apples

In a blender or food processor, combine the apple juice with the remaining ingredients. Blend for 2 minutes or until smooth. Serve immediately.

Yields 3 cups

CHOCOLATE SMOOTHIE

1 orange (⅓ cup juice)

1 tangerine (¼ cup juice)

¼ banana

2 tablespoons unsweetened cocoa

(raw chocolate powder)

½ teaspoon pure vanilla extract

¼ teaspoon ground cinnamon

1 serving protein powder

1 cup ice

Separately juice orange and tangerine.

In a blender or food processor, combine orange juice and tangerine juice with the remaining ingredients. Blend for 2 minutes or until smooth.

Serve immediately.

Yields 2 ½ cups

CELERY PURPLE CABBAGE TONIC

4 stalks celery (½ cup juice)

½ head purple cabbage (½ cup juice)

1 apple (⅓ cup juice)

2 lemons (2 tablespoons lemon juice)

1 serving protein powder

Separately juice celery, cabbage, apple, and lemons.

In a blender or food processor, combine the juices with the protein powder.

Serve immediately.

Yields 2 cups

CRANBERRY GINGER JUICE
Fresh pear (to yield 1 cup juiced)
½ cup cranberries (2 tablespoons juice)
2 inch piece ginger root (1 teaspoon juice)
Lemon (to yield 2 tablespoons juice)

Separately juice pear, cranberries, and ginger.

In a blender or food processor, combine pear juice, cranberry juice, ginger juice, and lemon juice.

Serve immediately.

Yields 1 cup

CELERY APPLE JUICE
6 stalks celery (1 cup juice)
Fresh apples (to yield 1 cup juice)
Fresh grapefruit (to yield 1 cup juice)

Separately juice celery, apples, and grapefruit. Combine all the juices in a blender.

Serve immediately.

Yields 3 cups

CITRUS DELIGHT
Note: *May have a whole grapefruit 1 hour after this breakfast drink if necessary.*
1 orange
½ grapefruit
2 lemons

½ cup club soda
1 cup ice

Separately juice orange, grapefruit and lemon.

In a blender or food processor, combine the juices with club soda and ice. Blend for 2 minutes, or until smooth.

Serve immediately.

Yields 1 cup

CHERRY AND MELON SHAKE
1 cup honeydew melon chunks, peeled
1 banana
¼ cup pitted cherries, frozen
1 tablespoon unsweetened coconut flakes
½ cup unsweetened rice milk
1 serving protein powder
1 cup ice

Juice melon.

In a blender or food processor, combine melon juice with remaining ingredients. Blend for 2 minutes or until smooth.

Serve immediately.

Yields 1 cup

PAPAYA PINEAPPLE SHAKE
1 apple
1 slice papaya
1 lemon
¼ cup mashed avocado
½ cup rice milk
1 serving protein powder
⅓ teaspoon cinnamon
1 cup ice

Separately juice apple, papaya, and lemon.

In a blender or food processor combine the juices with the remaining ingredients. Blend for 2 minutes or until smooth.

Serve immediately.

Yields 1 cup

FROSTY PEAR AND POMEGRANATE JUICE
1 pear
1 cup raw pomegranate seed
1 banana
1 serving protein powder
1 cup ice

Separately juice pear and pomegranate.

In a blender or food processor, combine pear and pomegranate juice with remaining ingredients. Blend for 2 minutes or until smooth.

Serve immediately.

Yields 1 ½ cups

GINGER CELERY SPLASH
2 oranges (½ cup juice)
1-inch piece of ginger root (1 teaspoon juice)
¼ cup cranberries (1 tablespoon juice)
1 serving protein powder
1 cup ice

Separately juice oranges, ginger, and cranberries.

In a blender or food processor, combine orange juice, ginger juice, and cranberry juice.

Blend for 2 minutes or until smooth.

Serve immediately.

Yields 1 ½ cups

GARLIC AND SWISS CHARD JUICE

1 apple
1 cucumber
1 stalk celery
1 small bunch Swiss chard
1 clove fresh garlic

Juice the apple, cucumber, celery, chard, and garlic. Blend together in a food processor.
Serve immediately.
Yields 1 ½ cups

LEAFY BEET VEGETABLE JUICE

2 apples
2 carrots
1 small bunch beet greens
1 beet
1 serving protein powder
1 ½ cups ice

Separately juice apples, carrots, beet greens, and beet.
In a blender or food processor, combine the juices.
Serve immediately.
Yields 2 ¼ cups

KIWI LEMON MELON TONIC

1 cup watermelon chunks, peeled
4 peeled kiwis
1 lemon
1 serving protein powder
1 ¼ cups ice

Separately juice watermelon, kiwi, and lemon.

In a blender or food processor combine the juices with the remaining ingredients. Blend for 2 minutes or until smooth.

Serve immediately.

Yields 1 ½ cups

GREEN MACHINE JUICE

1 cup parsley

3 cucumbers

1 small bunch Swiss chard

2 red bell peppers

2 inch piece ginger root

1 cup watercress

Juice all items together.

Serve immediately.

Yields 2 ¼ cups

PINEAPPLE CRANBERRY SMOOTHIE

1 cup peeled pineapple

2 cups watermelon chunks, peeled

½ cup cranberries

1 lemon

1 cup seltzer

1 serving protein powder

½ cup ice

Juice pineapple, watermelon, cranberries, and lemon.

In a blender or food processor, combine the juices with the remaining ingredients. Blend for 2 minutes or until smooth.

Serve immediately.

Yields 3 ¼ cups

WALNUT PROTEIN SHAKE

1 apple

¼ banana

⅓ cup ground or whole pecans or pecan butter, unsalted
1 serving protein powder
½ teaspoon pure lemon extract
1 cup seltzer
1 cup ice

Juice apple.

In a blender or food processor, combine the apple juice with the remaining ingredients.

Blend for 2 minutes or until smooth.

Serve immediately.

Yields 2 ½ cups

ROMAINE LETTUCE AND APPLE REFRESHER
3 apples
1 head romaine lettuce
1 lemon

Together, juice apple, lettuce, and lemon.

Serve immediately.

Yields 1 ½ cups

STRAWBERRY BANANA SPLIT
2 apples
1 pear
2 cups strawberries
2 stalks celery
½ banana
2 tablespoons protein powder
1 cup ice

Separately juice apples, pear, strawberries, and celery.

In a blender or food processor, combine the juices with the remaining ingredients.

Blend for 2 minutes or until smooth.
Serve immediately.
Yields 2 ½ cups

SUNFLOWER PAPAYA SHAKE

1 papaya
2 tablespoons unsweetened flaked coconut
4 tablespoons hulled sunflower seeds, unsalted
1 teaspoon pure almond extract
1 cup rice milk
1 cup ice cubes

Juice papaya.

In a blender or food processor, combine papaya juice with remaining ingredients.

Blend for 2 minutes or until smooth.

Serve immediately.

Yields 2 ¼ cups

SUNFLOWER SPROUT APPLE JUICE

1 apple
3 cups sunflower or alfalfa sprouts
1 lemon
1 cup water

Separately juice apple, sprouts, and lemon.

Combine the juices in a blender with the water.

Serve immediately.

Yields 1 ½ cups

TANGERINE KIWI COCKTAIL

1 tangerine
2 peeled kiwis

1 serving protein powder
¼ cup ice
1 cup water

Juice tangerine and kiwi.

Blend the juice with the remaining ingredients for 2 minutes or until smooth.

Serve immediately.

Yields 1 ½ cups

TANGY STRAWBERRY SHAKE

4 apples
½ cup cranberries
2 cups strawberries, fresh or frozen
1 cup plain rice milk
1 serving protein powder
1 teaspoon ground cinnamon
1 cup ice

Juice the apples and cranberries.

In a blender or food processor, combine the juices with the remaining ingredients.

Blend for 2 minutes or until smooth.

Serve immediately.

Yields 3 cups

WATERMELON LEMON SPRITZER

2 cups peeled watermelon cubes
2 peeled kiwis
2 lemons
1 cup sparkling water
½ cup ice

Juice watermelon, kiwis, and lemons.

In a blender or food processor, combine the juices with the remaining ingredients.

Blend for 2 minutes or until smooth.

Serve immediately.

Yields 2 cups

LUNCH

Tips

Rice, soy, or almond cheese can be substituted in any of these recipes for any regular kind of cheese. Sour cream, yogurt, cream cheese, and cottage cheese all can be obtained from nondairy choices.

Be careful, some lactose-free, rice, and soy-based products contain casein, which is a dairy ingredient.

Look for labels that say dairy free, wheat free, gluten free, and vegan.

Note: Extra Virgin Olive Oil is abbreviated EVOO in the recipes below.

SPICY PASTA AND BLACK BEAN SOUP
4 cucumbers
1 head cauliflower, steamed and chilled
1 cup diced yellow onions
4 tablespoons EVOO
½ cup unsweetened rice milk
1 ½ cups chopped tomato
1 cup cooked black beans
½ cup chopped escarole or kale
¼ cup chopped celery
¼ cup sliced carrots
2 teaspoons chopped fresh dill
4 teaspoons chopped fresh basil
½ teaspoon sea salt

½ teaspoon black pepper

⅓ teaspoon cayenne pepper

4 cloves garlic, crushed

1 cup uncooked whole grain "rice-macaroni"

Juice cucumbers and cauliflower.

In a large saucepan, sauté onion in oil for 5 minutes.

Add 1 ½ cups cucumber juice, cauliflower pulp, and rice milk. Bring to a boil over high heat, then reduce the heat to medium.

Add remaining ingredients except for macaroni, and simmer, uncovered for 15 minutes.

Boil macaroni, drain, and add to mixture.

Serve hot or cold.

Serves 3–4

EGGPLANT PARMIGIANA SANDWICH

1 (¼-inch thick) circular slices eggplant

4 tablespoons EVOO

1 clove garlic

4 plum tomatoes

½ cup filtered water

¼ teaspoon basil

¼ teaspoon sea salt

2 slices sprouted spelt bread

2 oz. soy or rice mozzarella

Preheat oven to 375 degrees F. Oil pan with 2 tablespoons of the oil.

Bake eggplant slices in oiled pan for 20 minutes or until tender. Set aside.

In a saucepan, sauté garlic in remaining 1 tablespoon of the oil for 2 minutes.

Dice tomatoes. Add to saucepan with water, basil, and sea salt. Simmer for 20 minutes, stirring frequently.

Toast spelt bread.

Place eggplant on 1 slice bread and cover with tomato sauce. Top with sliced soy cheese.

Cover with another slice of bread and bake for 5 minutes.

Remove and serve immediately.

Serves 2

BEAN SALAD WITH MACADAMIA AND MUSTARD

2 cups steamed fava beans

¼ cup soy mayonnaise with dill to flavor

¼ cup raw macadamia

1 tablespoon mustard

1 tablespoon flax seeds

¼ cup fresh dill sprigs for garnish

In a medium-size mixing bowl, toss beans with mayonnaise and mustard.

Sprinkle macadamia nuts and flax seeds on top of bean mixture.

Serve cold or at room temperature, garnish with the dill sprigs.

Serves 2

VEGGIEBALL STEW

1 teaspoon sea salt

⅓ teaspoon black pepper

2 tablespoons Worcestershire sauce

1 teaspoon grated lemon peel

1 teaspoon dried basil

1 tablespoon curry powder

1 teaspoon wheat-free tamari sauce

1 stalk celery, chopped

1 onion, chopped

2 tablespoons egg substitute

4 ounces tempeh

¼ cup spelt flour
1 tablespoon EVOO
4 cups water
1 cup yellow squash, sliced
1 small turnip, boiled and cubed
1 medium red potato, boiled and shredded
1 cup fresh tomato, peeled, cored, and chopped
1 leek with top sliced off
Vegetable broth bouillon, for 1 quart
1 tablespoon chopped fresh basil

In a medium size bowl, combine salt, pepper, Worcestershire, lemon peel, basil, curry, celery, scallion, egg substitute, and chopped soy tempeh.

Shape into 1-inch balls and roll in spelt flour.

Heat oil in skillet and brown the balls, turning gently between a fork and spoon.

Set aside. Save any drippings.

In a large saucepan, with 4 cups of water, place squash, turnip, potato, tomato, leek and vegetable bouillon.

Boil on medium heat for approximately 30 minutes.

Add veggieballs to soup and reheat for 5 to 7 minutes.

Sprinkle with dill on top.

Serve with sprouted bread.

Serves 3–4

PRIMO PASTA
½ pound quinoa pasta
5 artichoke hearts
¼ teaspoon sea salt
¼ teaspoon cayenne
1 lemon
4 tablespoons EVOO

4 cloves garlic, minced

3 ounces sun-dried tomatoes

½ pound seitan, cubed

1 sprig fresh basil, chopped

15 olives, pitted and sliced

¼ cup grated soy or rice parmesan, optional

Cook pasta. Steam artichoke hearts until tender. Season seitan with salt, cayenne, and lemon.

In a skillet, sauté garlic with sundried tomatoes in olive oil for 3 minutes.

Add seitan, basil, and olives and cook until seitan flakes when tested with a fork, about 5 minutes or more.

In a large bowl, toss seitan mixture with the pasta, and parmesan, and serve.

Serves 2

BROCCOLI STIR FRY

1 cup firm tofu

2 cups broccoli florets

2 tablespoons hot sesame oil

2 tablespoons tamari sauce

2 teaspoons fennel seeds

1 teaspoon grated fresh ginger

3 cloves garlic, minced

2 teaspoons lemon juice

In a medium saucepan, sauté tofu and broccoli in oil for 3 minutes over medium heat. Remove from pan and place mixture in bowl.

Combine remaining ingredients in saucepan. Cook on medium heat until mixture simmers for 1 minute. Add broccoli mixture and cook, covered, for 2 minutes.

Stir well. Serve with short grain brown rice or Far East rice noodles.

Serves 1

DYNAMITE VEGGIE SAUSAGE

¾ cups uncooked orzo

1 cup water

¾ teaspoon fresh oregano, finely chopped (or ½ teaspoon dried)

2 tablespoons finely chopped Italian parsley

3 tablespoons Extra Virgin Olive Oil, divided

1 tablespoon balsamic vinegar

2 cloves garlic, pressed

3 tablespoons hazelnuts, finely chopped

Sea salt to taste

Freshly ground black pepper to taste

6 Greek olives, green and black, pitted and chopped

4 soy sausage links

6 cups (9 oz.) spinach leaves, washed, dried, and steamed until just wilted

¼ cup crumbled tempeh

Parsley for garnish

Cook orzo according to package directions.

In glass jar, mix water, oregano, parsley, 1 ¾ tablespoons Extra Virgin Olive Oil, vinegar, garlic, hazelnuts, salt, and pepper. Cover tightly and shake well.

Combine chopped olives and cooked orzo in a bowl. Pour dressing over mixture and toss.

Lightly brown sausage links in remaining olive oil.

Arrange steamed spinach leaves with soy sausage on two plates. Fill with orzo and olive mixture and sprinkle with tempeh on top. Garnish with parsley.

Serves 3–4

CREAM OF PUMPKIN SOUP
2 tablespoons coconut oil
1 small onion, chopped
2 cloves garlic, chopped
½ cup apple, peeled, cored, and chopped
½ cup pumpkin flesh, grated
½ cup celery chopped
1 cup silken tofu
1 teaspoon mild curry powder
¼ teaspoon ground turmeric
¼ teaspoon ground cumin
1 tablespoon chopped basil
1 tablespoon rice flour
1 teaspoon arrowroot powder
3 cups vegetable broth or 3 cups water plus 2 vegetable bouillon cubes
2 servings protein powder

In a saucepan, heat oil and sauté onion, scallion, garlic, apple, pumpkin, and celery for about 5 minutes.

Stir in tofu and cook for 2 minutes.

Add remaining ingredients, except broth, and cook and stir an additional 3 minutes.

Slowly add broth and bring to a boil.

Cover, lower heat, and simmer for 15 minutes.

Place half the soup in a blender with the protein powder and puree.

Return puree to the pot.

Cook an additional 3 minutes.

Serve hot.

Serves 2

TEMPEH WITH RICE AND PEPPERS

½ pound tempeh

1 ½ cups cooked brown rice (warm or at room temperature)

¾ tablespoon chopped fresh marjoram

½ teaspoon chopped fresh tarragon

2 tablespoons diced red bell pepper

2 tablespoons diced yellow bell pepper

2 tablespoons diced green bell pepper

1 teaspoon sea salt

¼ teaspoon cumin

1 ½ tablespoons EVOO

Steam peppers for 1 minute only, to keep them crisp.

Grill tempeh for 5 minutes.

Combine all ingredients in a bowl and mix well.

Serves 1–2

SALADS

Note: In the recipes below, Extra Virgin Olive Oil is abbreviated EVOO.

CAESAR SALAD WITH CROUTONS

3 carrots (¾ cup pulp)

4 ½ cups chopped romaine lettuce

½ cup spelt croutons

1 ½ tablespoons grated soy cheese

Natural Dijon salad dressing (available at health food stores)

Juice carrots.

In a large mixing bowl, toss ¾ cups carrot pulp with lettuce.

Toss salad with the desired amount of Dijon salad dressing, spelt croutons, and soy cheese.

Serve cold or at room temperature.

Serves 2

ENDIVE OLIVE SALAD

½ pound endive, washed

1 medium sweet onion

Olive oil for sautéing and dressing

2 large cloves garlic

½ cup mixed olives

1 teaspoon grated fresh or powdered ginger

¼ teaspoon turmeric

Sea salt to taste

Place dried endive in a bowl and spread the leaves out.

Cut onion into rings and mix into endive.

In a lightly oiled pan over medium heat, sauté garlic cloves until slightly brown.

Allow a few minutes for garlic to cool, then cut into strips or rings and add to dish.

Add olives, and sprinkle with sprouts as a garnish.

Add turmeric and salt to taste.

Drizzle on olive oil, as desired.

Serve immediately or refrigerate and serve cold.

Serves 2–3

HOT DULSE BROWN RICE SALAD

2 cups cooked brown rice

½ cup diced sweet onion

2 tablespoons chopped dulse leaves

3 teaspoons EVOO, plus extra oil for sautéing

1 ½ tablespoons Bragg's liquid amino

⅓ cup hot water

1 garlic pickle or cucumber, diced

1 tablespoon ground fennel seeds

2 teaspoons lemon juice

2 sprigs fresh parsley, chopped

Sea salt
Fresh ground pepper

Cook brown rice.

Sauté onion and dulse in small amount of oil over medium heat. Mix amino with water and pour over cooked rice.

Add onion, dulse, pickle, fennel. Mix all ingredients well.

Add olive oil and sprinkle with lemon juice and parsley.

Add small amount of water if dry.

Serve hot, adding salt and pepper to taste.
Serves 2

BROCCOLI PASTA SALAD

2 cups cooked whole grain brown rice pasta (bowtie, shell, ziti, or penne)
3 cups tomato salsa
1 cup broccoli florets, steamed
½ cup mixed olives
1 cup whole pine nuts
3 tablespoons EVOO

In a large bowl, toss pasta with the remaining ingredients.

Serve cold as a salad (or main dish).
Serves 2

RED PEPPER POTATO SALAD

½ pound red potatoes
3 medium celery stalks, minced
½ small onion, minced
¼ cup finely chopped yellow and red bell peppers
1 tablespoon minced parsley
1 tablespoon minced mint
1 teaspoon tarragon

½ cup soy mayonnaise

2 tablespoons sour pickle relish (optional)

Sea salt to taste

Fresh ground pepper to taste

Steam potatoes until cooked but firm, about 15 to 18 minutes. Drain, peel, and allow to cool.

Place celery, onion, and peppers in a large bowl.

Add parsley, mint, and tarragon.

When potatoes have cooled, dice them, and add celery and onion mixture.

Add mayonnaise a little bit at a time until mixture is well coated, but not too wet.

Add relish, sea salt, and pepper to taste, and mix well.

Cover with plastic wrap and refrigerate.

Serve cold.

Serves 2

ARUGULA AND SPINACH SALAD

½ pound washed arugula

½ pound washed spinach

1 medium size red onion

1 ounce dandelion leaf

Olive oil for sautéing and dressing

2 large cloves garlic

1 teaspoon grated fresh or powdered ginger

Broccoli sprouts

¼ teaspoon turmeric

Sea salt to taste

Place dried spinach and arugula into bowl and spread leaves out.

Cut onion into rings and mix into spinach.

Cut dandelion leaves into 1-inch strips and add to dish.

In a lightly oiled frying pan over medium heat, sauté garlic cloves until slightly brown.

Allow a few minutes for garlic to cool before adding to the dish. Then cut into strips or rings and add to dish.

Add sprouts, and sprinkle on turmeric and sea salt to taste.

Drizzle with EVOO.

Serve immediately or refrigerate and serve later.

Serves 2–3

SPICY HUMMUS AND CUCUMBER SALAD

1 large cucumber sliced
1 ½ teaspoons EVOO
1 teaspoon sea salt
1 clove garlic, cut in half
2 tablespoons chopped fresh dill
1 cup fresh hummus
2 tablespoons chopped fresh mint
2 teaspoons freshly squeezed lemon juice
¼ teaspoon jalapeno or Tabasco sauce
2 teaspoons apple cider vinegar
Dash paprika

Combine all ingredients except the cucumber and paprika in a blender.

In a serving bowl, mix together cucumber slices and blender mixture.

Garnish with paprika and serve immediately.

Serves 2

ADZUKI VEGETABLE SALAD

3 oz. adzuki beans, cooked (chilled)
3 oz. onion, chopped
3 oz. tomato, chopped

3 oz. green pepper, chopped

1 ½ oz. almonds, blanched and slivered

2 tablespoons sesame oil

½ teaspoon minced garlic

½ teaspoon tarragon

¼ teaspoon basil

1 teaspoon salt

Combine all ingredients.

Serve at room temperature.

Serves 2

APPLE, WALNUT, AND TOFU SALAD

¼ cup onions, minced

¼ cup celery, minced

2 teaspoon raw apple cider vinegar

½ cup Nayonaise

¼ teaspoon ground, cumin

1 apple, ½ inch diced

1 pound firm tofu, drained and crumbled

¼ cup raw walnuts

Combine onions, celery, vinegar, Nayonaise, cumin and apple and mix well.

Mix in tofu and walnuts.

Serve or refrigerate for up to three days.

Serves 2

BROCCOLI TORTELLINI SALAD

2 cups uncooked vegan tortellini

½ cup broccoli florets, steamed 3 to 4 minutes

¼ cup sliced black olives

½ cup marinated artichoke hearts (jarred)

3 tablespoons apple cider vinegar
1 tablespoon tamari

Place the tortellini in boiling water for 15 minutes, then drain and let cool for 10 minutes.

Combine with the other ingredients in a medium size bowl, then refrigerate for 2 hours before serving.
Serves 2

ORIENTAL SEAWEED SALAD
3 oz. hijiki (1 oz. dry)
3 oz. carrots cut in long thin strips
3 oz. daikon, cut in long thin strips
3 oz. scallions, chopped
2 tablespoons safflower oil
1 teaspoon minced garlic
½ teaspoon caraway seeds
½ teaspoon salt
3 oz. amaranth, cooked (chilled)

Soak and rinse hijiki three times and place in bowl.

Lightly sauté carrots, daikon, and scallions in skillet with safflower oil for about 5 minutes, then add to the hijiki.

Add garlic, caraway seeds, and salt.

Combine with amaranth.

Mix well.
Serves 2

PASTA SALAD
4 oz. of quinoa macaroni swirls, uncooked
1 cup vegan cottage cheese
½ teaspoon dry mustard
⅔ tablespoon plain vegan yogurt (no added sugar)

1 bell red pepper, coarsely chopped
4 scallions, chopped
1 tablespoon parsley flakes
1 teaspoon dill
1 teaspoon tamari (soy sauce) or
Braggs's Amino Acids
Salt and pepper to taste

Cook the quinoa according to the directions on the package. Drain well and chill.

In a large mixing bowl, combine the vegan cottage cheese, mustard, and yogurt.

Add the quinoa, toss well, and add the remaining ingredients.

Toss again.

Serve on a bed of lettuce.

Serves 4

BITTER-SWEET
3 oz. butternut squash
3 oz. arugula
3 oz. alfalfa sprouts
1 ½ oz. currants
2 tablespoon sunflower oil
½ teaspoon dill
½ teaspoon parsley
½ teaspoon salt

Peel the butternut squash.

Cut in half and remove the seeds.

Discard the seeds.

Place the squash, cut side down, in a baking pan with ⅓ inch of water.

Bake for 40 minutes at 400 degrees.

When squash is cool enough to handle, cut into bite-sized pieces.

Place in a medium mixing bowl.

Rinse arugula carefully to get all of the dirt off.

Tear off the stems and discard.

Add the arugula to the squash.

Add the remaining ingredients.

Toss gently so as not to mash the squash.

Serve hot or cold.

Serves 2

DINNER

Tips

The average diabetic gets most of his or her protein from animal sources that include beef, pork, veal, chicken, lamb, and dairy. Most of their carbohydrates come from refined breads with partially hydrogenated fat that include bagels, white bread, sandwich bread, pizza crust, muffins, and donuts.

All of the above contribute to the development of diabetes and exacerbate symptoms in individuals who already have the disease.

In the recipes below, you will find healthy dinner alternatives. These include foods rich in protein, fiber, tofu, beans, nuts, whole grains, and vegetables.

PISTACHIO CHOP SUEY

For the sauce

1 teaspoon honey

1 cup vegetable broth or 1 vegetable bouillon cube

1 teaspoon tamari

1 tablespoon rice vinegar

1 ½ tablespoons arrowroot powder

1 tablespoon apple cider vinegar

For the vegetables

4 leaves bok choy

2 teaspoons toasted sesame oil

3 cloves garlic, minced

½ cup canned heart of palm, rinsed, drained, and sliced diagonally

1 cup cauliflower

1 celery stalk

1 cup sliced shiitake

1 cup sprouts, preferably mung beans, rinsed

½ cup toasted pistachios

To prepare sauce, in a small saucepan, heat honey, broth, tamari, and rice vinegar.

In a bowl, whisk together arrowroot and cider vinegar.

To prepare vegetables, separate bok choy leaves from stems. Heat sesame oil in wok.

Add garlic, bamboo shoots, bok choy stems, cauliflower, and celery, and stir fry for 4 minutes.

Add mushrooms, bean sprouts, and bok choy leaves.

Stir fry 2 more minutes.

Empty wok into a large bowl.

Combine honey-tamari mixture with arrowroot sauce in middle of wok.

Stir constantly until sauce thickens and loses its cloudiness.

Gently stir in vegetables and reheat for 2 minutes.

Garnish with roasted pistachio.

Serves 2

CURRY CHICKPEAS

12 ounces or 1 can chickpeas

1 cup water

3 tablespoons toasted sesame oil

½ cup finely chopped onion

4 cloves garlic

2 scallions

1 teaspoon freshly grated ginger

3 tablespoons lemon juice

¼ cup roasted pecans

4 tablespoons ground curry

1 teaspoon sea salt to taste

Finely chopped radicchio for garnish (optional)

Fresh green salad (premix available in grocery)

Simmer chickpeas in water with sesame oil, onion, garlic, scallion, ginger, and lemon juice for 15 to 20 minutes, until chickpeas are soft.

Add pecans, cumin, and salt.

Let cook 5 or more minutes.

Be careful not to overcook or it will become mushy.

Drain.

Garnish with radicchio or cilantro and serve with a fresh green salad.

Serve immediately.

Serves 2

EGGPLANT MOZZARELLA

2 small to medium eggplants, peeled

Sea salt to taste

4 tablespoons EVOO blended with

2 sprigs chopped saffron

⅔ cup tofu cream cheese

¼ pound fresh soy mozzarella, thinly sliced

1 (8 ounce) can tomato sauce

1 teaspoon dried tarragon

¼ teaspoon cayenne pepper

2 tablespoons fresh chopped basil

¼ cup rice or soy parmesan cheese

Cut eggplant into slices ¼ inch thick.

Sprinkle slices with salt and weight them down with a heavy plate.

Let stand for 1 hour or overnight.

Drain and rinse slices and pat them dry.

Mix chopped basil into tofu cream cheese.

In a heavy skillet, heat oil over medium heat.

Sauté eggplant slices until golden brown on both sides.

Drain on paper towel.

Preheat oven to 350 degrees F.

In a round casserole dish, layer eggplant, tofu cream cheese mixture, soy mozzarella, tomato sauce, oregano, and cayenne.

Continue to build layers until you have used up all of the ingredients. The final layer should be tofu cream cheese mixture sprinkled with parmesan.

Bake for 20 minutes, until top is golden brown and bubbly.

Serve warm.

Serves 2

YOU GOTTA LOVE IT

1 cup finely chopped chard, steamed 5 minutes

1 cup diced pears

1 cup sliced mushrooms

½ cup sliced leeks

1 teaspoon sea salt

1 teaspoon freshly ground black pepper

2 tablespoons EVOO

4 ½ teaspoons apple juice

½ cup black eyed peas, steamed 15 minutes

½ teaspoon paprika (preferably Hungarian)

3 tablespoons ground allspice

1 teaspoon ground nutmeg
½ cup cashews

In a large saucepan, sauté chard, pears, mushrooms, leeks, salt, and pepper in oil over medium-high heat for 7 minutes.

Add remaining ingredients and cook an additional 10 minutes.

Serve hot.

Serves 3–4

INDIAN CASSEROLE

2 ½ tablespoons coconut oil, divided
¼ cup oat flour
½ cup cooked split peas
⅓ cup curry powder
¼ teaspoon minced garlic
¼ teaspoon sea salt
¼ teaspoon oregano
¼ cup filtered water
½ cup coarsely chopped kale
½ cup bite-size broccoli pieces
1 cup cooked brown short, grain rice
½ avocado, sliced

Preheat oven to 375° F. Lightly grease 4 × 8 baking pan with coconut oil.

In a blender, combine oat flour, split peas, oil, curry, garlic, sea salt, oregano, and water.

In a separate bowl, combine kale, broccoli, and brown rice. Mix well.

Transfer to covered baking pan, top with flour and peas mixture. Bake for 15 minutes. Place avocado slices on top for garnish.

Serve hot.

Serves 2

VEGETABLE STIR FRY

2 tomatoes (½ cup juice)
1 extra firm tofu, cut into 1-inch cubes
2 tablespoons olive oil
1 cup chopped yellow onions
2 cups frozen peas
1 cup chopped tomatoes
¾ cup plain soy milk
3 teaspoons apple cider vinegar
½ cup finely chopped arugula
2 green chili peppers, finely chopped
3 cloves garlic, crushed
2 teaspoons grated ginger root
1 teaspoon ground coriander
1 teaspoon ground turmeric
¼ teaspoon chili powder
1 ½ teaspoons sea salt
Spinach or other leafy green salad

Juice tomatoes. Set aside ½ cup of the juice.

In a large frying pan, brown tofu in oil over high heat. Add onions. Sauté 2 to 3 minutes or until onions are soft.

Reduce heat to medium-low. Add the ½ cup of tomato juice and remaining ingredients except the salad, and simmer, uncovered for 5 minutes.

Serve with fresh green salad.

Serves 4

JASMINE RICE PILAF

2 tablespoons walnut oil
2 shallots, finely chopped
4 cloves garlic, minced

1 cup jasmine basmati rice, rinsed and drained

1 ⅓ cup vegetable broth (optional) or water

⅓ cup fresh spearmint

½ cup frozen peas

1 tablespoon Bragg's liquid aminos or to taste

Spinach or cooked arugula

3 tablespoons EVOO

In a stockpot, heat walnut oil over low heat. Sauté shallots and garlic for 3 minutes.

Add uncooked rice and stir 1 minute.

Add vegetable broth or water, spearmint, peas, and aminos. Bring to a full boil, then reduce heat to a simmer. Cover and cook over low heat for about 15 minutes or until water is absorbed and rice is tender.

Remove from heat.

Release steam by angling lid away from face and hands. Cover the pot with a towel to absorb excess water vapor without losing heat.

Serve on a bed of spinach or arugula sprinkled with olive oil.

Serves 2

ZESTY TOMATO SALAD

1 teaspoon sea salt

⅛ teaspoon cayenne pepper

½ teaspoon freshly ground black pepper

2 tablespoons lime juice

2 tablespoons fresh basil

½ cup chopped fresh rosemary

3 ripe tomatoes

1 bunch arugula

1 bunch watercress

In a small bowl, combine salt, cayenne, black pepper, lime juice, basil, and rosemary.

Cut tomatoes into thick slices; toss with arugula and watercress. Pour dressing over salad, and let marinate for 1 hour in the refrigerator.

Serve chilled.

Serves 2

ORIENTAL RICE NOODLES WITH SHIITAKE MUSHROOMS

3-inch piece ginger root

2 cups sliced, stemmed shiitake mushrooms

1 cup sliced red or yellow sweet pepper

3 tablespoons toasted sesame oil

1 cup mung bean sprouts, drained

3 teaspoons tamari

3 teaspoons sliced scallions

¾ pound rice noodles, cooked

Juice ginger.

In a large frying pan, sauté mushrooms in oil over high heat until soft.

Reduce heat to medium-low.

Add 2 tablespoons ginger juice, bean sprouts, soy sauce, and scallions.

Simmer for 1 to 2 minutes or until mixture has thickened.

Spoon the vegetable mixture over rice noodles and serve hot.

Serves 2

LENTIL BURGERS

4 carrots (½ cup pulp)

1 cup cooked red lentils

¼ cup lentil sprouts

¼ cup ground unsalted cashews or cashew butter

2 tablespoons chopped unsalted almonds

1 tablespoon diced yellow onion

2 teaspoons curry powder

½ teaspoon ground coriander

1 teaspoon sea salt

½ cup whole spelt bread crumbs

2 pita bread pockets (sprouted)

¼ teaspoon cayenne pepper

Juice carrots.

Preheat oven to 425 degrees F. In a small mixing bowl, combine ½ cup carrot pulp with remaining ingredients except bread crumbs and pita.

Mix well.

Shape mixture into 2 patties.

Coat patties with bread crumbs and place them on ungreased cookie sheet.

Bake patties for 10 minutes.

Turn patties over, and bake an additional 10–15 minutes.

Serve hot in pita bread pockets (add hummus flavored with lemon for a more exotic taste).

BROCCOLI MUSHROOM QUICHE

2 tomatoes (½ cup juice)

1 large bunch fresh basil (½ cup pulp)

1 cup silken tofu

1 cup avocado, crushed with 3 tablespoons lemon juice

¼ teaspoon finely chopped jalapeno peppers

¼ cup finely chopped tomatoes

¼ cup finely chopped Bermuda onion

¾ cup grated soy cheese

2 tablespoons EVOO

⅛ teaspoon sea salt

⅛ teaspoon black pepper
1 ½ cups broccoli florets
1 ¼ cup thinly sliced mushrooms
1 Spelt Crust (use pre-baked available at health food store)

Preheat oven to 375 degrees F.

Separately juice tomato and basil.

Set aside ½ cup of the tomato juice and ½ of the basil pulp.

In a blender or food processer, combine tofu, avocado, jalapenos, onion, cheese, oil, salt, black pepper, tomato juice and basil pulp mixture.

Blend for 1 minute or until creamy.

Arrange broccoli and mushrooms in the bottom of the Spelt Crust.

Layer the chopped tomatoes on top. Pour tofu mixture over vegetables.

Bake quiche, uncovered, for 25–30 minutes or until the top has set and begun to turn light brown.

Remove quiche from the oven.

Let stand for 5 minutes before cutting.

Serve hot with a salad.

Serves 4–6

MEDITERRANEAN OLIVE AND RICE PASTA
¾ teaspoon fresh oregano
⅛ cup finely chopped Italian parsley
3 tablespoons EVOO
2 tablespoons balsamic vinegar
1 clove garlic, pressed
1 tablespoon finely chopped macadamia nuts
Sea salt to taste
Freshly ground black pepper to taste

12 oz. to 1 pound rice pasta

8 Greek black olives, pitted and chopped

4 cups (about ½ pound) spinach leaves, washed, dried, and steamed until wilted

½ pound medium-firm tofu, cubed

¼ cup crumbled tempeh

Parsley for garnish

In a glass jar, mix oregano, Italian parsley, olive oil, vinegar, garlic, macadamia nuts, salt, and pepper.

Cover tightly, shake well, and set aside for flavors to meld.

Cook rice pasta in water according to package directions. Combine pasta and chopped olives in a bowl.

Pour dressing over mixture and toss.

Arrange steamed spinach leaves on a plate.

Add olive pasta mixture and cubed tofu.

Sprinkle tempeh on top. Garnish with parsley.

Serves 2

ORZO FOR DINNER

¼ pound orzo pasta

⅓ pound spaghetti squash, cooked then diced into ½-inch cubes

Water

½ cup chopped Swiss chard

2 teaspoons minced garlic

2 teaspoons thyme

½ teaspoon sea salt

Cook the orzo pasta according to package directions.

Drain and set aside.

Steam Swiss chard for 6 minutes.

Combine Swiss chard with squash, orzo, garlic, thyme, and sea salt in a baking dish.

Bake at 375 degrees F for 15 minutes.

Serve hot.

Serves 1

GLUTEN FREE VEGAN PIZZA

For the sauce

Organic Vegan Pizza Sauce (at health food stores)

For the crust

Wheat, Gluten, and Diary Free Rustic Crust (at health food stores look for the "Old World Napoli Gluten Free Rustic Crust" made with rice flour, tapioca flour, soy oil, soy flour, raw cane sugar, yeast, chia seeds, salt, and spices)

For the toppings

Wash and slice 3 medium size white mushroom caps, 1 small vine ripe tomato, and ½ cup white onion

Shred 2 cups of soy or rice mozzarella cheese (at health food stores look for "Vegan Gourmet Dairy Free, Gluten Free Mozzarella Cheese")

Preheat oven to 450 degrees F.

Brush both sides of the crust with EVOO.

Pour ⅔ cup of sauce onto crust and spread evenly with a spoon. Sprinkle 2 cups of shredded soy or rice mozzarella cheese on crust (more or less, depending on your taste).

Add mushrooms, tomatoes, and onions. (You can replace these with other veggies, including peppers, olives, eggplant, artichokes, and broccoli.)

Place in oven at 400 degrees F and let bake for 12–15 minutes or until crust is crisp and cheese has melted.

Sprinkle with oregano, salt and pepper to taste.

Drizzle with olive oil (optional).

Serves 1–2

TOFU DOGS ON SPROUT GRAIN BREAD

2 Tofu Hot Dogs (at health food stores look for "Tofu Dogs" made with soy protein, soy beans, beet powder, sunflower oil, natural smoke flavor, salt, paprika, vegetable gum, and tomato pulp)

Sprouted bread (at health food stores look for "Ezekiel Bread" made with all organic ingredients: sprouted whole wheat, sprouted barley, millet, lentil, soy beans, spelt, fresh yeast, and sea salt)

Place Tofu dogs in a skillet over medium heat for 5–7 minutes. Turn dogs over half way through the heating time.

Serve on top of bread (bread can be warmed, toasted or served at room temperature).

Toppings (optional)

Organic Sugar Free Ketchup (at health food stores)

Any variety of Organic Mustards (at health food stores)

Sauerkraut (at health food stores—heat over medium heat for 3 minutes or serve cold)

Organic Baked Beans (at health food stores)

Serving suggestions

Serve plain or with any variety of salads or Organic Frozen French Fries (obtained at health food stores, get ones that contain organic potato, canola oil, apple juice concentrate, and citric acid) or with side of brown rice and beans.

Serves 1–2

BEVERAGES

ALL GREEN

½ cucumber

1 leaf kale

½ bunch parsley

1 small romaine

3 stalks celery

2 oz. whole Aloe Vera juice from a bottle

Juice cucumber, kale, parsley, romaine, and celery, then add aloe juice.

Note: Buy whole leaf Aloe Vera juice. To preserve juice for 24 hours, add ⅛ teaspoon ascorbic acid.

Serves 2

FROZEN CHERRY SUPREME

3 cups orange juice
1 cup ice cubes
½ cup frozen cherries
1 banana
¼ teaspoon ground cinnamon

Combine all the ingredients in a blender and blend until smooth.

Serves 2

MANGO STRAWBERRY SMOOTHIE

1 ½ cups mango juice
1 pint strawberries
1 scoop protein powder
½ cup plain soy yogurt (with no added sugar)

Blend all ingredients until smooth.

Serves 2

RAW PEACH PECAN MILK

2 peaches
1 cup pecans
4 cups filtered water
1 teaspoon stevia

Dash of sea salt

Combine all ingredients in blender or food processor.
    Strain and drink.
    Keeps in refrigerator 1–2 days.
Serves 2

DESSERTS

CHILLED CANTALOUPE STUFFED WITH CHERRY CREAM
1 cup frozen cherries
¼ teaspoon lemon extract
2 cups silken tofu
1 cantaloupe, halved, seeded, and chilled

In a blender, combine the cherries, extract, and tofu, and blend for 3 minutes on medium speed until a creamy consistency is reached.
    Spoon into the cantaloupe halves and serve.
Serves 2

RAW HAWAIIAN HOLIDAY
½ cup raw tempeh cut to bite size pieces
½ cup zucchini chopped to bite size pieces
½ cup pineapple cut to bite size pieces

Combine in a bowl and set aside.

Marinade
1 tablespoon nama shoyu
2 teaspoons lemon juice
2 cloves garlic, minced
¼ teaspoon allspice

Combine all ingredients and pour over tempeh, zucchini and pineapple.

Set aside.

Serves 2

STICKY SWEET RICE ON PAPAYA

2 ¼ cup coconut milk

⅓ cup agave

¼ teaspoon sea salt

1 cup basmati short grain white rice, rinsed

2 ripe, seeded papaya, cut in half

1 teaspoon fresh lemon juice

1 teaspoon sunflower seeds

Thick coconut cream (optional topping)

4 mint leaves for garnish

Bring coconut milk and agave to a boil in a large saucepan, then add salt and cook for 5 minutes.

Add rice, stir, and reduce heat to simmer.

Cover and check after 20 minutes.

Remove from heat when all liquid has been absorbed. Sprinkle each papaya half with lemon juice and sunflower seeds.

Top with rice mixture.

Add a dollop of coconut cream (if desired), and garnish with one mint leaf.

Serves 2

DRESSING AND DIPPING SAUCES

CAULIFLOWER WITH GARLIC SAUCE

1 cup garbanzo beans or chickpeas (precooked and pureed)

3 tablespoons tahini

1 cup cauliflower florets

1 cup sliced red bell pepper

1 teaspoon lemon juice

¼ teaspoon turmeric

½ cup unsalted whole cashews

½ cup diced red bell peppers as garnish

4 sprigs fresh parsley, as garnish

2 bulbs garlic, crushed

3 tablespoons olive oil

Dash of cayenne pepper

Preheat the oven to 425 degrees F.

In a medium size mixing bowl, combine the garbanzo purée, tahini, cauliflower, broccoli, sliced red pepper, lemon juice, turmeric, and cashews, and toss to mix.

Pour the mixture into a greased 9 × 12-inch baking dish or other large glass or ceramic dish.

Cover with a glass lid or foil and bake for 25 to 30 minutes or until the cauliflower is just tender. (The other vegetables should still be crunchy.)

Garnish with the diced red pepper and parsley, and serve hot or cold with a rice dish or green salad.

For the garlic sauce:

Sauté garlic in olive oil and add a dash of cayenne pepper. Drizzle garlic sauce over cauliflower.

Serves 2

EXOTIC TOFU DIP

2 cups silken tofu

2 tablespoons chopped fresh chives

4 tablespoons prepared mustard

½ cup vegan mayonnaise

3 tablespoons balsamic vinegar

1 teaspoon freshly ground black pepper

2 tablespoons chopped fresh dill and paprika for garnish

Process all the ingredients, except the paprika/dill mixture, in a food processor or blender until smooth.

Sprinkle with paprika.

Serve chilled with raw carrot, celery sticks, broccoli, and cauliflower florets.

Yield: 2 ½–3 cups

MINT SAUCE

1 cup fresh mint or spearmint, no stems, finely chopped
¼ cup water
1 teaspoon white powdered stevia
(available in health food stores)
⅓ cup red wine vinegar

Boil mint in water for 5 minutes. Remove from heat and let steep, covered, for 15 minutes.

Add the stevia powder and vinegar. Stir and serve with new baby potatoes.
Serves 2

SPICY PEANUT SAUCE

1 tablespoon toasted sesame oil
1 clove garlic
¼ cup smooth peanut butter
1 teaspoon agave
1 teaspoon fresh lime juice
⅓ cup plus 1 tablespoon water
2 drops hot chili oil or Tabasco sauce

Combine all the ingredients in a blender and mix until smooth, 2 to 3 minutes.

Serve at room temperature over cooked noodles.

Yield: ⅔ cup

ENTREES

ANGEL HAIR MUSHROOM AND PEAS
2 tablespoons extra virgin olive oil
3 ½ cups sliced mushrooms
1 cup fresh or frozen peas
1 tablespoon salt
¾ teaspoon freshly ground black pepper
½ cup soy milk
1 cup sliced radicchio
⅔ cup grated vegan Parmesan cheese
3 cups cooked angel hair pasta

In a large saucepan, heat the oil over medium to high heat and sauté the mushrooms and peas for 5 minutes or until tender.

Add the salt, pepper, and soy milk, cover, and cook another 2 minutes.

Add the radicchio and cook 1 minute more.

Remove from heat and toss with the vegan Parmesan cheese and pasta.
Serves 2

BBQ COCONUT RIBS WITH BEET SPAGHETTI
4 Medjool dates, pitted
6 sun-dried tomatoes
1 cup coconut flakes (not sweetened)
⅛ cup onion
½ apricot
2 cloves garlic
1 tablespoon chipotle (deseeded to desired heat)
1 tablespoon extra virgin olive oil
1 tablespoon mushrooms

Combine all ingredients, except coconut flakes, in food processor. Blend till pleasantly chunky.

Spoon stuffing and form into rectangles strips or desired shape and roll in coconut flake.

Beet spaghetti
Place beet in Spiral Vegetable Slicer and make spaghetti noodles.

Serve coconut ribs on beet spaghetti and eat together. The sweet beet complements the spicy, savory coconut ribs.

Makes 6 Coconut Ribs

BROCCOLI AU GRATIN
1 bunch broccoli
2 tablespoons vegan butter
2 tablespoons whole spelt flour
1 ½ cup white wine
¼ pound vegan cheddar cheese, grated

Cut the broccoli into stalks and cut the stems into bite-sized pieces. Steam the broccoli until it is just tender.

While the broccoli is steaming, butter or oil a medium size casserole.

Put the steamed broccoli into the casserole.

Preheat oven to 350 degrees F.

Melt the butter in a saucepan and whisk in the flour.

Gradually add the white wine, whisking until well blended.

Add the grated cheese while stirring constantly.

Continue cooking over medium heat until the sauce thickens, about 15–20 minutes.

Pour the sauce over the broccoli.

Bake for 15 minutes.

Serves 4

BUTTERNUT SQUASH WITH TOASTED SESAME SAUCE

1 butternut squash, cut into ½-inch pieces

2 tablespoons toasted sesame oil

6–8 tablespoons tahini

3–4 tablespoons gomasio

2 teaspoon salt

Steam the squash for 15 to 20 minutes. Remove from the heat and divide into two or three portions. Combine the oil and tahini in a small bowl and mix well.

Pour the tahini mixture over the squash.

Sprinkle with gomasio.

Serves 2 to 3

CHICKPEA AND ZUCCHINI CURRY

1 cup dry chickpeas

2 tablespoons olive oil

1 large onion, sliced

1 ½ teaspoon turmeric

¼ teaspoon cayenne pepper or more to taste

2 teaspoons ground cumin

1 teaspoon mustard seeds

1 ½ teaspoon ground coriander

¾ teaspoon cinnamon

4 cloves garlic, pressed

1 or 2 thin slices of fresh ginger root

1 whole clove

1 large tomato, coarsely chopped

1 tablespoon tamari (soy sauce)

6 oz. tomato paste, thinned with ½ cup water

2 medium zucchini sliced

4–5 cups cooked brown rice

Soak the chickpeas in water to cover overnight.

Drain.

Cook the chickpeas in unsalted water for about an hour or until they are soft enough to mash with a fork.

Set aside.

Heat the oil in a large skillet.

When it is hot but not smoking, add the onion and all of the seasonings.

Cook until the mustard seeds pop.

Then add the tomato, tamari, tomato paste, and chickpeas.

Stir well to mix with seasonings.

Let it cook, covered with a lid, for about 15 minutes, stirring occasionally.

Add the zucchini, mix well, and continue to cook, covered. When the zucchini is cooked, about 10 to 15 minutes later, your meal is done.

Serve over brown rice.

Serves 4 to 6

CURRY MUSHROOM TOFU GRATIN WITH BUTTERNUT SQUASH

½ cup TVP (texture vegetable protein)

2 teaspoon safflower oil

1 teaspoon garlic, chopped

½ cup onions, ½ inch diced

3 cups mushrooms, washed, stems removed, and sliced

1 teaspoon Madras curry powder

½ pound firm tofu, drained and crumbled

In a food processor pound TVP to the consistency of bread crumbs, and put aside.

Heat oil in a non-stick skillet set to low.

Cook onions, garlic, and mushrooms on low for ten minutes, until mushrooms are cooked and moisture has cooked off.

Add curry and tofu, and cook on low for 10 more minutes.

Put mixture in a casserole dish and top with TVP.

Bake at 350 degrees F for 20 minutes until TVP has browned.

Serves 2

GREEN PLANTAIN BALLS

1 green plantain, left in its peel

4 teaspoons agave

2 teaspoons almond extract

2 teaspoons vanilla extract

Sea salt to taste

Callaloo or cooked spinach (optional)

Place the plantain in a pot of unsalted water with cover and bring to a boil.

Add the agave and extracts, and boil until tender, about 30 minutes.

Remove and let cool.

When cool enough to touch, remove and discard the peel.

Slice the flesh and season with sea salt.

Serve warm with Callaloo (or spinach if Callaloo isn't available), Jamaican Rum Down or the optional topping below.

Serves 2

LINGUINI WITH GARDEN VEGETABLES

½ cup extra virgin olive oil

3 tablespoons water

2 cups broccoli florets

4 cups sliced mushrooms

2 teaspoons salt

½ teaspoon freshly ground black pepper
1 cup chopped fresh tomatoes
¼ cup chopped fresh basil
3 to 4 cups cooked linguini or capellini
¾ cup grated vegan Parmesan cheese

In a large saucepan, combine the oil, water, and broccoli, and cook, covered, over medium to high heat for 5 minutes.

Add the mushrooms, salt, and pepper, and cook until tender. Remove from the heat and stir in the tomatoes, basil, pasta, and cheese.
Serves 2 to 3

NICE RICE
3 oz. basmati rice, cooked (chilled)
3 oz. amaranth, cooked (chilled)
1 oz. watercress, chopped
1 ½ oz. red pepper, diced
2 tablespoons safflower oil
1 teaspoon minced onion
½ teaspoon salt
Juice of 1 lemon

Combine all ingredients.
Toss and serve.
Serves 2

POPEYE'S PICK ME UP
3 oz. spinach, chopped
3 oz. okra, sliced
3 oz. red pepper, chopped
3 oz. split peas, cooked
1 ½ tablespoons sunflower oil

½ teaspoon soy sauce or Braggs Amino
Acids (as soy sauce replacement)
½ teaspoon tarragon
½ teaspoon salt
3 oz. brown rice, cooked

Steam spinach, okra, and pepper for 7 minutes or until tender.

Purée split peas in blender along with oil, soy sauce, tarragon, salt, and 2 oz. water until mixture achieves sauce consistency.

Pour split peas over vegetables and brown rice and serve warm.
Serves 2

PURPLE CABBAGE AND SPAGHETTI SQUASH STIR FRY

¼ cup toasted sesame oil
2 cups broccoli pieces
2 cups sliced purple cabbage
¼ cup sliced scallions
2 cups diced cooked spaghetti squash
3 cloves garlic, sliced
1 ½ cups cubed firm tofu
2 tablespoon tamari
1 teaspoon salt
¼ cup sesame seeds for garnish

Heat the oil until hot, but not smoking, in a large saucepan or wok over high heat.

Add the broccoli, cabbage, and scallions and stir fry for 5 minutes.

Add the remaining ingredients, except the sesame seeds, and cook an additional 5 to 7 minutes.

Garnish with the sesame seeds.
Serves 3

RICE AND LENTILS (DAHL)

2 cups basmati rice
1 cup washed red or yellow lentils
1 cup button mushrooms
3 cloves garlic, thinly sliced
1 yellow onion, chopped
4 cups water
1 tablespoon tamari
3 tablespoons toasted sesame oil
1 teaspoon cumin seeds
2 teaspoons sea salt
Orange wedge for garnish

Combine the rice, lentils, mushrooms, garlic, and onion in a large bowl.

Add enough water to cover.

Soak for 1 hour, then drain and rinse.

Place the mixture in a heavy oven-proof pan.

Add the water and tamari.

Bring to a boil over medium heat. Cover, reduce heat, and simmer for 20 minutes.

Preheat oven to 450 degrees F.

Turn the oven off and place the tightly covered pan of cooked rice and lentils in the oven.

Allow to sit for 20 minutes to absorb excess moisture.

In a small frying pan, warm the oil over medium heat.

Add the cumin seeds and salt, and sauté until brown and fragrant.

Serve rice and lentils hot, topped with cumin seasoning and garnished with orange wedges around the edge of the plate.

Serves 2

SASSY BEAN AND BULGUR

1 ½ tablespoons sunflower oil
3 oz. kidney beans, cooked
3 oz. bulgur, cooked
3 oz. brown rice, cooked
3 oz. mushrooms, sliced
3 oz. carrots, sliced
1 oz. scallions, chopped
1 oz. tomato sauce
½ teaspoon oregano
½ teaspoon salt
3 oz. spinach leaves

Preheat oven to 350 degrees F. Lightly grease 4 × 8 baking pan with sunflower oil.

Combine all ingredients together except spinach leaves.
Mix well.
Transfer to baking pan and place in oven for 20 minutes.
Serve on bed of spinach leaves.
Serves 2

SAUTÉED VEGETABLES OVER BROWN RICE

1 garlic clove, chopped
½ medium onion, sliced
2 tablespoons toasted sesame oil
1 carrot, peeled and sliced
1 medium parsnip, peeled and sliced
1 red pepper, chopped
1 medium zucchini, sliced
½ medium eggplant, sliced
Tamari (soy sauce) to taste
5–6 mushrooms, sliced
6–8 oz. of tomato, sliced

Sauté the garlic and onion in the sesame oil in heavy skillet. Add the carrot, parsnip, red pepper, zucchini, and eggplant. Put in the tamari and finally add the mushrooms.

Cook over medium heat for 20 to 25 minutes, mixing frequently.
Lower heat and simmer for 5 to 10 minutes.
Then add the tomato sauce and simmer for an additional 5 minutes.
Serve over brown rice.

Serves 2

SOBA NOODLE SUPREME

3 oz. asparagus, cut into 1-inch pieces
3 oz. butternut squash
3 oz. buckwheat noodles (soba), cooked
3 oz. spinach, cut into bite-size pieces
5 tablespoons sunflower oil
1 teaspoon dill
1 teaspoon salt

Preheat oven to 400 degrees F. Steam the asparagus until tender, approximately 8 minutes. Cut squash in half, remove the seeds and discard.

Place squash in a 4 × 8 baking pan, cut side down, with ⅓ inch water, and bake for 40 minutes.

When cooled, remove skin from squash and cut the squash into bite-size pieces.

Combine all the ingredients together and mix well.

Serve warm.

Serves 3

SQUASHED POTATO CASSEROLE

3 oz. sweet potato
3 oz. yellow squash, cubed

1 oz. green pepper, chopped

2 tablespoons olive oil

½ teaspoon thyme

½ teaspoon basil

½ teaspoon salt

3 oz. basmati rice, cooked

3 oz. amaranth, cooked

Preheat oven to 400 degrees F. Pierce sweet potato with fork and place in oven for 45 minutes. When potato cools, cut into ½-inch cubes.

Lower heat to 375 degrees. Steam squash and pepper until slightly tender.

Lightly grease 4 × 8 casserole pan with safflower oil.

Combine all ingredients and mix well.

Transfer to casserole pan and place in oven for 15 minutes.

Serves 2

TOFU NOODLE VEGETABLES

Olive oil cooking spray

1 small yellow onion, quartered and thickly sliced

1 scallion, diced

1 small carrot, thinly sliced

½ small red bell pepper

½ small green bell pepper

½ small fresh Anaheim chile, seeded and finely chopped

1 ½ teaspoon Dijon style mustard

1 clove fresh, crushed elephant garlic or 3 cloves regular garlic

¼ teaspoon cayenne or to taste

½ teaspoon soy sauce, plus additional to taste, or Bragg's Amino Acids

2 teaspoon sesame, peanut or olive oil

¼ cup water

Sea salt

Freshly ground pepper to taste

1 pound firm tofu sliced into ½ inch strips

Pinch cumin seed, crushed well

(use mortar and pestle)

1 tablespoon ground flax seed

5 ounces extra long Chinese noodles, cooked

Agave (optional)

In a large skillet sprayed with olive oil, sauté onion, scallion, carrot, peppers, Anaheim chile, mustard, garlic and cayenne. When carrot strips are crisp-tender, add ¼ teaspoon soy sauce, sesame oil, water, salt and pepper to taste.

Mix well and set aside.

Spray another large skillet with olive oil, and heat over medium heat.

Place the tofu strips in the pan with crushed cumin and ¼ teaspoon soy sauce.

Brown tofu lightly on both sides, approximately 2 minutes. Drain the oil and juices from the vegetable mixture into a small saucepan. Add flaxseed and heat until thickened; set aside.

Cover entire bottom of nonstick baking pan with vegetable mixture.

Lay tofu strips on the vegetables, with thickened mixture on top. Broil for 2 minutes.

Place cooked noodles (tossed with pinch of salt and freshly ground pepper, if desired) in a decorative dish.

Cover the center with the vegetable mixture, and top with tofu strips.

Serve immediately.

Use remaining thickened mixture as side sauce, with a little agave added, if desired.

Serves 2

VEGETARIAN LASAGNA

1 tablespoon safflower oil

½ cup onion, ¼ inch diced

1 teaspoon garlic, chopped

1 pound firm tofu, drained and crumbled

1 cup cooked and chopped spinach

3 cups marinara

½ box rice lasagna (no boil)

¼ cup vegan Parmesan, shredded

¼ cup vegan mozzarella, shredded

Heat oil on low heat in a large skillet.

Cook onion and garlic for five minutes and add tofu.

Cook tofu for ten minutes on low heat.

Add spinach and half of the marinara and heat throughout.

In a 9 × 9 glass baking dish, layer marinara, noodles, and tofu. Top with cheese and cover.

Bake at 350 degrees F for one hour.

Serves 2

VEGGIE-SKETTI

3 oz. spaghetti squash

3 oz. scallions

6 oz. tomato

3 oz. green pepper

1 ½ oz. onion

2 oz. mushrooms

2 tablespoons olive oil

¼ teaspoon basil

½ teaspoon rosemary

1 teaspoon fresh garlic, minced

1 teaspoon salt

Cut the squash in half, remove the seeds and discard them. Place the halves in a baking pan with ⅓ inch of water, with cut side down.

Bake for 40 minutes at 400 degrees.

When the squash is cool enough to handle, remove the pulp. Carefully wash the scallions, tomato, pepper, onion, and mushrooms.

Chop them medium fine.

In a large skillet, place the oil and sauté the vegetables along with the seasonings and salt for 5 minutes.

Combine all the ingredients in a large bowl.

Mix carefully and then transfer to a serving dish.

Serves 2

RAW PEANUT SAUCE OVER ZUCCHINI NOODLES AND ORANGES

1 zucchini (spaghetti cut in spiral vegetable slicer)
1 orange cut to small bite-size pieces
4 cloves garlic
3 tablespoons raw peanut butter
3 teaspoons sesame oil
3 teaspoons of nama shoyu
2 teaspoons agave
½ teaspoon sea salt
¾ teaspoon ginger
Dash of cayenne pepper

Combine all ingredients, except zucchini and orange, in food processor.

Serve sauce over zucchini spaghetti and orange.

Serves 2

PERSIAN DULSE

3 oz. chickpeas
½ oz. dulse, dry

3 oz. cauliflower

3 oz. tempeh

2 oz. onion

6 oz. tomato sauce

2 tablespoon olive oil

1 minced garlic clove

¼ teaspoon salt

½ teaspoon basil

2 oz. water

In a medium bowl, soak the chickpeas overnight in 16 oz. of water.

In the morning, rinse the chickpeas and transfer into a medium soup pot with 20 oz. of fresh water.

Cook for 1 ¾ to 2 hours, until done.

Rinse dulse 2 or 3 times in cold water.

Rinse cauliflower and cut into florets.

Cut tempeh into ½ inch cubes and put all the ingredients together in a medium mixing bowl.

Peel and slice the onion and add to the mixture.

Toss gently.

Add the remaining ingredients and mix well.

Transfer to a greased baking pan and bake for 20 minutes in a preheated 350 degree oven.

Serves 2

ALGERIAN CHILI

2 cups small dried navy beans

⅛ cup Extra Virgin Olive Oil

1 medium onion, finely chopped

1 scallion, finely chopped

1 ½ small dried red chiles

8 cloves garlic, minced

½ tablespoons sweet paprika

⅛ teaspoon freshly ground black pepper

1 tablespoon curry powder

2 teaspoons ground cumin

5 sun-dried tomatoes, reconstituted and puréed to generate ½ cup tomato paste

1 tomato, coarsely chopped

3 ½ cups water or vegetable broth

1 bay leaf

Pinch of cayenne

10 fresh flat-leaf parsley sprigs, half tied together with kitchen string, half minced

1 ¼ teaspoon sea salt

5 fresh cilantro sprigs, chopped

Soak the dried beans overnight.

Drain and set aside.

Over medium heat in a large soup pot, heat the oil and cook the onion and scallions, stirring occasionally, until tender, 6–8 minutes.

Add the chiles, garlic, paprika, pepper, green pepper, curry powder, and cumin.

Cook, stirring, for 2–3 minutes, and then add the sun-dried tomato paste and cook, stirring until the mixture thickens, 1–2 minutes.

Stir in the fresh tomato and 1 cup of the water or broth and bring to a boil.

Add the beans and the remaining 2 ½ cups water or broth, bay leaves, cayenne, sea salt, and the parsley bundle.

Lower the heat to medium-low, cover and cook until the beans are tender, 1–2 hours.

Discard the chiles, bay leaves, and tied parsley before serving. Stir in the minced parsley and cilantro. Serve warm.

Serves 2

SIDES

COOL GARDEN NOODLES

2 tablespoons sunflower oil

1 teaspoon chopped fresh parsley

½ teaspoon minced garlic

½ teaspoon basil

½ teaspoon salt

Pinch of ginger

3 oz. brown rice, cooked (chilled)

3 oz. buckwheat noodles, cooked (chilled)

3 oz. avocado, chopped into bite-size pieces

3 oz. marinated artichoke hearts, chopped into bite-size pieces

Combine all ingredients and mix well.

Yield: 2 Servings

CURLY ENDIVE WITH BERRIES AND SEEDS

1 cup torn curly or Belgian endive

¼ cup well-packed basil leaves

1 cup torn Bibb lettuce

½ cup sunflower sprouts

1 cup chopped fresh tomatoes or shredded carrots

1 cup blueberries

½ cup sunflower seeds

Combine the endive, basil, lettuce, sprouts, and tomatoes in a large salad bowl.

Garnish with the blueberries and seeds.

Serve with a favorite dressing like Orange Vinaigrette.

Yields: 2 Servings

HOLIDAY STUFFED MUSHROOMS

6 mushrooms de-stemmed (mince stems and set aside)
4 tablespoons Extra Virgin Olive Oil
1 avocado
2 tablespoon flax seed, ground
2 teaspoon parsley, chopped
½ teaspoon sage
½ teaspoon rosemary
½ teaspoon thyme
Sea salt and pepper

Coat mushroom caps with 2 tablespoons of Extra Virgin Olive Oil.
    Place in dehydrator for 1 hour.
    Combine all other ingredients in a food processor.
    Stuff dehydrated mushroom caps with mixture and serve.
    Yields: 6 mushrooms

PEANUTTY BUTTERNUT SQUASH

3 oz. butternut squash
1 ½ oz. shallots, chopped fine
1 ½ oz. peanuts
2 tablespoons sunflower oil
1 teaspoon chopped fresh dill
¼ teaspoon thyme
½ teaspoon basil
½ teaspoon salt
3 oz. avocado, sliced

Preheat oven to 400 degrees. Lightly oil 4 × 8 baking pan with sunflower oil.
    Cut squash in half, remove the seeds and discard them.

Place squash halves in a baking pan, cut side down, with ⅓ inch water.

Bake for 40 minutes.

Take squash out of oven, and lower heat to 350 degrees.

When cool enough to handle, remove skin from squash and cut the squash into 1-inch cubes.

Combine the shallots with the squash and transfer to baking pan.

In a blender, place peanuts, oil, dill, thyme, basil, and salt.

Purée until smooth.

Pour over squash and shallots, and bake for 20 minutes.

Top with avocado.

Yield: 2 Servings

CRUNCHY HERBED GREEN BEANS

1 pound green beans

1 ½ cups boiling water

2 teaspoons sea salt

¼ cup finely minced onion

½ cup chopped green pepper

½ teaspoon marjoram

¼ teaspoon crushed rosemary

½ teaspoon pepper

Snip off the ends of the green beans and steam the beans over salted water for 3 to 4 minutes or until they're tender but not overcooked.

They should be crunchy.

Mix the beans, the onion, green pepper, and seasonings in a large bowl.

Serve hot.

Yield: 4 to 6 Servings

SOUPS

PORTUGUESE KALE-POTATO SOUP

½ pound fresh kale or Swiss chard
1 medium potato, peeled
4 cups water
⅛ cup full-bodied Extra Virgin Olive Oil
Sea salt to taste
Freshly ground black pepper to taste
Pinch of nutmeg
3 teaspoons spearmint leaves

Wash kale and cut off stems. Twist leaves tightly in a circular fashion and slice into very thin shreds.

Set aside.

In a large soup pot, place potato, water, oil, salt, and pepper, and bring to a boil.

Reduce heat to a simmer.

Cover and cook slowly about 25 minutes or until potato is tender.

Purée soup in food processor or blender.

Return purée to soup pot and add kale strips, nutmeg, and spearmint.

Cook about 15 minutes more or until kale is tender.

Serve hot.

Serves 2

FAVORITE VEGETABLE SOUP

3 oz. mung beans
3 oz. onions, sliced
2 oz. celery, chopped
2 oz. red cabbage, sliced
1 teaspoon chopped fresh parsley
3 tablespoons macadamia oil

½ teaspoon salt

½ teaspoon oregano

½ teaspoon basil

6 oz. basmati rice, cooked

Soak beans overnight in water. In the morning, rinse the beans, pour into saucepan, and add 32 oz. water.

Bring beans to a boil and lower to medium heat.

Place cover on the pot.

Allow to cook for about 1 ½ hours.

When the beans have cooked for 1 hour, add the vegetables, oil, and seasonings.

Purée half the mixture in blender for 15 seconds or until coarsely ground.

Return to the soup along with the basmati rice.

Mix well and allow to cook for an additional 10 minutes.

Yields: 4 to 5 cups

PENNE PASTA AND WHITE BEAN SOUP

3 cucumbers (1 ½ cups juice)

½ head cauliflower, steamed and chilled (½ cup)

¼ cup diced yellow onions

3 tablespoons Extra Virgin Olive Oil

¾ cups water

1 ½ cups chopped tomatoes

¾ cup cooked white beans

½ cup chopped escarole or kale

¼ cup chopped celery

¼ cup sliced carrots

¼ cups uncooked whole grain macaroni

2 teaspoons chopped fresh parsley

2 teaspoons chopped fresh basil

½ teaspoon sea salt

½ teaspoon black pepper

1 clove garlic, crushed

Separately juice the cucumbers and cauliflower.

Set aside 1 ½ cups of the cucumber juice and ½ cup of the cauliflower pulp.

In a large saucepan, sauté the onion in the oil for 2–3 minutes. Add the cucumber juice and water, and bring to a boil over high heat.

Reduce the heat to medium-low, add the remaining ingredients, and simmer uncovered for 15 minutes or until the pasta is tender.

Serve hot or cold with bread.

Serves 2 to 4

THICK AND HEARTY BORSCHT

4 tablespoons olive oil

2 onions, chopped

5 beets: 3 grated, 2 chopped

1 large carrot, sliced

2 leeks, sliced (optional)

2 cups shredded red cabbage

2 cups shredded green cabbage

2 teaspoons caraway seeds

1 teaspoon salt

2 tablespoons apple cider vinegar

1 bay leaf

2 cloves garlic

2 quarts vegetable stock

2 potatoes, boiled and diced

Heat the oil in a very large soup pot.

Add all the vegetables and cook over low heat for 10 minutes, stirring constantly, making sure all pieces get cooked.

The vegetables should be tender but not overcooked.

Add the seasoning and stock.

Bring to a boil and simmer for 1 hour until everything is very tender.

Add boiled potatoes.

Serves 4

VENICE NOODLE SOUP

5 tablespoons Extra Virgin Olive Oil

½ cup sliced zucchini

½ cup sliced potatoes

½ cup sliced celery

1 cup diced onions

¼ cup sliced mushrooms

¼ cup chopped fresh parsley

½ cup broccoli florets

1 teaspoon salt

¼ teaspoon freshly ground black pepper

2 bay leaves

¼ cup chopped fresh dill

6 cups water

2 cups uncooked noodles

4 cloves crushed garlic

In a large saucepan, heat the oil over medium heat and sauté the vegetables about 10 minutes.

Add the remaining ingredients, except the noodles, and let simmer over medium-low heat for 25 to 35 minutes.

Add the noodles 10 minutes before finishing.

Serves 2

Chapter 10

No More Excuses

After the grim reality of diabetes hits people, who are shocked when they receive this diagnosis, I have heard them ask, "How did I get here?" or "How did this happen?"

This book has given a whole list of reasons, but one so far unspoken has yet to be voiced. The truth is that we are unhappy. Dissatisfaction with our lives leads to disease. It leads to the behavior that inevitably causes serious harm to our health. And that is why it is so difficult for people to change, because even when they have supposedly "fixed" their medical issues, they still haven't fixed the underlying conditions that made them sick in the first place.

So, why are we dissatisfied? Think for a moment of the experiment I did when I contrasted five groups who were trying to lose weight. The manifest insight from the examination was that those who lost and kept off the pounds were ones who grounded their health changes in a solid, thoughtful philosophy. Yet, there's one other thing you might take away from that discussion. I run my get-well programs for groups, not by designing individualized programs for single dieters. There's a reason for that. I've found repeatedly that people can reverse health-endangering behavior and get on a health-enhancing path in the most efficient manner if they do so surrounded by others who are also fighting to regain or build their health.

After all, as I emphasized especially in relation to young people with eating disorders, it is often a disadvantageous, self-esteem-weakening home or peer environment that pushes a young person into negative actions. Then, it stands to reason if a person is, say, working on weight loss, then being surrounded by others who are diligently working on improving the same reduction—others who are sharing their feelings, and opening their hearts to each other about triumphs and setbacks—will be just what the doctor ordered for a sustained and successful effort.

Let's take another leaf from Dewey's books. I mentioned his idea of education, which involves learning to see more connections and acting on what one has found out, but I haven't noted one thing about this phase of his thought. He feels this is the preeminent type of education for democracy. But what is democracy? It is not the actually existing version in the United States or in any other nation. It is the ideal held up by my health improvement groups. Let me quote from Dewey's *The Public and Its Problems,* and then I will show its relevance to the argument made in this book.

> Wherever there is conjoint activity whose consequence are appreciated as goods by all singular persons who take part in it, and where the realization of the good is such as to effect an energetic desire to and effort to sustain it in being just because it is a good shared by all, there is insofar a community. The clear consciousness of a communal life, in all its implications, constitutes the idea of democracy.

Thus, to translate this into terms of health-sustaining groups, they can to be democratic in the sense meant, but only if the members come to two awarenesses, two consciousnesses. Each participant has to see that the positive changes he or she is making are not the result of personal effort alone, but are participatory rewards of being in the community. By the same measure, though, each individual has to know that his or her fellows in the group are making positive lifestyles changes not only because this other person has forcefully chosen health, which is part of the reason, of course, but that in a very real sense it is because others around him or her made that same choice. In other words, if you are in the group and are making positive changes, you discover you are only partly responsible for them, but you are also partly responsible for the positive steps being taken by those around you. This is where community starts, the same place happiness does.

We are in a new decade, and it's time to wake up to these new visions of self, health, and community. Sadly, many are still clinging to the self-destructive thoughts and behavior they acquired twenty, thirty, and forty years ago.

So let me add one last thought to these considerations. It's one provided by any vacation guide. Plan ahead.

We frequently fail to make changes we want to make because we don't approach change with a goal and a game plan on how to reach that goal.

I said goal, not goal post, but I think a football metaphor would be helpful here. Bill Belichick is the most successful coach in professional football, having coached the New England Patriots to three Super Bowl victories. Can you imagine Belichick going into a game without a game plan?

Yet, we often stumble through life without one. How much more valuable are our lives than a football game?

In the health-improvement groups I sponsor, there are people of all different ages, which has led me to see that the changes they need to make and how they are setting up a game plan can be categorized, in part, by generation. How each of us grew up and the world that we have known has everything to do with who we are. So, to change who we are, we need to look at what we have been through. For the baby boomer, that is a very different world and life than someone born in the 1980s. Each generation has a way of approaching issues and of interaction. Each has a separate approach to forming and being in a community. And, that means everything you have read in this text has to be molded to fit your own particular strengths and weaknesses.

You've almost finished the book. I will end with a set of testimonies from people like you, who have dared to drop old, unhealthy habits and move into a new space of healthy living. Let me repeat once more Dewey's point about education. It doesn't end with learning material, but with applying what you learned. Those who are willing to make that step and begin putting into practice the protocol, eating recommendations, exercise, and deep relaxation techniques provided in this book will find that life is exciting when you are consciously living a natural way. This is the kind of life in which, as Dewey said in my epigraph, healthy "action becomes an adventure in discovery of a self which is possible but as yet unrealized, an experiment in creating a self which shall be more inclusive than the one which exists."

Testimonials

Introduction

For my entire adult career in public health, I have been perplexed and concerned about how primary care physicians, as well as public health authorities, scientists, and scientific journals, treat patients' experiences with disease. Two things were especially troubling and have to do with not listening to patients or allowing them the freedom to try their own ways of recuperating health.

The first point is this. When a person walks into a doctor's office, one of the first things the doctor inevitably asks is, "How are you doing?" followed by, "Any changes?" The patient then will explain how his or her current treatment is either helping or hurting. As a result of this exchange, if necessary, the doctor will make some adjustments in the treatment.

In other words, the whole thing is very cut and dried. Half the time, having left a full waiting room, the patient feels his or her physician is in a rush to get to the next client. Yet, ask any patient and he or she will tell you that the more time each can spend discussing health with their physician, the better he or she feels about the treatment. Indeed, many doctors believe that quality time with a patient is essential for understanding all the variables that can impact (in a positive or negative way) the outcome of a patient's healthcare. Hence, feedback from the patient is crucial.

And there's a second problem. The doctor wants to dictate every step a patient takes. However, say a female patient decides to work on her own health and without "doctor's orders," changes her diet, begins supplementing and exercising, and no longer has elevated blood sugar, high blood pressure, elevated cholesterol, pain, fatigue, insomnia, or weight gain. When she reports to the doctor with improved results, in that they were achieved without drugs or medical intervention, this change is dismissed by the doctor as a "fluke" and statistically insignificant.

These two problems represent the dark side of medicine today. This explains how we can have a 2.5 trillion dollar medical complex that is unable to either prevent any illnesses, or successfully reverse (in any relevant numbers) any major disease. The patient doesn't count, except as an income stream for the pharmaceutical industry and for-profit hospitals. Sadly, the situation is only getting worse.

There is good news, however. When patients become empowered they realize they are more than just a broken part, a mechanical failure that needs correction. Rather, every part of their being, everything they think and how they approach the choices they make, will directly impact their health. Here are the voices of those individuals who chose positive empowerment. These are the stories of real people who have made real changes and today are enjoying good health. These people count.

1. Frank, Male

I used insulin and glucophage for severe diabetes. My blood pressure was high. I had asthma, but most frightening was the diagnosis of prostate cancer. I could not imagine a class of people changing without medications, but my conditions were not changing with medications so I decided to join [one of the groups Null organized]. My life changed tremendously. I learned to balance my job and personal life. Energy increased. I require less sleep. My blood pressure decreased. No more asthmatic episodes. I do not have to take diabetic medication. My weight went from 240 to 205 pounds. I keep to the protocol so I will never go back to those illnesses.

2. Viola, Female

I was afraid and confused. I was overweight and stuck in an unhealthy home situation. The hours stuck in self-doubt left me with a fear of being crazy. There was no one to talk to and nowhere to turn. At first I felt [when I joined a Null self-help group and heard about the dietary changes that were being advocated] "How can I give up all the food I ate my whole life?" Then I remembered how stuck I was, so I vowed to go on Gary Null's program totally. I lost weight and became a vegetarian.

My children and I thrive on the program. I will not ever again tolerate verbal abuse. I set firm boundaries. My children and I recently moved to another state and now we have a peaceful home. Uncluttering the past brought new friends into our lives.

3. Veronica, Female

I ate junk food and was a heavy coffee drinker. I was hypoglycemic and fainted frequently. My skin had ugly eruptions. I cried easily and had low energy. I had several allergies. I lost 15 pounds in this period. Eventually [as I changed my life] all my respiratory infections and skin problems disappeared. I follow the diet and juice during the day, eat fruits in the evening, and make one well planned meal a day. I am now a marathon runner. My energy is without limit. I am healthy.

4. Dora, Female

I developed cysts in my breasts and was diagnosed hypoglycemic. I did not feel well and wondered if my diet impacted on my physical system. Motivated by fear of future illnesses, I joined a health support group. The teachings and protocol gave me the answers I needed. I quickly lost 8 pounds. The lumps in my breast are gone, no more pain. I am vegan and organic. I do not test hypoglycemic; I can skip meals. With daily yoga and exercise, I have wonderful energy. My skin is moist. People compliment my glow and happier attitude. My hair and nails are healthy. I sleep well and am aware of potential toxic people and situations. My family is beginning to follow the protocol.

5. Robert, Male

I developed intestinal problems. My blood pressure was low, there was a tightness in my chest, and I suffered with a chronic, painful skin condition on my hands for 30 years. I am now on the protocol. My first improvement was a rush of energy after eliminating wheat and corn. My hand condition improved; the nails are not pulling away from my skin. My thinning hair is growing. I feel focused and aware of others around, and I aid street people. Writing letters [and thus opening routes of communication] eliminated the pressure in my chest.

6. Jozana, Female

I was overweight and could not slim down. I had acute heartburn, acid reflux, and angry outbursts. Coping with my teenage son was unbelievably stressful. I wanted to change my life and clear my mind. Since following the protocol, my body is alive and energetic. I unclutter my mind and home daily. I handle coworkers and my son without anger. The incredible homework questions made me think as I never did. I am optimistic, more open and accepting, patient, and less critical. I have traded anger for self-love.

7. Zara, Female

I am a juvenile diabetic. I used coffee and ate junk food, sodas, etc. I had ongoing diabetic retinopathy; fatty deposits in my eye. I sought healing with a mind-body-spirit approach.

It [health support group] opened me to spiritual meditation and finding strength within. I am delighted to report the retinopathy stopped developing, no more fatty deposits. I consulted with my physician three months into the protocol. My exam revealed my eye vessels are stronger and a thicker membrane is growing. I feel vital and energetic since eliminating negative, toxic people in my life.

8. Etta, Female

I had arthritis, psoriasis, low energy and uterine cancer. I had a hysterectomy, however, the cancer returned. I wanted to heal and experience total health. I found the right place at the right time. My cancer seems to be in full remission. I lost 20 pounds, the psoriasis cleared and my hair and skin look great. No more arthritic symptoms. I am aware of being hard on myself in the past and forgave myself and others. My immune system is strong.

9. Medina, Female

I am truly a survivor. I had breast cancer 11 years ago and refused chemotherapy and radiation but used Tamoxifen which impaired my vision and emotions. I developed polyps, an inflammatory digestive problem, and an ulcer. This was too much. Medication was making me sick. I sought a natural approach to healing and immune enhancement. I gained weight without cause; my abdomen bloated. After 3 months on the protocol, my immune system shot up. Digestion improved without bloating, and I eliminated many foods. The weight is slowly coming off. I feel radiant and wake up at 5:00 each morning with phenomenal energy to do breathing and meditations. All aspects of my life have fused. I am where I should be.

10. Scott D., Male

I am a construction worker. I felt I was losing stamina and did not know if I could handle my work. I felt my body age. Today I can keep up with younger coworkers, my physical endurance increased. Injuries and pulled muscles heal quickly. My forgiveness letters allowed me true introspection, and I focus on myself avoiding all toxic situations.

11. Jay D., Male

I have been a holistic dentist and vegetarian for 32 years. I had mood swings and problems concentrating at times, most likely due to sugar and dairy. I was negative on occasion. My hair was graying. My energy increased massively after the protocol and mood swings are gone. I maintain a good positive mental attitude for long periods of time. My concentration stabilized. I notice less gray hair in new growth. I now recommend the protocol to my patients.

12. Alexandra M., Female

I was dissatisfied with my body. My energy was low and I was very overweight. My acquaintances and friends were depressing me to the point of irritability. I had a fear of public speaking and did not know where to turn for guidance.

I joined a health support group. Gary Null was informative on the radio, but I could not apply this information in a constructive way [until I joined a group].

I lost 16 pounds without dieting. My increasing energy made me feel young again. I need less sleep and find I am not distracted with people's petty, unimportant issues. My house was uncluttered; having fewer objects gave me space, a feeling of freedom. My toxic relationships were dismissed; my self-esteem replaced them.

I learned to be the real me, healthy and vital.

13. Alice, Female

I was concerned about my health. My blood pressure and cholesterol were elevated. I had a stressful life and could not control these feelings. I disliked my varicose veins. I suffered with an acid reflux condition that I assumed was caused by my job. My body was falling apart.

I detoxed and carefully followed Gary's protocol. I felt stronger each week and released stress each day. My blood pressure is normal today. My digestion improved, no more acid reflux. I lost 15 pounds. My blood tests are good and my figure is leaner. I am shapelier. I feel cleaner. I do aerobics at home in the morning, yoga during evening hours, bike, walk, and run. My uncluttered environment and journal writing give me a new constructive outlook. I use green juices, and green and red powders with supplements. My water is pure. I am organic. I am goal-oriented.

14. Andrea, Female

I weighed 300 pounds and wore size 24–26 clothing. I was not diagnosed with illnesses, but I felt exhausted, had painful varicose veins, back problems, was nauseated after meals, lactose intolerant, and had bad digestion. I ate flesh foods and dairy. I listened to *Natural Living* [radio show] and joined a support group.

Today I weigh 225 pounds and wear a size 18. I developed a sense of value in the group and can say "no." I feel centered and empowered. I juice and take supplements. By discovering a new world of health food stores, I choose products carefully. As a creative cook, I enjoy translating old recipes into vegan meals using grains. I created a dance area at home and enjoy biking, skiing, kayak class, and swimming lessons.

15. Angelo, Male

I weighed 300 pounds, had high cholesterol and blood pressure, hepatitis B, discoloration around my eyes, used an inhaler, suffered from eczema, and bleeding knuckles and elbows. I also had hemorrhoids, felt extremely sluggish and fatigued, and had pain with simple movements.

I listened to *Natural Living* and joined a support group with my wife in 1999. Since then, all of my ailments are gone. I lost 100 pounds. I have constant energy: I run, race walk, power walk, skate, do aerobics, and train in a gym. I lost one width shoe size. My skin and hair improved. I need more frequent haircuts, and my hair is no longer graying.

I follow the protocol: juice and use green and red powders. My wife and I create organic vegetarian menus. I find it easy to complete tasks and am on a wild, uncluttering spree.

I work in image consulting today. My children are beginning to appreciate our new, healthy diet.

16. Connie, Female

I am 65 years old and thought fatigue, arthritis, high blood pressure, high cholesterol, cataracts, osteoporosis, and overweight were part of aging. My hair and nails were weaker and I was sensitive to the opinions of others.

I decided to go with Gary's research and knowledge. I wanted to be well and happy.

I no longer am tired and sluggish. I have no more aches and pains. I lost 20 pounds and look younger. My hair and nails grow in strong, and most of all I am indifferent to the opinions and criticisms of other people. Look what I did! Bravo for me.

17. Damon, Male

I felt frustrated and I could not muster up energy. I overslept, my hair was graying, my sinus infections drove me mad, and my cholesterol and blood pressure were elevated. This was not me, and I had to find a method of true reversal.

I went on Gary's protocol carefully. It was easy. I enjoyed new foods. I learned to understand body mechanisms. My elevated blood levels are normal now. My sinus problems are gone. I sleep less and awake with energy. My hair texture has improved and I have less graying. I am determined to achieve and have relationships with my family.

18. Doug, Male

I ate flesh foods, dairy, sugar; the everyday junk food, and was overweight. I actually did consider myself healthy even though I was scheduled for gall bladder surgery to relieve chronic heartburn. My pre-op EKG was abnormal, and I had a quadruple bypass. It was time to change everything. I listened to Gary Null's show and signed up for a support group.

The group members, Luanne and Gary's teachings, and the homework had a dramatic effect. I lost weight, no more heartburn, and enjoy a sense of good health. I am vegan, strictly on protocol. I shop in health food stores and continually learn all I can about healthier lifestyles. I begin the day with thirty minutes of exercise by power walking, and eat my big meal midday.

19. Ernestina, Female

I was unhappy with my lifestyle and uncomfortable in my body. Fatty tumors under my arm and thighs combined with excess weight made walking difficult. I was sluggish, used pain relievers for joint pain, and dwelt on past angers. I lived with exhausting tension and could not control my life or the situation I lived with. Without looking for excuses, I entered a support group.

We all sat in the room anxious to begin but not knowing how. Everything was explained to us. How we became sick, how we can clean out our bodies and rebuild our health. I looked forward to each meeting and followed the protocol. As I detoxified and switched to organic food, my anger and tension dissipated. Eventually the fatty tumors disappeared. I lost 30 pounds and no longer need pain relievers. I intend to continue this healthy lifestyle and spread the word.

20. Fatimah, Female

I was a sugar addict and ate two pounds of it per day, creating a sick, uncomfortable body. I over-ate using junk food. My energy was low, my skin was bad, and my blood pressure and cholesterol were high. This inability to control myself stressed me. As I listened to Gary, I thought about freeing myself from these habits. I joined a support group.

It is wonderful to be free of compulsive eating. I lost 50 pounds. I do not crave sugar. My cholesterol and blood pressure are lower, and I have real, vital energy. Problem solving comes easily, my marriage is happier, and I meditate. The foods I eat are healthy and so is my outlook.

21. Fran, Female, age 65

My skin condition embarrassed me. The sagging moles and dark age spots on my body saddened me. The energy I used to enjoy decreased with age. Tests indicated high LDL and HDL levels. I watched my hair change color and noticed my mental functions decrease.

The reasons for these unpleasant changes were explained to us in meetings of the support group. The foods we eat, water we drink, and thoughts we think all contribute to body malfunctions. I learned reasons for detoxification: why we need it and what we will experience as we begin. I realized I suffered from years of bad eating. Today I follow the protocol and always will. The result is a new healthy and optimistic me. Facial moles are gone, my skin is tighter and age spots faded. My attitude and body are more youthful. New hair grows in dark brown.

Also my blood tests went from high risk to normal. I am full of energy and open to change without fear. The support group gave my life back to me.

22. James R., Male

I procrastinated myself into a severe cardiac condition. After my angioplasty, I took blood pressure medication and joined Gary's Walking Club. I was amazed that the walkers and runners, some of whom overcame serious illnesses, were fit and healthy. They made major lifestyle changes. I looked at my life, working 7 a.m. to 9 p.m., without exercise. I was a coffee addict and felt stuck. A change was in order. I joined a group.

If you're going with the protocol, go with it all the way as I did. Organic, juicing, powders, vegan, and life changes. We were a great team, the support group people and me. We are different people today. That's what knowledge does. I am aware of labeling and chemicals. I no longer crave caffeine for energy. I ran in two marathons and confronted my procrastination. I believe in the power of actualization. "Speak the words, live by the words."

23. Bob, Male

My life was unmanageable and my stress was overwhelming. I had many allergies and frequent upper respiratory infections. My blood pressure and cholesterol were elevated. I heard about Gary Null's support groups and detoxification. I needed to change and decided to enter a group. That was the beginning of the best part of my life.

How could green juices clean toxins from one's body? Well, that's exactly what happened with good results. My energy built, my headaches stopped and cholesterol and blood pressure lowered. I have a new body since exercising, using weights, doing chi gong, and deep breathing. I feel calm, more patient, and less irritable. I love my food and progressive life.

24. Glen C., Male

I wanted an improved future without illness. My cholesterol was high and I had great pain from herniated discs, which prevented exercise. I was a compulsive eater and chose an unhealthy diet. I snored and simply did not care for myself. When Gary Null talked about a support group on his radio show, I did not hold back and joined in 2000.

I was a student again. The entire time was amazing to me. I learned why my body had problems and what I can do to reverse them. I understood the impact of mediation and forgiveness. I lost 18 pounds and am pain free. I exercise three times a week, practice martial arts, and do not snore. I recover quickly from illness, and feel happy and alert.

25. Glenroy, Male, age 65

I am diabetic and developed cellulites while serving in the military. I had severe knee and lower back disc pain. I could not climb stairs and used crutches and a cane for two months. Eventually I was paralyzed and confined to a wheelchair. Although my blood pressure and cholesterol were elevated, I ate the typical American diet of flesh foods, wheat, and dairy but beneath it all I desired health.

Since following Gary Null's juicing and detoxification diet, my body went from pain and illness to recovery and joy. My legs are not swollen with cellulites. My backache subsided and circulation is normal. I easily climb three flights of stairs to my apartment. I eat organic foods and use fish, use green and red powders and supplements. Life is active. Today I am retired and work with a veteran's council. I love babysitting my granddaughter since I became lighter and energetic. All past symptoms are gone. I am tolerant and learned humility. I focus myself. My body and life are mine.

26. Irene, Female

I was overwhelmed by possessions. My home was very large and cluttered. It became too much for my husband and me. My weight, cholesterol, and blood pressure went up. I developed cardiac arrhythmia and lost energy. My nails became weak. We were lost in indecision.

Joining a support group gave us the tools to create a new life and future. Detoxing returned my body to health. I lost 30 pounds, which normalized my cholesterol and blood pressure. I am no longer a cardiac patient. My nails are growing in strong. We are energetic and most of all we sold our large home, dividing the unessential items among our family, and now live in a four-room house and love it.

27. Jane, Female

My life was sluggish. I was overweight and always tired, which caused me to sleep too long. My eyesight was impaired with floaters and there were spots on my facial skin. I became an exhausted, negative woman.

I joined Gary Null's support group and through the detoxing cleaned up my life. I lost weight and am two dress sizes smaller. I enjoy renewed energy and require less sleep. After being post menopausal for five years, I began menstruating again. This makes me feel normal and happy. Facial spots are fading, hair is growing in healthy, eye floaters have diminished, and I have a positive attitude.

28. Janice, Female

I had a ten-year old son, but was diagnosed infertile. I miscarried and could not become pregnant. My periods were heavy. I had Lyme disease with headaches and joint pain. I was exhausted from all these conditions, plus allergies. We ate the typical American non-organic diet.

Good changes came with a Gary Null support group in 2000. I see a 95 percent improvement in all areas of health and life. My periods are normal, my vision improved, and allergies lessened. We eat an organic diet and follow the protocol using Gary's green and red powders. Our family relationships are better because we are healthy and optimistic.

29. Peggy, Female

I was slightly overweight. My symptoms were uncomfortable: skin out-breaks, cysts and eruptions on my arms, and premenstrual syndrome. These conditions did not fit into my projection of a happy future. That is why I joined a support group and learned a totally new way of life.

Today my facial skin is clear, the eruptions on my arms are gone, and the annoying sinusitis is over. It is a pleasure to be healthy. I intend to remain so.

30. Bill, Male

I am no longer sluggish and feel stronger both mentally and physically. I sleep less. My face is more colorful, much less pale. I lost 10 pounds and have better tone in my muscles. People comment on how much my appearance has improved.

31. Rainy, Male

I feel more focused and less toxic. I have a healthier, positive attitude towards life in general, and dealing with "problems" has become much easier. I feel much less depressed than usual. I feel more empowered. I do not take life too seriously anymore, and make time for friends and social activities.

32. Albert, Male

I feel like a new man. I lost 7 pounds. I can walk 10 miles. I sleep less. I help more people on the street and on the job, which feels great. I no longer eat at night.

33. Alexandria, Female

I lost 16 pounds and gained much more energy. My feelings of deep anger that would eventually depress me have subsided. My friends and family have all commented on the change. I am more muscular. I never thought I would love exercise but now I do!

34. Felicia, Female

I can focus much better. My indigestion is gone. My joint pain is gone. My skin cleared up. I am much slimmer and tight now but not too skinny. My face is not puffy anymore. My arms are toned. I don't worry about getting sick all the time like I used to.

35. Lavy, Male

I am more aware of myself. I no longer overreact to others. I feel more confident. No need to smooth things over with people anymore. I simply feel better.

36. Jennifer, Female

I have so much more energy. The cysts I used to get on my back and chest are gone. I feel like I am standing taller. I feel slender. I feel great. I lost 10 pounds!

37. Mary Ann, Female

I gave up wheat, dairy, and sugar. I lost 5 pounds. My relationship to myself and others has transformed. I feel balanced and self assured. I feel emotionally strong. I am no longer afraid. I feel less controlling of situations and people. I feel less victimized. My bouts with depression are gone. I feel kinder and more compassionate. I don't think before this I was ever aware of how grateful I am. I am able to realize more dreams. They don't seem so out of reach as they used to.

38. Leda, Female

I used to get serious sinus infections three times a year, and now I rarely do. My skin was very dry and has become very smooth. I was diagnosed with rheumatoid arthritis and I hardly have any symptoms anymore. My sense of hearing has increased dramatically.

39. Karen, Female

I learned that my mental limitations take my life away. I convinced myself that I have physical limitations. I learned I have the brain power to bust through these barriers and live to my fullest potential.

40. Ellen, Female

I learned that I am still in there somewhere under all the stuff that has accumulated over the years. I learned it is never too late to get to the things I want to do that I have put off. I remember how good it feels to feel good.

41. Olive, Female

All of my adult life I have been preparing for tomorrow and the future. I have taken my life so seriously, I did not allow myself time to "play." I have learned to live in the moment, to live for today and to make time for play. It, too, is important.

42. Liz, Female

I have learned to forgive myself if I make a mistake, and to keep trying.

43. Wanda, Female

I have learned how to apply discipline, focus, patience, and common sense to all aspects of my life.

44. Linda, Female

I suffered from loss of muscle, my skin was thinning, and my hair was gray. I had no energy, I was extremely forgetful, and my vision was obstructed by floaters. I also felt hungry all of the time because I was hypoglycemic. After following Gary's protocol, I felt like a new person. I was stronger, my skin tone improved, and I had more energy and focus. My eyesight has cleared up and I am now able to control my hypoglycemia through my diet.

45. Iris, Female

Before joining Gary's support group, I was overweight, which caused pain in my knees and joints. I felt anxious all of the time, angry and overworked. I would also grind my teeth at night and wake up with jaw pain. After being in Gary's support group, I lost weight. My knees and joints no longer ache. I no longer grind my teeth, and I have a more positive outlook on life without the anxiety and anger that was plaguing me.

46. Patty, Female

I had no energy. My skin was dry and thinning, and I was gaining weight and losing muscle. My body felt stiff, and I had floaters blocking my vision. Gary's protocol helped me build muscle and lose weight. My joints no longer feel stiff, and my vision has improved greatly now that the floaters have disappeared. I have much more energy now and I feel great.

47. John, Male

Before I improved by joining a support group, I suffered from rosacea [facial redness], hair loss, dandruff, skin dryness, muscle wasting, over stimulated adrenals, low energy, herpes simplex, elevated cholesterol, kidney weakness, lack of focus, stress, and tinnitus [ringing in the ears].

48. Karin, Female

I was nearsighted and experienced severe premenopausal symptoms the week before my period, including night sweats, insomnia, and mood swings. Gary's support group helped relieve these symptoms and improve my vision.

49. Delia, Female

When I started with Gary's support group, I was constantly tired, my hands and feet were itchy, and my skin was extremely dry. I was a smoker and experienced frequent bronchitis, a chronic cough, and I could not breathe deeply. I also had high blood pressure and sciatica in my right leg, experienced constipation, and lost my night vision. After following Gary's protocol, I feel so much better. I have lost weight and learned to eat well and exercise, and now have much more energy. My skin has become much suppler and no longer itches. My blood pressure has decreased, and my sciatica has improved. A lot of my issues related to my smoking have eased. I am able to breathe better; I no longer get bronchitis; and my cough is gone. My eyesight and digestive issues have also improved greatly.

50. Raymond, Male

I was tired all of the time, my hair was gray, and I also suffered from irritable bowel syndrome, bloating and weight gain. After following Gary's protocol, I was able to lose weight, and I no longer have a pot belly. My digestive issues have greatly improved and I no longer feel bloated or have irritable bowel syndrome. I have much more energy, and my hair has stopped growing in gray.

51. Mark, Male

I joined Gary's support group because I wanted to have more energy. I had gray, thinning hair and osteopenia [low bone density]. I also had abdominal fat, fuzzy vision, and pain in my shoulders. After following his protocol, my hair has begun to grow in darker and thicker, and my bone mass has increased. I also lost weight, and the pain in my shoulders is gone. My vision has also greatly improved.

52. Deborah, Female

I always had irregular periods and had not menstruated in almost two years. I had been on the pill for years, but went off of it in 2000 due to a 35-pound weight gain. I went off the pill and gradually stopped getting a period. My libido was gone, it was impossible to lose weight around my mid-section, and I got occasional hot flashes. I also experienced depression at the thought of being infertile and the long-term effects of lacking estrogen. All my diabetes was reversed.

53. Michael, Male

I lost 15 pounds, my skin and hair color improved.

54. Elizabeth, Female

I had candida and a cystofibroid breast. Today I am free of these conditions and feel completely healthy and full of energy. My skin has improved. My hair is thicker. I am happier and have more focus and clarity.

55. Adele, Female

I was unhappy about my weight and double chin and darkening complexion. After following the protocol, my memory improved. The most wonderful difference this program gave me is seeing my body change. I lost 25 pounds and gained muscle.

56. Peter, Male

My food sensitivities were treated with antibiotics in the past. Now after following Gary Null's allergy protocol, I find I can tolerate almost all foods. My depression, lethargy, and poor complexion have reversed. I feel vital, healthy, and alive.

57. Steven, Male

I lost 25 pounds. My hair and skin have rejuvenated. I use meditation, hypnosis, affirmations, and creative visualization to de-stress.

58. Didi, Female

I increased my body fat to a healthier level and enjoy sex again. My cholesterol dropped 50 points and HDL went up. I no longer crave sweets.

59. Kevin, Male

I lost 60 pounds in 14 days. Exercise is primary on my agenda.

60. Winston, Male

I suffered from a lack of energy, insomnia, and flatulence caused by a spastic colon. My skin looks great, and the liver spots on my neck and chest are barely visible. Hair, nails, and toenails grow quickly and with strength. Constipation, bloating, and indigestion are greatly reduced.

61. Mimi, Female

I lost 10 pounds.

62. Barbara, Female

The head of gastroenterology at a major NY hospital told me, "Get rid of your colon and get on with your life." Since I followed Gary's protocol, my colon is perfect. The last colonoscopy revealed a pink and pretty large intestine.

63. Iris, Female

Chronic fatigue and gastro-intestinal problems are less active, and I no longer require naps.

64. Amy, Female

I lost 12 pounds. I no longer have menstrual cramps. My facial skin has never been better. I have a regular exercise routine.

65. Juliet H., Female

I had chronic cysts on my ovaries. Within three months all symptoms of ovarian cyst disease disappeared. My eye bulging is reduced. I no longer have soreness in my throat area and I breathe with comfort.

66. Frank, Male

Eight months after a 20-hour long brain surgery that left me in intensive care for three days, I joined Gary's health support group and running club. I soon after discontinued steroids, seizure pills, synthroid, laxatives, and antacids. My physician does not understand my physical, emotional and mental recovery in so short a time.

67. Andrew, Male

My hair was thinning. {Since joining a group,} I lost 20 pounds and built great muscle tone. My hair loss stopped, the bursitis in my knee diminished. I no longer need naps in the afternoon. I sleep less and recover from colds quickly. I cured pharyngitis without antibiotics.

68. Muriel, Female

I feel fantastic. I have more energy, I think more clearly, and my husband and I both quit smoking.

69. Charlotte, Female

I lost 35 pounds. I feel really strong. I have a happier, more content attitude about my life.

70. Dimitrios, Female

I lost 15 pounds and retained this loss. I work out three times a week. I hardly watch television. I love running and walking.

71. Andrea, Female

My allergies improved. I have fewer colds and better elimination. My energy increased and I lost some weight.

72. Beatrice, Female

My hair was thinning. I had a fungal infection on my right heel. I barely had enough energy to get through my daily tasks. I noticed ridges on my fingernails. Now my hair is growing in healthier, the nail ridges have lessened, and I do not have arthritic pain. The heel fungus disappeared. My energy level is high.

73. Susan, Female

I lost 20 pounds. My skin is smooth, nails strong, and my hair is shiny.

74. Patrick, Male

My recall and memory is sharp. My skin is clear. I have less nasal mucous, an improved resting heart rate. My tonsil size decreased. No longer do I have dark circles under my eyes and pain from peripheral neuropathy in both legs has diminished as has arthritic pain. I have not been ill since I started the program.

75. Elaine, Female

I lose one pound a week. My blood pressure dropped. My hair is shiny. I am not dehydrated nor do I get headaches.

76. Sigrid, Male

I lost 30 pounds.

77. Trelline, Female

[Before the program] Stress, weight, hypertension, anemia, and a heavy menstrual period. [With the program] my hair, skin, and nails are strong and healthy. The anemia was life threatening. Today I no longer have this condition, and my periods are normal.

78. Gary, Male

I was 35 pounds overweight. My blood pressure was 180/110, my cholesterol 240. I lost 18 pounds, and now I run the NY marathon.

79. Eugene, Male

I was diagnosed with a small melanoma in my right eye. I am legally blind in my left eye. The cancer has not grown for eight months. Migraine headaches virtually disappeared. I lost 35 pounds and my back has improved. Other minor conditions have also improved.

80. Nevea, Female

I no longer have sinus infections or colds, my skin looks great, and my menstrual periods are normal.

81. Natalie K., Female

I no longer have tension headaches and the severity of cold sores has diminished.

82. Stacey T., Female

I lost more than 60 pounds. I sleep less. My skin cleared up, and I have bladder control. I practice yoga and meditation.

83. Eleanor H., Female

Before the support group, I had physical disorders. My adrenal and thyroid functions were low, leaving me exhausted, stressed, cold, and tired. I did not have energy to exercise. The protocol reversed these problems. I have not had a sinus infection in ages. My hypoglycemia is practically gone. I wake up early without stress, feeling happy and alert. I no longer use prescription medications. My body will heal itself.

84. Rich V., Male

My skin tone improved. I lost weight and now run eight miles a day. My sense of smell is improving. My hair grows less gray. I no longer feel a slump of energy at 3 p.m. each day.

85. Liz M., Female

I lost 20 pounds. I have incredible energy and no exhaustion. I sleep fewer hours, but have restful sleep. I am not depressed.

86. Liza S., Female

I am a teacher and would get angry at my students. [On the program] I lost 25 pounds and have more strength and less pain. My skin looks good. I can tolerate my students without anger. My new viewpoints and positive energy seems to be rubbing off on them.

87. Chris M., Male

My strength and endurance increased. My complexion is clearer.

88. Florence H., Female

I lost weight and feel more energetic. I follow the protocol with enjoyment.

89. Moishe, Male

Shyness, guilt, and low self-esteem were replaced with self respect and personal control. An acne condition and weak nails have cleared. The arthritis that hampered me is 70 percent improved. I no longer need drops for dry eyes. I used to take injections two or three times a week without improvement for several allergies. I had difficulty walking in the toxic city air. These problems either diminished or are completely gone. I look 10 years younger. My facial skin is clear and healthy.

90. Patricia B., Female

I was diagnosed with myelogenouos leukemia during my separation from my abusive husband of 28 years. I was in remission with chemotherapy and attended a Gary Null lecture on "Who you really are." Today I power walk and run three miles five times a week. I do 200 crunches daily. I could not believe I would find the energy to make myself well but I did.

91. Kristi A., Female

My attitude and body transformed. I lost 83 pounds.

92. Josephine, Female

Since starting Gary's protocol, my candida has greatly improved without allergy-like symptoms, my fibroid cysts disappeared, and my adult acne went away.

93. Angela, Female

I lost 5 pounds. Eczema improved and flexibility improved. I have more energy and feel less self-centered.

94. Monica, Female

I lost 3 pounds. I require less sleep. My bronchial condition is corrected. My vision at 71 years of age has remained stable without the need of eyeglasses. Gum health has improved, and nails are stronger and growing more rapidly. My hair roots' color has become speckled brown, black, and gray where it was previously white, and it also grows more rapidly. Skin wrinkles are lessened and skin texture is smoother and softer. Sexually my aging process has been reversed. I am pre–menopausal again. My breasts are fuller and firmer, and my reproductive organs are now self lubricating.

95. Patricia F., Female

I have a psychiatric history that spans more than 30 years. I have a goiter and an inflamed thyroid from lithium and mild tardive dyskinesia [involuntary movements] from Stelazine. Today I am off all psychiatric drugs. I am off lithium and Wellbutrin and Stelazine. I feel balanced, happy and excited by life. I am less confused and clearer in my thinking, with improved recall.

96. Pat, Female

I feel better now than I did in my 20s. I am 42 now. I lost 20 pounds. My skin is clearer, my energy increased. I feel greater mental stability. Dry skin on my feet cleared up, thinning hair improved, allergies are gone. I have not had a cold or flu since I started the protocol. I need less sleep yet wake up refreshed.

97. Joel, Male

I lost 8 pounds. I lost 2 inches off my waist line. 2 percent body fat is gone. My hair and skin look better, and my eyes are clearer.

98. Natalie, Female

I lost 50 pounds. I have increased energy. I feel more awake and alert and less fatigued. My hair is shinier. The redness on my face has faded. I no longer need medication for my menstrual cramps.

99. Tara, Female

My arthritis has improved and my joints are less painful. Shingles and genital herpes are gone. My allergies have improved and my periods are more regular. I have very little lower back pain and I am not constipated.

100. Peter, Male

I lost 8 pounds. Thyroid problems are gone. No more depression. I have lots of energy. I need no crutches.

101. Stanley, Male

I feel like I did 10 years ago. I have reduced blood pressure. I have a better ability to concentrate. I have increased physical strength. I have increased stamina, and I have an increased interest in sex.

102. Jennie, Female

Depression has diminished and I have less pain in general. I have more control over my emotions.

103. Sandy, Female

I came to the program overweight, short of breath, and diabetic. I lost 29 pounds. I walk 2 miles a day without being short of breath, and my diabetes is under control.

104. Patricia, Female

My skin cleared up. It is smooth and soft now. I have more energy. My varicose veins are lightening up. I lost 10 pounds. I am down a size and a half. I feel so good exercising.

105. Eva, Female

I lost 35 pounds. I am no longer depressed and bloated. Pain has subsided. My back never hurts anymore.

106. Susan M., Female

I lost 20 pounds, my skin is smoother, my hair is shinier, and my nails are stronger. I am much stronger with much more muscle tone.

107. Nick, Male

I no longer feel bloated, and my energy level has increased. I lost 20 pounds. I have packed on 5 to 7 pounds of muscle. I run three to four miles a day three to four times a week.

108. Liza, Female

I have lost 25 pounds and have less pain from fibromyalgia and arthritis. I am mentally clearer and much more focused. I have more energy yet I sleep a lot less.

109. Gary M., Male

I have clearer thinking. I lost 11 pounds. I have more energy. My skin tone glows. My breathing is much better. My attitude towards life is much more positive.

110. Nancy, Female

I am no longer constipated, and my overall body pains have subsided.

111. Joel, Male

I have more energy and overall get more done from day to day.

112. Hyacinth, Female

My cholesterol was high. I had dizzy spells. Arthritic fingers, skin and hair showed signs of early aging. My skin is firmer and young looking; the cholesterol level has dropped. My hair is growing back; my nails are firm and pink. The arthritis in my fingers diminished, and I do not have dizzy spells. I think clearly, and I am alert.

113. Maria Q., Female

I had fatigue and edema. I could not tolerate heat and had migraine headaches, arthritis, and an irregular heartbeat. I lost 15 pounds, and now my energy is very high and so is my optimism.

114. Neville, Male

I have better clarity of my thoughts. My cholesterol dropped, so did my weight, and my muscle tone has improved.

115. Michael, Male

[In the past] seizures began with Alzheimer-like symptoms. Abnormally severe edema in my legs incapacitated me. I was in a coma for 60 days. Nursing home care was considered. My health took an upward turn on the Gary Null protocol. Today I no longer need a compressor for leg edema. My leg size decreased 30 percent. I sleep less and lost 23 pounds. I exercise with hand weights. My blood pressure is lower. My brain speed seems to be faster.

116. Nellie, Female

My blood pressure was 140/90, and cholesterol read 268. I had large fibroids and was warned about cancer. Excess stress created chest pains and angina. I lost 15 pounds. My cholesterol is now 198 and blood pressure is 120/80. My last medical exam was excellent, no trace of fibroids. I power walk and feel energetic. People compliment my healthy skin. I handle stress with humor and do not react to other people's indifference. All and all, life is healthier.

117. Oliver, Male

I weighed 238 pounds. My cholesterol and blood pressure were elevated. I had pain in my chest, pain in my knees and ankles, and frequent heartburn. I was embarrassed by brown age spots on my skin and my eyesight was off. My weight went from 238 pounds to 188 pounds within 5 months. Blood pressure and cholesterol values were lower. I exercise one to two hours daily, meditate, and use juices and supplements with great enthusiasm. No longer do I have chest pains or heartburn. I feel energetic, less astigmatic, and my hair and nails are healthier. The support group ended but my life just began.

118. Ricardo, Male

I was constantly sick with colds and the flu, my hair was thinning, I lost my energy, and I was getting fat. I overreacted to people who were critical of me and never dealt with situations correctly. I changed my eating habits and followed Gary's protocol. I no longer get the cold and flus anymore, my hair is thicker, and I have the energy of my youth. I did not diet, I just followed the protocol and lost weight. I feel clarity and handle people effectively. That's maybe because I found my self-esteem. It was a major improvement for me.

119. Richard, Male

I noticed I got a lot of upper respiratory infections when I gained weight. Also, my energy dropped, and I needed more sleep. My skin was dry and often was problematic. I lost 20 pounds and have good energy because of it. I do not need to sleep as long as I used to. I no longer cough up phlegm. My skin is smooth and moist.

120. Rose, Female

My blood pressure shot up. That was just one of the frightening aspects of aging that hit me. I was tired during the day and wanted my vitality back. The best way was to go into a Gary Null Health Support Group. The body is remarkable. In a short amount of time my blood pressure normalized. I feel much more energetic as well.

121. Ruben, Male

I did not like the way I felt or looked. My skin broke out with infectious cysts. I needed long nighttime rests. My weight gain coincided with frequent outbreaks of colds and flu, and my hair developed a dry unpleasant texture. In a short amount of time, I lost 12 pounds and the skin cysts cleared up. My hair is soft and healthier. I do not have respiratory infections anymore. I sleep less and enjoy waking hours more. The protocol really worked for me.

122. Susie, Female

The night my son brought me to the emergency room I was told I would not wake up the next day. I had three bleeding ulcers and felt angry at my illness. The anemia caused extreme fatigue, and the daily weight loss I experienced was somewhat of a joke to me. I was told I might lose 30 percent of my stomach if the condition persisted. I was sent home with medications. Gary mentioned on his radio show that aloe and cabbage juice are good for ulcers. I bought a juicer and aloe and drank the combination. All medication was discarded that day. Eventually, I joined a health support group. Aloe, cabbage, and sometimes sauerkraut soothed my problem, but it was the green juices and elimination of dairy, wheat, and other products that really built me up. My endoscopy revealed no ulcers. I think that is remarkable. I lost 15 pounds on the protocol; my body began to reshape. At this point never straying from the program, I have reversed my aging, and I am emotionally stronger.

123. Job, Male

Before I joined the support group, I weighed 210 pounds, smoked three packs of cigarettes a day, drank alcohol, felt depressed, had knee pains and upper respiratory infections. One day I looked at the very aged man in the mirror and was shocked.

Today I follow Gary Null's protocol and use his green, red, and protein powders. The shakes keep me feeling full and satisfied all day. I drink purified water, use supplements and feel terrific. I haven't had a cold in five years, no more upper respiratory infections.

124. Joe, Male

I follow an organic, vegan diet and do not take vaccines. My neighbors tell me I look 45 years old. They admire my changes. I appreciate my healthy lifestyle. It makes me quite aware of the tremendous amount of obesity today. I am confident and pleased with my life.

125. John F., Male

I developed psoriatic arthritis 30 years ago. I underwent surgery to fuse my right wrist. My knees and neck were deteriorating, so I used heavy medications and over-the-counter analgesics. My blood pressure elevated, and I was advised to change careers.

My daughter motivated me to join a health support group. Today I am vegan, and eat no sugar or wheat. After I began the protocol and juicing, I became pain free in four weeks. I take no more medications, and all swelling subsided. My doctor commented that the condition of my knee joints is the best he has observed and my blood pressure is normal. I am able to take long walks. I have reclaimed my life. Neighbors who have observed my improvement now follow the protocol. One couple, a diabetic and his wife who has multiple sclerosis, report physical improvements. By following the protocol, my cousin lost ten pounds in two weeks and no longer has heartburn.

126. Karen, Female

I would often have swollen glands and frequent upper respiratory infections. My energy was low, my hair began to gray, and I was overly tired before my period. My life was complicated with people I today call toxic.

I joined a support group and decided to give it all I had. I juiced and became organic, very careful with my food plan. I did the homework and carefully listened to lectures and guest speakers. Today I am in excellent health without colds, pre-menstrual discomfort or [being bothered by] the impact of annoying people. My energy is high, and I forgive past errors.

127. Karina, Female

I was quite ill before I learned how to detoxify. My skin condition was unsightly, my gums bled, I had neuropathy in my hands and knees, pains from arthritis, and was diagnosed with kidney disease. Floaters and retinopathy caused sight problems. Tests showed abnormal thyroid levels, and my blood pressure and cholesterol were high.

Today, after completing the support group, following Gary's directions, and carefully going with it day by day, I do not have bad skin. My teeth and gums are fine. Pain from neuropathy and arthritis is gone.

Tests determined my kidney disease is reduced. My eye problems have disappeared. My thyroid tests read normal as do the blood pressure and cholesterol blood tests. I have a normal life and am thankful for the experience, education, and caring I received.

128. Kenneth, Male

I carried around too much weight on my body. I was uncomfortable with pain in my shoulder from an injury. My asthma often held me back. These problems made me angry and pessimistic. I often had temper tantrums, sometimes with violence. My confidence and esteem were low.

The juicing, homework, vegetarian diet, lectures and confidence the people in the group showed me got me through the first few weeks. I am vegan and enjoy my lifestyle now. I learned a lot about myself by answering the questions. I thought about my relationships. I lost over 35 pounds. My nose no longer runs all day, my asthma seems to be controlled, and I do not try to keep up with others. My life is uncluttered and so is my head.

129. Keith, Male

I was quite unhappy about my life. I had to lose weight and thought that was the problem. I did not feel I could accomplish much. I didn't know where I was going, wasn't doing anything constructive. I was not sure lectures and change of diet would help. Things were that bad, so what did I have to lose? I joined a support group.

Many group participants entered that door wondering if this would work. We knew the information and teaching would be correct but wondered could we do it. I did it and so did everyone else. What a change from day one to graduation. I lost ten pounds and maintain it. I don't feel alone and look forward to planning a better future. I actually feel happy and have learned to listen to my inner voice. The experience has reshaped me. I know I have self determination, and I am wild about the protocol.

130. Larry, Male

Carrying around a heavy body caused exhaustion and fatigue. I never exercised and ate the typical American diet. I often had heartburn probably from sugar in sodas and bad food.

It took some time to get used to drinking juices, but the explanations and respect shown to the people in the group made us enthusiastic. I began to feel the energy growing. I went with it totally: organic, vegan, exercise. I run and power walk. My hair is growing in darker, I lost 20 pounds, and my digestion improved. I still follow the protocol, use the powders and supplements, and love my new body and lifestyle. Thank you Luanne and Gary for helping us understand our lives are in our hands.

131. Luis, Male

At the time I joined a support group I weighed 155 pounds. My blood pressure was high and so was my cholesterol. I was not "sharp" anymore. My memory was not as good as it once was. My hair was growing in thinner and I felt tired. I listened to Gary Null on the radio and read his books, and when a new support group began I joined immediately. I was enthusiastic and optimistic. I stayed after class to pass my good feelings on to the group members. I knew I could improve my health and help them improve theirs. Today I weigh 145 pounds. I am totally organic, juice, use pure water, and I have great energy. My hair and eyebrows are thicker. Blood pressure and cholesterol tests are normal. My memory improved, my skin looks great, and I can read without glasses. I eat my last meal before 6 p.m. This experience gave me a new lease on life.

132. Marina, Female

I had several problems and wanted a solution. The medical community did not have that solution. I was overweight and that sapped my energy. After menopause, my hair and nails became weak, and I felt very depressed. I was given Prozac for "Multi-Menopause Syndrome." I was still depressed. Wasn't there anyplace to help people like me? Finally I heard about a health support group and without knowing exactly what it was, I signed up.

I joined the group, and it was so interesting, and it was an intelligent class, which respected the people attending. I learned how diet affects mood and the body. I followed the protocol and lost weight. I kept it off. I have lots of energy. My hair and nails are coming back to their premenopausal thickness. I stopped Prozac when I began the protocol and feel great. I sleep well, no more depression.

133. Marlene, Female

I was overweight, which caused a knee joint to swell and become damaged. My blood pressure was high. I always caught colds and flu, and had difficulty recuperating from them. Environmental allergies made me feel sick. I ate dairy and meat. When I had my hair analysis, I was told there was uranium, arsenic, titanium and commercial dyes in my system. My health diagnosis was so bad I knew I had to do something and that something was announced on Gary Null's radio show. I joined a group.

I learned how we damage our body with food and exposure. I was fascinated. Most of the people in the group grew their own illnesses. I followed Gary and Luanne's instructions carefully, one day at a time. Today I am 40 pounds thinner. I can walk freely. I discovered new foods and grains, new breads. I have less sinus discomfort, less allergies, no more upper respiratory infections. A sense of well being is in me. The forgiveness letters and homework gave me insight. I deal with past angers. The classes gave me freedom. I am grateful.

134. Mary Ann C., Female

I began to display the signs of aging. My weight went up with my fatigue, my hair was weaker, and my skin was wrinkling. I was pessimistic about losing my looks. I was in pain because of herniated disks in my neck. I noticed my muscle tone was not as it was just a few years ago. I was determined to turn these conditions around and joined a support group after I heard group members speak about their positive experiences.

The group experience was exciting. The group participants were wonderful, optimistic, and helpful to me and each other. We were a family. I lost 20 pounds and have fewer wrinkles today. My hair is healthier. I have less pain in my neck, and with exercise my muscle tone improved. I do not get colds or flu, and I feel stronger, calmer, more positive. It's a miracle, but not really. It's cleaning out, building up, and keeping to the protocol.

135. Monty, Male

I was an overweight semi-vegetarian. I used dairy and had digestive discomfort. I felt healthy, but angered easily. I am a trained psychologist, studied Chinese medicine, herbology, and German electro acupuncture. I lived in Italy for many years.

I joined Gary's support group to learn the protocol for myself and my patients. I recognized my defensive anger. Today living vegan, juicing, and enjoying changed eating patterns I find life quite different. I meditate, am self empowered, set boundaries, and will not expose myself to abuse. My career is beginning to be successful. I make contacts easily. Recalling my former behavior and anger, I realize the support group and detox protocol remolded my life.

136. Barbara, Female

I weighed 168 pounds and gained weight without overeating. I used pain medication for a spinal disk injury and was in rehab, badly stressed with anxiety attacks. I was swollen after eating my usual meat, wheat, sugar, coffee, and dairy. My cholesterol was high and migraine headaches caused me to be bedridden. I was labeled disabled for four years. Candida plagued my body. I threw up after meals. One day after reading one of Gary's books, I saw him on PBS. I joined a support group in 1994.

I attended classes open to change, and after two weeks on the protocol, being vegan, organic, and never returning to toxic foods, the change began. I exercise in a rehab center for my back problem. Probiotics and sensible eating eliminated throwing up. I am a vegetarian cook and intend to study vegetarian meal preparation. Back pain is sporadic and not as acute. I am still in recovery but use no medication. I never looked at life as I do now.

137. Rick, Male, age 80

I had surgery for an aortic hernia. I also had a hiatus hernia, high cholesterol, herpes, and stress.

I entered a support group, became vegan and organic. I completed all assignments, listened to the lectures, and found health and satisfaction. My body healed well after very dangerous surgery. I now own my business and compete successfully with people much younger who treat me as an equal. I have a stress-free, self-motivating life. My family relationships healed with strategies developed in the group writing assignments. All things considered, the support group gave me the health to revitalize my body and enter a long, satisfactory future.

138. Eileen, Female

I was overweight. My hair and nails were weak. I had a swollen knee because of three automobile accidents. I suffered with skin eruptions. I could not sleep well and was tired all day long. I wanted to be healthy and change my work. I decided to join a support group. I heard members of Gary's groups speak of their successes. I intended to change my work and life.

The group had a wonderful effect. I became friends with several people and spoke to them during the week. We motivated each other. Today, I am 25 pounds thinner. My hair and nails grow rapidly. The swelling in my knee has lessened. I no longer have skin eruptions. My energy is high all day long because I sleep well. I have also actualized a new career.

139. Joseph I., Male, age 63

I read Gary Null books and listened to *Natural Living* for many years with good results. I have hepatitis, high blood pressure, diabetes, damaged nerves, and recently had a bout of Bell's Palsy. I also have three bulging disks on my spine. With all of these problems, I sought relief and healing.

I decided to follow the protocol. The people that stick to it had good results. Today I juice, no longer use eyeglasses during the day, and am delighted that my blood pressure and diabetes are controlled, and that the Bell's Palsy did not return for two years. I discontinued weight lifting when my back was injured 10 years ago. I recently resumed lifting weights. I have a lot of energy, and the skin on my face is strong. My nails are healthy and pink. As a senior on a fixed income, I cannot afford a nutritionist, however, I study nutrition with Gary's shows and books. Thank you.

140. Pat, Female, age 63

I was hospitalized three times for congestive heart disease. I was on oxygen 24 hours a day for emphysema. I weighed 225 pounds. I had arthritis, diabetes, sciatica, glaucoma, and used steroids.

I came to support group meetings in a wheelchair with oxygen hook ups. Today I call myself "A Walking Miracle." I follow the protocol, walk daily, no longer use steroids, and even traveled to New York City. It took awhile to clean my system out, but vegan organic living was the answer. My neighbors are happy to see me as I leave for my daily stroll. Detoxification works.

141. Alice D., Female

My immune system was weak. I caught many upper respiratory infections. I required long hours of sleep each night. Many years ago a physician injected cortisone into my scalp. We soon discovered I was allergic to the drug and I developed alopecia [bald spots]. My eyes were dry, and I was generally uncomfortable with myself.

I began support group sessions and stuck to the protocol and affirmations. I soon noticed I no longer had colds and flus. I slept less and awoke refreshed. My eye condition is improving and I am aware of the relationship between un-cluttering and getting my life in order. I am happy to report my life is indeed satisfying. The protocol and teachings brought success.

142. Ken S., Male

I work in a prison. This is very stressful work. The impact of this job set me up for tense evenings at home. I felt guilty about my work; it drained my energy. My hair was thinning. I felt this was part of aging. My energy was low. I did not know what to do to rebuild my stamina and change my life. When a support group was formed, I joined it.

I follow the protocol and eliminated all allergic foods. I juice, which cleans out my system and gives me energy. I am aware of environmental toxins that can reshape my body and mind. I lost 20 pounds. New hair is growing on my head. My stamina increases daily. The job stress that pulled me down does not impact on my personal life as much as it did. I do not feel guilt about my work. Lately, I think about and question religious doctrine. Things are opening up.

143. Maria R., Female

I was prescribed Prozac for Multi-Menopausal Syndrome by my gynecologist. I gained weight and lost energy. My hair and nails were weak. I had difficulty sleeping and felt depressed. I thought I followed a sensible eating plan. I did not connect food and aging.

I began the detox protocol carefully and followed it diligently. I wanted to reverse my aging and clean my system out. I lost weight and am keeping it off. I have good energy. My hair and nails are growing to pre-menopausal thickness and strength. I discontinued the Prozac when I began the protocol and am not depressed. I sleep well, look well, and get healthier each day.

144. Moishe, Male

I was not energetic at all. My skin was rough. I had fungus infections on my nails and several allergies. A chronic, dry, burning eye problem persisted. I feared loneliness and did not travel. I isolated myself. I heard support members speak of their improvements when I visited Gary Null's office and decided I would enter a support group.

Initially, after a short time of detoxing, my energy and endurance shot up. As I continued, my skin and nails healed. I do not have allergic reactions today. My eye problems have healed, and my hair grows quickly. The lectures and homework made me look deep within. I live alone today. I do not fear loneliness. I attend activities and feel open to people.

145. Dorothy, Female

During the program, I lost 50 pounds and many inches. My bra and shoe sizes are reduced, and I am five dress sizes smaller. My skin tone and elasticity improved, and my energy level increased. I had several hair cuts in the past month. I handle stress and negativity, and this increased my self-esteem. Mediation time is important as is reading and reflection, not only at the end of the day but whenever I require it. I set future goals, focusing on solutions and personal needs. I use affirmations in the present tense during the day, accepting myself without denial. I am confident of positive solutions without negative factors. My strengths are far greater than I once thought. I am a work in progress, and forgive, learn my lessons, and leave the garbage.

146. Gloria, Female, age 78

I came into a support group with several physical ailments. I was somewhat overweight. My hair was graying. I had macular degeneration, hypoglycemia, periodontal disease, varicose veins in my legs, and a spinal curvature, which, I was told, could become degenerative. I joined a support group.

I shed 10 pounds and am filled with renewed self confidence. My sparse hair is fuller and growing back with dark color. There is an improvement in the macular degeneration problem I feared would be permanent. I do not have hypoglycemia or periodontal disease. The leg varicosity decreased, and my spinal curvature feels less acute. My amalgam fillings were removed. I returned to school for a degree and, best of all, my family is proud of these reversals. They prepare my special protocol foods when I visit and respect my choices.

147. Bob, Male

I was curious about this thing called a detox protocol. I did not feel unhealthy, but I decided to attend a group and see if it impacts in any way. I wanted to lose some weight, but did not like dieting. My blood pressure was a bit high, and I did get headaches.

I came to each meeting and listened and learned. I lost weight without dieting. My waistline is smaller. My blood pressure is normal. I need less sleep and my headaches are gone. The protocol and science behind it are valid. It was a wonderful experience.

148. Paul P., Male

I wanted to feel healthy. Medications did not do the trick. They could not make me feel healthy but only relieved discomfort for a short period of time. I had high blood pressure and frequent muscle pulls. If a health support group worked for so many other people, I decided to give it a try.

The dietary changes created physical improvements in three days. I follow the protocol and writing exercises. I listened to the lectures, and then one day I am told my blood pressure medication is [to be] cut in half. I no longer have muscle pulls. The spiritual aspect of our teachings had an impact, and I decided to slow my pace and un-clutter my home. It made me feel free. I now consider myself as important as my clients and am beginning to understand myself.

149. Maria T., Female

I was depressed and overweight, uncomfortable with the extra pounds. I held anger in and did not discuss, understand or share my feelings with anyone. I was afraid to take risks, such as asking for a raise. Being timid and angry was not a good place to be. I knew and trusted Gary Null, so I joined a group to see if I could be happy and make changes.

I am on the protocol and love it. My depression lifted as my health increased. I exercise without fear of injury. I lost 20 pounds, and my energy is high. I cope, do not hold anger in, and speak my mind. I spoke up at work and got a raise.

150. Joyce C., Female

My energy level has gone up. I can get through the day without feeling drowsy. The eczema and constipation improved. Tinnitus symptoms greatly diminished. I lost weight after two months in the program, and my body fat went down almost 10 percent. I did not gain any weight back. My memory has significantly improved. I can now connect the names and faces of friends. I am calmer and more relaxed.

151. Gary L., Male

My blood pressure improved significantly. My triglycerides dropped to normal range. I raised my good cholesterol and lowered the bad cholesterol. The homocysteine levels are better and lower than before. [High homocysteine levels are related to cardiovascular disease.] I am less depressed, and have a more positive outlook on life with more energy. I also lost 15 pounds so far.

152. Edwin M., Male

My hepatitis C viral load is greatly reduced from 7 million to 4 million since following Gary Null's protocol. I think clearer. Brain fog, mental, and physical fatigue are reduced. The aches and pains in my knees and ankles are gone. My weight is reduced by 40 pounds. I find my mental and physical clarity enhanced, and I have more energy and strength. I seem to need at least two hours less sleep.

153. Michael C., Male

My results following Gary's protocol are phenomenal. I lost 23 pounds, and trimmed over five inches from my waist. I eliminated two blood pressure medications. I sleep at least an hour less and experience a strong feeling of well being. My rate of hair loss decreased. I have strength and energy. The joint aches and back pains disappeared. I breathe easier, and my sinuses have cleared up.

154. Lillian R., Female

I have had remarkable results since going on Gary Null's detoxification protocol. My energy level is greatly increased. My blood pressure dropped to a stable, measurable reading. I am no longer constipated. I am totally motivated to heal myself, body and mind, and bringing joy into my life.

155. Ruth K., Female

To date, I can happily report wonderful changes on Gary's protocol. I lost 18 pounds, and my blood pressure returned to normal. My energy level increased, and I am not sluggish after meals. Feeling and thinking in a positive mode have increased my self-esteem. I feel good about myself. I did not regain weight because I am determined to continue the program.

156. Dow R., Male

My energy levels have improved. My skin is clearing up. My toenails and skin feel softer. I lost several pounds with no effort.

157. Don, Male

The detoxification protocol worked very well for me. My blood pressure dropped to 120/90. I no longer have warts on my hands, and my energy increased tremendously. I walk and climb stairs without getting out of breath. New black hair is growing in without any falling out. My memory has improved and is becoming sharper.

158. Tim, Male

I no longer have problems sleeping. I have more energy. My eating habits improved. I worry less and have hope for the future. I lost weight without effort and kept it off.

159. Eloise H., Female

My arthritis and knee stiffness subsided. Inflammation and swelling subsided. My blood pressure is significantly lower. Cholesterol levels are reduced to 159. I lost six pounds, and all my pants fit me. I sleep better and enjoy abundant energy and a sense of well being.

160. Allen C., Male

Since I began Gary's protocol, I lost 10 pounds. My arthritis is greatly alleviated, particularly in my knees. I see a considerable improvement in my chronic fatigue condition. I have good energy and require less sleep. My blood pressure dropped, and I now have a positive outlook on life.

161. Lyn W., Female

My energy levels are up since I started the program. I think more clearly and can better cope with depression. I have a smoother, more regular elimination. Communication with my family is open and positive.

162. Alexandre, Female

One morning I woke up filled with energy.

When I started the program, I had a real lack of energy. I was sleeping 10 to 12 hours a night and was always tired by 4 p.m. Now my sleep is down to six to eight hours each night. I still can't believe it.

I also lost 10 pounds just from the elimination of sugar, dairy, and wheat. I also maintain a regular exercise program.

163. Molly, Female

I feel sexy (at 59!), and I'm thinking about companionship. People who haven't seen me blurt out, "My God what have you done to yourself? You look fabulous!"

I lost 16 pounds, went down two sizes in clothing, and my abdomen went from 44 to 39 inches. I am much more relaxed, am more able to handle stress, and I need less sleep. My vision is clearer, my hair has gone back to its original color, and I feel 20 years younger. My meditation is now much deeper and richer, and I have less anger and depression. Most days I do 20–30 stretching exercises, and I am now willing to challenge my values and beliefs.

164. Charles, Male

I have distanced myself from members of my family who are hostile and negative.

I have made many changes on the physical level due to the Reversing Aging Study. I have much less muscle soreness, less lower back pain, which has bothered me for years, and an increase of energy throughout the day. I have better digestion, my skin looks better, and my eyes are clearer. I didn't consider myself overweight, but I went from 192 to 186 pounds, and I am physically stronger. If I get a rare cold, it is of short duration. I have a marked diminishment of allergic reactions.

On the emotional and mental level, an improvement in mental alertness. My mind feels stronger, and I have fewer periods of brain fog, and an improved outlook on life because I am proactive. I have more belief in my abilities. I must not only know, I must actualize.

165. Bruce, Male

Reflecting on my life choices, I have discovered a pattern in the types of women I've had relations with. It spoke volumes about my motivations.

I believe my energy level has increased, and I have fewer stomach pains. My dry skin has subsided. I have had only one outbreak of herpes. I find that I am sleeping more regularly.

I've decided to take charge of my fate. To do this, I've enrolled in a graduate program at Columbia University where I've met several entrepreneurial students with whom I am in the process of beginning a technology venture.

166. Donna, Female

I dove right into the protocol. I have lost about 25 pounds.

Being overweight only became a problem for me in my adult life. In my thirties I went through a difficult divorce. I was emotionally devastated. I had been smoking and drinking to numb the pain. I decided that I would stop smoking and cut back on the wine. But this became more of a hurdle than I had envisioned. I guess I turned to food to fill the void I felt in my gut. I gained weight steadily and kept it on for over ten years. I was unhappy with the way I looked, but I didn't have the will to do anything about it.

I tried a couple of techniques to lose the weight. I tried food combining and met with some success. Shortly after that, I joined the health support group. My general health was not bad, but I was terribly uncomfortable with the extra weight.

I dove right into the protocol. I juice every morning. I have eliminated meat, dairy, and wheat. I take all of the supplements and meditate every morning. I also have read books and listened to several tapes recommended by Gary. The one aspect of the protocol that I have been less than consistent with is exercise. Focusing on being positive, setting boundaries, and detaching from toxic relationships has been very liberating.

I have been in the program for nine months and I have lost about 25 pounds. I am a new energized person. I have taken control of a situation where I felt dissatisfied and helpless. The protocol has become a way of life.

167. Elaine, Female

I feel energetic, attractive, and strong.

The changes I was able to make during this protocol were more marked than any changes I have been able to make in several years. When I followed the protocol closely, I lost 12 pounds, several inches from my hips and waist, and my blood pressure dropped to 102/60. My self-confidence and energy level rose to a new high. I received many comments on my shiny hair and people commented on how nice my skin was. I no longer get headaches, whereas before I usually got at least one severe headache a month. I feel more confident, positive, clear headed, and able to focus on other life goals. I feel like a different person: stronger, happier, and enthusiastic. The homework questions keep me focus and practical. I believe they are critical to reversing the aging.

168. Marina, Female

I have more energy, so I am more active.

I started gaining weight at 47 years old. When I joined, I felt tired and had many medical complications. I started drinking juice and changed my way of eating. I walk three to five miles a day. I lost 27 pounds in five months. I have more energy, so I am more active.

169. Jacob, Male

I like loving myself a little.

Before I began the program, I had a very low energy level. I needed a sugar boost through the day. My digestion was not great, and the sugar cycle confused my thinking.

I have been on the program only three months and have lost 10 pounds. Overall, my energy level is greatly increased. My thinking is much clearer, and I am much more conscious of my interaction with people throughout the day. My body functions have become more regulated. I am much more aware of what and when I choose to eat. Generally, my attitude is much better.

I like that I am able to listen better and hear what it is people are saying to me. I am more patient with people and have become more aware of my own needs. I am even able to express them sometimes.

Before the program, I was upset with my work, feeling trapped by myself. I felt that my work controlled me and that I had no power. I felt as if I always had to get things done but was never able to feel joy in doing them.

Now, after following the program, I am beginning to take more control of my work time. And I have started to take control of my non-work time. I am able now to step back and congratulate myself on small steps taken. I have a more positive view of the future. I like feeling better. I like loving myself a little.

170. Ted, Male

Fifty pounds of fat is gone.

I lost 50 pounds, my body is stronger, my heart is stronger, and my blood pressure is down. I find that my head is clearer. I have not had chronic bronchitis or any colds, and there is a recognizable reduction of mucus in nasal passages. I no longer suffer from heartburn. I feel great! I am energetic and happy.

The best part of all of this is that I feel in control of my life. I no longer drink champagne. I've continued the walking program, and I feel my body changing. I've achieved self-esteem, self-reliance, and the notion that I'm the hero in my life. I'm becoming clearer and clearer about how I live my life, and I see how the old ways don't work. I now question why I have certain beliefs. I've reclaimed myself and my life, and I have hopeful and exciting feelings about my future.

171. Wanda, Female

A 20-year-old friend I hadn't seen in a year, sees me and says, 'Wow! What have you done?' I told him the 'Gary Null Thing.'

Since starting Gary's protocol, I lost 25 pounds, and went from flab to muscle tone. I am well defined, and I get stares in the park now! My joints are limber, and I am more flexible. My blood pressure went down 20–30 points, I have more endurance, and I can take mental and physical stress better. My digestion has also improved and I have five bowel movements a day. I need less sleep, my hair is much richer, with better texture, and I am vital and horny!

My cognitive functions are also much better, especially my memory. I am less scattered. I am calm. I really like running, swimming, and power walking. These activities are wonderful and invigorating. It's almost like a spiritual retreat. I have a much greater thirst for spirituality, to find that "something."

172. Renee, Female

A big accomplishment for me was giving up my nicotine addiction (two packs daily) and an addiction of 10 to 15 cups of coffee a day. It was difficult in the beginning, but now I feel much better physically and mentally!

My energy level has greatly improved, my blood work has improved, and my cholesterol has improved, going from 214 to 187. My triglycerides and PSA levels have also improved. I've incorporated new foods into my diet. I've eliminated dairy entirely, and have less congestion, bloating, and nasal drip. I am currently working on giving up wheat 100 percent. My siblings want to institutionalize my mother. However, I would not allow this to happen and have taken big steps legally and emotionally to avoid this.

173. Sharon, Female

After one year on the program, I have lost 20 pounds and reduced my cholesterol level by over 30 points.

Upon hearing Gary was having an orientation for weight management, I finally said to myself, "That's it, no more excuses." The major issue I was faced with was being "slightly overweight" most of my life. But "slightly overweight" turned into "very overweight" after the birth of my three children. I was very lazy, not exercising, and eating everything. Hips and backside became wider, arms were heavier, and my nickname was "thunder thighs."

I wondered if I could really follow Gary's healthy protocol. Could I go through the detox and change to a completely different lifestyle? I needed the support of the group. But I also needed the support of my family. Our meals would be taking a whole different turn. I took a deep breath and decided to take it one day at a time. I made a six month commitment. It is now one year later, and I am thrilled to say that I made it.

After one year on the program, I no longer suffer with the excruciating pain from heel spurs. The protocol has helped me immeasurably. After losing 20 pounds, the spurs are almost completely cleared up. I have also reduced my cholesterol level by over 30 points. I started at 190, and at the six-month blood workup it read 157.

174. Keith, Male

At the age of 51, I am finally starting to live and understand my life.

I lost 10 pounds; my mucus drainage has stopped completely; and allergic reactions completely diminished, especially since I changed my diet. I no longer eat meat or dairy.

I feel that I am gearing myself to be more positive and see myself as a whole, complete, independent person. I now feel that I am in control of my own needs and destiny.

175. Cynthia, Female

Being angry at people and being concerned with how they feel about me is no longer my concern.

Since starting on Gary's protocol, I lost 10 pounds, and I got my cholesterol level down. I have a lot of energy, and my hair is much better. I now exercise and meditate daily.

176. Toby, Female

My blood pressure stabilized. I was hospitalized for a diagnosis of appendicitis. I stopped medication and began drinking green juices and taking supplements. A CAT scan two weeks later ruled out appendicitis. I lost 15 pounds. I am less fearful of trying new things and more willing to work towards creating future projects.

177. Joan, Female

By the fourth month, I lost 12 pounds.

When I had the opportunity to get into Dr. Null's program, I made the decision to do it. By the fourth month, I lost 12 pounds.

I drink five glasses of organic vegetable juices a day. My family and I eat organically now. I feel things are starting to go in the right direction.

My big lesson is learning to take time for myself. Now I'm learning to get out in the sun and exercise. I am learning to have patience with myself. I do attribute the weight loss to the diet, the love I have for myself, and the pride I have in what I'm doing.

178. Marilyn, Female

Cholesterol dropped from 300 to 215.

I have experienced more loving feelings toward my husband, and less anger about taking care of him. I am more understanding and less fearful regarding the future.

179. Rudy, Male

Chronic pains in my penis finally dissipated. I think this pain was related to the toxic state I was in prior to the program.

My waistline has been greatly reduced, and my muscle mass has increased. I actually began having a 30ish body instead of a 47-year-old body. I have more energy, and my premature gray hair is more natural and brown. I had a fungus on my toes for years, which is beginning to clear up. My joints are moving more freely, my skin is smoother, and I have lessened my propensity for worry and reduced the fear level. I feel more self-assured and confident. This program has helped me become more centered, and enhanced my belief that this [form of natural] happiness is so important. This class is also beginning to restore my belief in spirituality.

180. Joan, Female

Depression is much less.

Gary's support group and protocol helped me battle depression. I gained 5 pounds, and I now wake up with more energy. I require less sleep, and there are noticeably fewer muscle-lethargy headaches. I feel wonderful.

181. Frank, Male

I am so glad that I joined Gary's support group. Following his protocol, I lost 9 pounds; my muscle tone, cardiovascular capacity, and digestion have improved. I require less sleep, my allergies are much better and not clogged up. I meditate after work; it clears my head. Exercise has been the easiest part. After doing my cardio exercise, I feel great. I work out at the gym in the mornings and sometimes after work. I walk the golf course instead of riding. Now I trust myself to make decisions, and I go with my gut. My home is less cluttered. I have more of a sense of order. I no longer judge or at least am very aware of doing so if I must. I am now considering moving to a warmer climate. I no longer worry what people think of me. I will not let anyone stop my connection to "my joy." I have disconnected from a lot of negative friends. My faith is even stronger. The positive voice is beginning to overpower the bad.

182. Bella, Female

For 20 years I've had purple spots on my tongue. Now, my tongue has returned to its original color.

The vision in my left eye has increased, and I no longer wear a contact lens in the left eye. All of my non-accomplishments in life I blamed on my father, because he mistreated me as a child. I blamed my mother for not going to college after high school. After writing the forgiveness letter, I no longer blame my father. I no longer blame my mother.

My personal challenge was the exercise program. In the beginning, it was the hardest thing for me to do. Now I exercise six days a week. I've also overcome my fear of public speaking. In January, I was the moderator for a fashion show. A year ago I could not have done that.

I forever shall be grateful.

Since the beginning of my participation in this program, the following has occurred: increased mental clarity, a better sense of overall calm and relaxation, a much-improved outlook on life, an even broader sense of consciousness and self, less crankiness, less fatigue, improved recall and memory, a much improved ability to cope with stress, faster and more graceful movement, overall improvements in my level of energy, clearer skin, clearer nasal passages, less excess mucous, improved resting heart rate, decrease in the amount of sleep needed for rejuvenation, improved workout recovery times, a noticeable increase in lean muscle tissue, improved bowel movements, which are also more regular, less sluggishness, more patience, and a decrease in my tonsil size.

No longer do I have dark shadows under my eyes. There is a significant decrease in pain from peripheral neuropathy in both legs, and an extremely remarkable decrease in arthritis pain, both resulting from multiple trauma suffered July 7, 1997. The surgeon who operated on my crushed right leg stated that posttraumatic arthritis was inevitable, and that I may have to consider fusion in the future. I haven't gotten sick since I began the program, and that is without a spleen.

183. Paula, Female

I had cystic breast disease for the last 20 years. Four months after becoming a vegetarian and following the detox program, the fibroids are all gone. I lost 5 pounds, my eyes are not dry anymore, and I don't get chest pain after eating certain foods. I have more energy and can get by with fewer hours of sleep per night. I am no longer "righteous."

184. Maria, Female

At the beginning of the program, I was very tired all of the time. It was difficult for me to get up in the morning. I was tired all day long. My skin had a dark sickly look to it. I had dark circles under my eyes, and my skin would always break out with pimples. My hair was falling out. My body was very thin, and I had no muscle tone. [Now] I have integrated exercise by getting a membership to the YMCA. I also go for walks and ride my bicycle. I have also begun to play the drums in a rock band and have found it to be a fun way to get a great workout.

My skin is now much clearer and healthier looking. My body has more muscle tone now that I work out regularly. I also haven't had a cold in the six months of this program. My nose used to be clogged all of the time, but now it is always clear. I have also had my mercury fillings taken out, which has resulted in a dramatic increase in energy.

I have a more positive outlook on life than I used to have. I still fall into negative slumps sometimes, but I am more aware of them so I can get myself out of them.

I had a job that I absolutely hated. It was a "go nowhere" job in an office in a field that I had no interest in. Luckily for me, I was laid off, which has given me a lot of time to focus on music. My band has been traveling and playing shows with such a great response every place we play. This has given me a sense of satisfaction in being able to do what I love to do.

I am a much more happy person spiritually now than ever before. I only surround myself with warm, loving, nurturing people, and I don't tolerate any negative thoughts of my own or from other people. I used to feel that my best days were behind me, but now I feel that they're way ahead of me.

185. Bill, Male

Before I started the program, I had gallstones and dryness on my fingers. I no longer have any symptoms of gallstones. I lost 3 pounds and my skin is 50 percent less dry, including on my fingers. My immune system is stronger, and I have not had any colds this winter. I see the light at the end of the tunnel. I feel less guilty about saying no. I know what is correct, and I will not be bullied by others. I am also getting less depressed in regards to money.

186. Miranda, Female

Since working with Gary, I generally feel better about me. I really have a better attitude. I lost 5 pounds, my energy level is higher, and I feel more alert and rested in the mornings. My cravings for sweets diminished, my ingrown toenails healed, and my scalp dryness eased. I've become more open and confident.

187. Rona, Female

I joined the Reversing Aging Group, because I was unfit. I had extremely high blood pressure, and I suffered from occasional swelling of the soles of the feet, which had been diagnosed as an unspecified allergic reaction. Every afternoon I became tired, and I had chest pain. Now, my skin tone has improved, I have stronger nails, my blood pressure is lower, my stamina and fitness level have improved, and I don't have chest pain anymore. The allergic reaction has not occurred since I joined the support group. I am no longer tired in the afternoon.

My behavior has also changed. Before I joined the group, I was very angry and stressed, tended to fight fire with fire, and was very confrontational. Now I am a much happier person. This has been noted by numerous colleagues. I no longer allow people to push my buttons. I have a more positive outlook, and I am proactive in attaining career objectives.

188. Liz, Female

I am choosing relationships that are positive.

In the six months since beginning the program, I have changed physically, losing 20 pounds and working out four to five days a week. I have incredible energy and am not tired. I sleep less, but the sleep I get is restful.

Mentally, I am more clear-thinking, making decisions regarding my life and business quicker, as opposed to laboring over them. I have no depression, but a general feeling of grounding and balance. Affirmations work.

I love work! I own my own business, an organic vegan, home-delivery service. Since being a member of the group, I am more organized. No procrastination. Our company has tripled its business. The company has become an extension of my being.

I have much more quality play in my life, and I choose very carefully who I'd like to play with. My time is important. Most important, because work is demanding, I truly enjoy my "playtime." As far as relationships go, once again, time is valuable, [and knowing that] made it easy to shed relationships that were toxic and draining. I moved out of a six and-a-half year relationship to a studio apartment that belongs to me, [and is] serene, peaceful, and beautiful. I am choosing relationships that are positive.

Although not every day moves gracefully through my life, each day is growing more enjoyable and fun. This support group has helped change my life to a positive peaceful state of being. A definite catalyst.

189. Angelo, Male

I am ecstatically happy now. And so is my family!

It is my wife who discovered the Gary Null detox program. She is the inspiration for the success we are both experiencing. I was ready for a major change, whatever it was. I'm glad it was this protocol. I had always believed that I was eating properly in the past. However, I was blind to reality. I was getting fatter and fatter, and my health was declining quickly.

Since beginning the program five months ago, I have lost approximately 105 pounds. My blood pressure is 120/80, and my cholesterol level has dropped to 158. I feel superb. As I walk, I feel like I am on air, and that I could walk for as long as the day is long. I have much more flexibility. I can perform many of the physical tasks that I could not do before. Before, I could not cross my legs or even tie my shoelaces. Now I can bike, jog, or power walk for long periods of time.

I have learned to laugh every chance I get. I still get the job done, but now I am able to enjoy myself at the same time. I will not tolerate any negativity at all. If I am wrong, I have learned to apologize.

190. Diane P., Female

Prior to seeing Gary on PBS, I never heard of him. A dark spot on my mammogram was suspicious. The specialist wanted to biopsy my breast. I objected and bought one of Gary's books. This began a tremendous education in all areas of my life.

My diet, life, and relationship with animals changed. I followed the detox in one of Gary's books. My breast specialist was quite distressed. I soon entered a support group and followed the protocol carefully.

After one year, I returned for another mammogram. The spot was gone. My blood pressure medication was lowered, and I will soon discontinue it altogether. I meditate, use yoga, power walk, exercise, and attend cardio exercise. Spirituality and self empowerment are very effective motivators for change and self improvement. My family had an attitude shift, and we reclaimed power by home schooling our child and not returning her to the atmosphere created by 9/11. My mother went through cardiac surgery and is on the protocol. Her cardiologist is amazed with the improvement in her walking stress test, cholesterol level and blood pressure. My husband's hair no longer falls out and appears thicker than it was originally.

191. Michael, Male

I joined Gary's support group because I wanted to eliminate medications for anxiety and depression. My hair was graying and my complexion was dry and bumpy. I had nervous twitches.

I am now vegan and organic, and I juice and exercise without a need for medications. I am aware of mind/body connections. My colitis dissipated as my behavior created changes in body chemistry. The psychological and emotional changes empowered me to study the negative impact of toxic foods and people. I stopped fighting life. Now life supports me.

My twitching also stopped from ozone therapy treatments, and my hair is long and healthy. Today I enjoy the new career I have actualized: teaching others self-empowerment.

192. John B., Male

My blood pressure was elevated. It was difficult getting out of bed in the morning. My energy was low, and I felt tired upon awakening. My tongue was coated, and I was slightly overweight.

I followed the protocol without question. My blood pressure is lower, I feel great in the morning, my tongue is not coated, and I lost about 8 pounds without dieting. I see improvement in my hair and skin, and acknowledge the protocol to be life restoring.

193. Olivier, Male

My cholesterol and blood pressure were elevated. I felt pain in my chest, knees, and ankles in addition to gastric distress. I weighed 238 pounds and was unhappy with brown age spots on my skin. Astigmatism caused discomfort. An internet acquaintance suggested that I listen to Gary Null to motivate direction. I began psychotherapy.

The protocol was successful. I lost 50 pounds in five months and was inspired to continue. My blood pressure and cholesterol lowered. I now exercise one to two hours daily and meditate. Juicing and using supplements improved my endurance. Life is positive without pains. Age spots faded, my astigmatism improved, and my skin texture, nails, and hair are healthy. I learned to let go, not get involved in details or hang on. Today I am involved in research, I live a vegan lifestyle, I am organic, and I put health first for my family and the planet.

194. Marcia C., Female

I made changes 47 years ago with Dr. Max Warmbrand, [but more recently] I entered a Gary Null support group overweight, with low libido, and white hair. I rarely exercised. My nails were weak, and my energy was low.

I was delighted with the protocol. My energy increased, my nails became stronger, and my once-white hair grew in thicker and in its original brown color. I lost weight in a slow, consistent manner.

Today, I am a healthy, energetic woman. I am involved in several new careers; songwriter—one song was recorded—and I am the author of a book based on life-motivating therapy. I am in the process of submitting ideas for an impending radio show for seniors. Life is more fun than it ever was. Part of that is motivating people to jump right in.

195. Carol J., Female

I listened to *Natural Living* before entering a support group. I had been to Paradise Gardens [where Gary Null hosts retreats in Naples, Florida] twice, but was not totally vegetarian.

Being overweight most of my life caused painful arthritis. My turning point came attending Florida retreats and joining a support group. I quickly adapted to the new lifestyle but hardly exercised. It was when I began yoga lessons that power walking tempted me. It caused joint pain until arthritic symptoms subsided. My energy increased when wheat and dairy were eliminated, and juicing increased. At this point, I became a serious power walker.

I lost 15 pounds the first month on the protocol and felt terrific. Doing support group homework kept me committed to future goals. I moved to a new home, which is uncluttered, and was satisfied to disassociate with the people I felt were obnoxious. I lost 75 pounds. I now belong to a rowing team and race walk with the Gary Null Running and Walking Club.

196. Nelly P., Female

I was slightly overweight. My blood pressure and cholesterol were elevated. I had large fibroids and was given a possible cancer warning by my physician. Excess stress caused chest pain diagnosed as possible angina. Business tension caused worry as I tackled difficult tasks to fulfill my mission helping people in Peru. My husband and I adopted two children but tension affected my family. Then I watched Gary on PBS.

I joined a support group and lost 15 pounds. My cholesterol and blood pressure normalized. My family is now vegan. Medical examinations confirmed that I no longer have fibroids. I learned power walking at Paradise Gardens, and I am energetic and patient at home with my children, less of a perfectionist, and I handle stress with humor. I work out in a gym. Friends admire my lovely skin. Life is fulfilling and easier.

197. Joseph M., Male

When I began attending support group meetings, I was chronically tired. It was difficult getting up in the morning. My skin had a dark, sickly look with pimples, and there were dark circles under my eyes. My hair was falling out. My body was very thin and lacked muscle tone.

My health is much improved today. I integrated exercise by getting a membership to the YMCA. I walk and bicycle. I began playing drums in a rock band.

198. Miriam R., age 66

I was an unhappy widow living in a cluttered environment without future goals. I discovered *Natural Living* and began to evolve into the vibrant woman I am today.

I sold my large home, which uncluttered my life and opened the door to new experiences. Today I live a happy life. I exercise my body, I am vegan, I ran a five-mile marathon, and I attend track meets with high energy. I am no longer depressed. Life has changed into a positive experience without depression or anger.

199. Wilma, Female, age 69

I had a radical hysterectomy at age 38 and was later diagnosed with chronic fatigue for many years. I refused to take pharmaceutical female hormones and used vitamins for fatigue. My body began to ache with arthritis. I didn't realize I was in a state of acute depression, and I continued to follow the typical American diet. It was difficult to listen to *Natural Living* while I was working, but I had heard the show over the years, and nine years ago I joined a support group.

I used biofeedback to prevent blackouts, and medical examinations diagnosed acute angina attacks. Because I was aware of alternative solutions, I decided to have vitamin C drips. The blackouts ceased after chelation.

Today I follow the protocol using green and red powders. I attended a Florida retreat. My cardiac, chronic fatigue, and cancer are in total remission. I reject immunizations. I am a life-loving woman who is healthy and in complete control of my life!

200. Kenneth, Male

I've been diagnosed with probable MS, and joined the health support group for people with neurological disorders. It has been a life-changing experience. For me to be a part of this health support group, I needed to first ask myself one question, "Do I want to get well?" I would retreat to this question whenever anything I had to do to get me well took me out of my comfort zone. Being able to answer "YES" made it easier to make changes.

Because I've answered yes to everything, I am much better today. The heavy metals that plagued my body are almost completely eradicated compared to six months ago. My cognitive functions have also improved greatly. I no longer have any symptoms. This is not about symptom suppression for me anymore. I will follow through with the protocol to the point of elimination. Reverse the lesions in the brain, and remove the worry about the protein in the spine that triggers MS symptoms. My original neurologist will wonder what happened, and what I did. The protocol is a series of therapies and lifestyle changes working in chorus to get you better than well.

For help finding a holistic practicioner near you, please contact Gary Null & Associates at 1-877-627-5065.

References and Resources

Chapter 1—"Pushing Back Against Diabetes"

Abidoff MT. Special clinical report on effects of glucose-6-phosphatase on human subjects. Russian Ministry of Health, Moscow, 1999. Unpublished study.

Al-Thakafy HS, Khoja SM, et al. Alterations of erythrocyte free radical defense system, heart tissue lipid peroxidation, and lipid concentration in streptozotocin-induced diabetic rats under coenzyme Q10 supplementation. *Saudi Med J.* 2004 Dec;25(12):1824–30.

Ametov AS, Barinov A, et al. The sensory symptoms of diabetic polyneuropathy are improved with alpha-lipoic acid: The SYDNEY trial. *Diabetes Care.* 2003 Mar;26(3):770–6.

Anderson JW, Randles KM, et al. Carbohydrate and fiber recommendations for individuals with diabetes: A quantitative assessment and meta-analysis of the evidence. *J Am Coll Nutr.* 2004 Feb;23(1):5–17.

Anderson RA, Broadhurst CL, et al. Isolation and characterization of polyphenol type-A polymers from cinnamon with insulin-like biological activity. *J Agric Food Chem.* 2004 Jan 14;52(1):65–70.

Anderson RA, Cheng N, et al. Elevated intakes of supplemental chromium improve glucose and insulin variables in individuals with type II diabetes. *Diabetes.* 1997 Nov;46(11):1786–91.

Antoniades C, Tousoulis D, et al. Vascular endothelium and inflammatory process, in patients with combined type II diabetes mellitus and coronary atherosclerosis: The effects of vitamin C. *Diabet Med.* 2004 Jun; 21(6):552–8.

Auer W, Eiber A, et al. Hypertension and hyperlipidaemia: Garlic helps in mild cases. Br J Clin Pract Suppl. 1990a Aug;69:3–6.

Bahijiri SM, Mira SA, et al. The effects of inorganic chromium and brewer's yeast supplementation on glucose tolerance, serum lipids and drug dosage in individuals with type II diabetes. *Saudi Med J.* 2000 Sep; 21(9):831–7.

Basu R, Chandramouli V, et al. Obesity and type II diabetes impair insulin-induced suppression of glycogenolysis as well as gluconeogenesis. *Diabetes.* 2005 Jul;54(7):1942–8.

Bone K. Bilberry: The vision herb. *MediHerb Prof Rev.* 1997;59:1–4.

Boudou P, Sobngwi E, et al. Hyperglycaemia acutely decreases circulating dehydroepiandrosterone levels in healthy men. *Clin Endocrinol* (Oxf). 2006 Jan;64(1):46–52.

Breithaupt-Grogler K, Ling M, et al. Protective effect of chronic garlic intake on elastic properties of aorta in the elderly. *Circulation.* 1997 Oct 21;96(8):2649–55.

Cameron NE, Cotter MA, et al. Effects of alpha-lipoic acid on neurovascular function in diabetic rats: Interaction with essential fatty acids. *Diabetologia.* 1998 Apr;41(4):390–9.

Centers for Disease Control and Prevention. *National diabetes fact sheet: general information and national estimates on diabetes in the United States, 2007.* Atlanta, GA: US Department of Health and Human Services, Centers for Disease Control and Prevention, 2008.

Chandalia M, Garg A, et al. Beneficial effects of high dietary fiber intake in patients with type II diabetes mellitus. *N Engl J Med.* 2000 May 11;342(19):1392–8.

Charles-Bernard M, Kraehenbuehl K, et al. Interactions between volatile and nonvolatile coffee components. 1. Screening of nonvolatile components. *J Agric Food Chem.* 2005 Jun 1;53(11):4417–25.

Cheng JT, Liu IM. Stimulatory effect of caffeic acid on alpha1A-adrenoceptors to increase glucose uptake into cultured C2C12 cells. *Naunyn Schmiedeberg's Arch Pharmacol.* 2000 Aug;362(2):122–7.

Cohen-Boulakia F, Valensi PE, et al. In vivo sequential study of skeletal muscle capillary permeability in diabetic rats: Effect of anthocyanosides. *Metabolism.* 2000 Jul;49(7):880–5.

Corti A, Ferrari SM, et al. UV light increases vitamin C uptake by bovine lens epithelial cells. *Mol Vis.* 2004 Aug 6;10:533–6.

Crespy V, Williamson G. A review of the health effects of green tea catechins in vivo animal models. *J Nutr.* 2004 Dec;134(12 Suppl):3431S–3440S.

Dhawan V, Jain S. Effect of garlic supplementation on oxidized low density lipoproteins and lipid peroxidation in patients of essential hypertension. *Mol Cell Biochem.* 2004 Nov;266(1–2):109–15.

Diabetes Prevention Program Research Group. The Diabetes Prevention Program: Baseline characteristics of the randomized cohort. *Diabetes Care.* 2000 Nov 1;23(11):1619–29.

Diabetes Prevention Program Research Group. Reduction in the incidence of type II diabetes with lifestyle intervention or metformin. *N Engl J Med.* 2002 Feb 7;346(6):393–403.

Diabetes Prevention Program Research Group. Within-trial cost-effectiveness of lifestyle intervention or metformin for the primary prevention of type II diabetes. *Diabetes Care.* 2003 Sep 1;26(9):2518–23.

Doggrell SA. Alpha-lipoic acid, an anti-obesity agent? *Expert Opin Investig Drugs.* 2004 Dec;13(12):1641–3.

Doly M, Droy-Lefaix MT, et al. Effect of Ginkgo biloba extract on the electrophysiology of the isolated diabetic rat retina. In: Funfgeld EW, Ed. Rokan *(Ginkgo biloba)—recent results in pharmacology and clinic.* New York: Springer-Verlag; 1988:83–90.

Dewey, John, *Human Nature and Conduct.* New York, Modern Library, 1957 (Original 1922).

Durak I, Kavutcu M, et al. Effects of garlic extract consumption on blood lipid and oxidant/antioxidant parameters in humans with high blood cholesterol. *J Nutr Biochem.* 2004 Jun;15(6):373–7.

Ebbesson SO, Risica PM, et al. Omega-3 fatty acids improve glucose tolerance and components of the metabolic syndrome in Alaskan Eskimos: The Alaska Siberia project. *Int J Circumpolar Health.* 2005 Sep;64(4):396–408.

Efendy JL, Simmons DL, et al. The effect of the aged garlic extract, 'Kyolic,' on the development of experimental atherosclerosis. *Atherosclerosis.* 1997 Jul 11;132(1):37–42.

Eibl NL, Kopp HP, et al. Hypomagnesemia in type II diabetes: Effect of a 3-month replacement therapy. *Diabetes Care.* 1995 Feb;18(2):188–92.

Elamin A, Tuvemo T. Magnesium and insulin-dependent diabetes mellitus. *Diabetes Res Clin Pract*. 1990 Nov;10(3):203–9.

Elkayam A, Mirelman D, et al. The effects of allicin on weight in fructoseinduced hyperinsulinemic, hyperlipidemic, hypertensive rats. *Am J Hypertens*. 2003 Dec;16(12):1053–6.

Fagot-Campagna A, Pettitt DJ, Engelgau MM, et al. Type II diabetes among North American children and adolescents: an epidemiologic review and a public health perspective. *J Pediatr*. 2000;136 :664–672.

Farvid MS, Jalali M, et al. The impact of vitamins and/or mineral supplementation on blood pressure in type II diabetes. *J Am Coll Nutr*. 2004 Jun;23(3):272–9.

Forbes JM, Cooper ME, et al. Role of advanced glycation end products in diabetic nephropathy. *J Am Soc Nephrol*. 2003 Aug;14(8 Suppl 3):S254–S258.

Furukawa Y. [Enhancement of glucose-induced insulin secretion and modification of glucose metabolism by biotin]. *Nippon Rinsho*. 1999 Oct;57(10):2261–9. Review.

Gardner CD, Chatterjee LM, et al. The effect of a garlic preparation on plasma lipid levels in moderately hypercholesterolemic adults. *Atherosclerosis*. 2001 Jan;154(1):213–20.

Ghosh D, Bhattacharya B, et al. Role of chromium supplementation in Indians with type II diabetes mellitus. *J Nutr Biochem*. 2002 Nov;13(11):690–7.

Hemmerle H, Burger HJ, et al. Chlorogenic acid and synthetic chlorogenic acid derivatives: Novel inhibitors of hepatic glucose-6-phosphate translocase. *J Med Chem*. 1997 Jan 17;40(2):137–45.

Hodge AM, English DR, et al. Glycemic index and dietary fiber and the risk of type II diabetes. *Diabetes Care*. 2004 Nov 1;27(11):2701–6.

Hodgson JM, Watts GF, et al. Coenzyme Q10 improves blood pressure and glycaemic control: A controlled trial in subjects with type II diabetes. *Eur J Clin Nutr*. 2002 Nov;56(11):1137–42.

Holzgartner H, Schmidt U, et al. Comparison of the efficacy and tolerance of a garlic preparation vs. bezafibrate. *Arzneimittelforschung*. 1992 Dec;42(12):1473–7.

Hounsom L, Horrobin DF, et al. A lipoic acid-gamma linolenic acid conjugate is effective against multiple indices of experimental diabetic neuropathy. *Diabetologia*. 1998 Jul;41(7):839–43.

Hsu FL, Chen YC, et al. Caffeic acid as active principle from the fruit of Xanthium strumarium to lower plasma glucose in diabetic rats. *Planta Med.* 2000 Apr;66(3):228–30.

Huang SY, Jeng C, et al. Improved haemorrheological properties by Ginkgo biloba extract (Egb 761) in type II diabetes mellitus complicated with retinopathy. *Clin Nutr.* 2004 Aug;23(4):615–21.

Hung PF, Wu BT, et al. The antimitogenic effect of green tea (-)-epigallocatechin gallate on 3T3-L1 preadipocytes depends on the Erk and Cdk2 pathways. *Am J Physiol Cell Physiol.* 2005 May;288(5):C1094–108.

Imparl-Radosevich J, Deas S, et al. Regulation of PTP-1 and insulin receptor kinase by fractions from cinnamon: Implications for cinnamon regulation of insulin signaling. *Horm Res.* 1998 Sep;50(3):177–82.

Institute of Medicine. Food and Nutrition Board. Dietary Reference Intakes: Calcium, Phosphorus, Magnesium, Vitamin D and Fluoride. National Academy Press. Washington, DC, 1999.

Isaacsohn JL, Moser M, et al. Garlic powder and plasma lipids and lipoproteins: A multicenter, randomized, placebo-controlled trial. *Arch Intern Med.* 1998 Jun 8;158(11):1189–94.

Isley WL. Hepatotoxicity of thiazolidinediones. *Expert Opin Drug Saf.* 2003 Nov;2(6):581–6.

Jacob S, Henriksen EJ, et al. Enhancement of glucose disposal in patients with type II diabetes by alpha-lipoic acid. *Arzneimittelforschung.* 1995 Aug;45(8):872–4.

Jacob S, Ruus P, et al. Oral administration of RAC-alpha-lipoic acid modulates insulin sensitivity in patients with type-2 diabetes mellitus: A placebo-controlled pilot trial. *Free Radic Biol Med.* 1999 Aug;27(3–4):309–14.

Janssen B, Hohendel D, et al. Carnosine as a protective factor in diabetic nephropathy: Association with a leucine repeat of the carnosinase gene CNDP1. *Diabetes.* 2005 Aug;54(8):2320–7.

Johnston KL, Clifford MN, et al. Coffee acutely modifies gastrointestinal hormone secretion and glucose tolerance in humans: Glycemic effects of chlorogenic acid and caffeine. *Am J Clin Nutr.* 2003 Oct;78(4):728–33.

Joshi SR. Metformin: old wine in new bottle—evolving technology and therapy in diabetes. *J Assoc Physicians India.* 2005 Nov;53:963–72.

Jovanovic L, Gutierrez M, et al. Chromium supplementation for women with gestational diabetes mellitus. *J Trace Elem Med Biol.* 1999;12:91–7.

Kahler W, Kuklinski B, et al. [Diabetes mellitus—a free radical-associated disease. Results of adjuvant antioxidant supplementation]. *Z Gesamte Inn Med.* 1993 May;48(5):223–32.

Kannar D, Wattanapenpaiboon N, et al. Hypocholesterolemic effect of an enteric-coated garlic supplement. *J Am Coll Nutr.* 2001 Jun;20(3):225–31.

Kapoor D, Malkin CJ, et al. Androgens, insulin resistance and vascular disease in men. *Clin Endocrinol* (Oxf). 2005 Sep;63(3):239–50. Review.

Kawabata T, Packer L. Alpha-lipoate can protect against glycation of serum albumin, but not low density lipoprotein. *Biochem Biophys Res Commun.* 1994 Aug 30;203(1):99–104.

Keen H, Payan J, et al. Treatment of diabetic neuropathy with gamma-linolenic acid. The Gamma-Linolenic Acid Multicenter Trial Group. *Diabetes Care.* 1993 Jan;16(1):8–15.

Khaw KT, Barrett-Connor E. Dietary potassium and blood pressure in a population. *Am J Clin Nutr.* 1984 Jun;39(6):963–8.

Kim MJ, Ryu GR, et al. Inhibitory effects of epicatechin on interleukin-1betainduced inducible nitric oxide synthase expression in RINm5F cells and rat pancreatic islets by down-regulation of NF-kappaB activation. *Biochem Pharmacol.* 2004 Nov 1;68(9): 1775–85.

Kohn RR, Cerami A, et al. Collagen aging in vitro by nonenzymatic glycosylation and browning. *Diabetes.* 1984 Jan;33(1):57–9.

Koscielny J, Klussendorf D, et al. The antiatherosclerotic effect of Allium sativum. *Atherosclerosis.* 1999 May;144(1):237–49.

Kris-Etherton PM, Etherton TD, et al. Recent discoveries in inclusive food-based approaches and dietary patterns for reduction in risk for cardiovascular disease. *Curr Opin Lipidol.* 2002 Aug;13(4):397–407.

Krone CA, Ely JT. Ascorbic acid, glycation, glycohemoglobin and aging. *Med Hypotheses.* 2004;62(2):275–9.

Kucharska J, Braunova Z, et al. Deficit of coenzyme Q in heart and liver mitochondria of rats with streptozotocin-induced diabetes. *Physiol Res.* 2000;49(4):411–8.

Kudolo GB. The effect of 3-month ingestion of Ginkgo biloba extract (EGb 761) on pancreatic beta-cell function in response to glucose loading in individuals with non-insulin-dependent diabetes mellitus. *J Clin Pharmacol*. 2001 Jun;41(6):600–11.

Lum H, Roebuck KA. Oxidant stress and endothelial cell dysfunction. Am *J Physiol Cell Physiol*. 2001 Apr;280(4):C719–C741.

Luque RM, Kineman RD. Impact of obesity on the growth hormone (GH) Axis: Evidence for a direct inhibitory effect of hyperinsulinemia on pituitary function. *Endocrinology*. 2006 Mar 2, 147:2754–2763.

Mader FH. Treatment of hyperlipidaemia with garlic-powder tablets: Evidence from the German Association of General Practitioners' multicentric placebo-controlled double-blind study. *Arzneimittelforschung*. 1990 Oct;40(10):1111–6.

Mahesh T, Menon VP. Quercetin alleviates oxidative stress in streptozotocin-induced diabetic rats. *Phytother Res*. 2004 Feb;18(2):123–7.

Manzella D, Barbieri M, et al. Chronic administration of pharmacologic doses of vitamin E improves the cardiac autonomic nervous system in patients with type II diabetes. *Am J Clin Nutr*. 2001 Jun;73(6):1052–7.

Marcy TR, Britton ML, et al. Second-generation thiazolidinediones and hepatotoxicity. *Ann Pharmacother*. 2004 Sep;38(9):1419–23.

Medina MC, Souza LC, et al. Dehydroepiandrosterone increases beta-cell mass and improves the glucose-induced insulin secretion by pancreatic islets from aged rats. *FEBS Lett*. 2006 Jan 9;580(1):285–90.

Melhem MF, Craven PA, et al. Alpha-lipoic acid attenuates hyperglycemia and prevents glomerular mesangial matrix expansion in diabetes. *J Am Soc Nephrol*. 2002 Jan;13(1):108–16.

Mensink M, Blaak EE, et al. Lifestyle intervention according to general recommendations improves glucose tolerance. *Obes Res*. 2003 Dec;11(12):1588–96.

Meriden T. Progress with thiazolidinediones in the management of type II diabetes mellitus. *Clin Ther*. 2004 Feb;26(2):177–90.

Meyers CD, Kamanna VS, et al. Niacin therapy in atherosclerosis. *Curr Opin Lipidol*. 2004 Dec;15(6):659–65. Review.

Mingrone G. Carnitine in type II diabetes. *Ann NY Acad Sci*. 2004 Nov;1033:99–107. Review.

Monnier VM, Kohn RR, et al. Accelerated age-related browning of human collagen in diabetes mellitus. *Proc Natl Acad Sci* USA. 1984 Jan;81(2):583–7.

Montonen J, Knekt P, et al. Dietary antioxidant intake and risk of type II diabetes. *Diabetes Care*. 2004 Feb;27(2):362–6.

Mullan BA, Ennis CN, et al. Protective effects of ascorbic acid on arterial hemodynamics during acute hyperglycemia. *Am J Physiol Heart Circ Physiol*. 2004 Sep;287(3):H1262–H1268.

Mullan BA, Young IS, et al. Ascorbic acid reduces blood pressure and arterial stiffness in type II diabetes. *Hypertension*. 2002 Dec;40(6):804–9.

Muniyappa R, El-Atat F, et al. The Diabetes Prevention Program. *Curr Diab Rep*. 2003 Jun;3(3):221–2.

Murase T, Nagasawa A, et al. Beneficial effects of tea catechins on diet-induced obesity: Stimulation of lipid catabolism in the liver. *Int J Obes Relat Metab Disord*. 2002 Nov;26(11):1459–64.

Nagamatsu M, Nickander KK, et al. Lipoic acid improves nerve blood flow, reduces oxidative stress, and improves distal nerve conduction in experimental diabetic neuropathy. *Diabetes Care*. 1995 Aug;18(8):1160–7.

Nawale RB, Mourya VK, Bhise SB. Non-enzymatic glycation of proteins: a cause for complications in diabetes. *Indian J Biochem Biophys*. 2006 Dec;43(6):337–44.

Neil HA, Silagy CA, et al. Garlic powder in the treatment of moderate hyperlipidaemia: A controlled trial and meta-analysis. *J R Coll Physicians Lond*. 1996 Jul;30(4):329–34.

Neri S, Signorelli SS, et al. Effects of antioxidant supplementation on postprandial oxidative stress and endothelial dysfunction: A single-blind, 15-day clinical trial in patients with untreated type II diabetes, subjects with impaired glucose tolerance, and healthy controls. *Clin Ther*. 2005 Nov;27(11):1764–73.

Norbiato G, Bevilacqua M, et al. Effects of potassium supplementation on insulin binding and insulin action in human obesity: Protein-modified fast and refeeding. *Eur J Clin Invest*. 1984 Dec;14(6):414–9.

Okuda T, Kimura Y, et al. Studies on the activities of tannins and related compounds from medicinal plants and drugs. I. Inhibitory effects on lipid peroxidation in mitochondria and microsomes of liver. *Chem Pharm Bull* (Tokyo). 1983 May;31(5):1625–31.

Paolisso G, D'Amore A, et al. Daily vitamin E supplements improve metabolic control but not insulin secretion in elderly type II diabetic patients. *Diabetes Care.* 1993a Nov;16(11):1433–7.

Paolisso G, D'Amore A, et al. Pharmacologic doses of vitamin E improve insulin action in healthy subjects and non-insulin-dependent diabetic patients. *Am J Clin Nutr.* 1993b May;57(5):650–6.

Paolisso G, Di Maro G, et al. Pharmacological doses of vitamin E and insulin action in elderly subjects. *Am J Clin Nutr.* 1994;59:1291–6.

Peponis V, Bonovas S, et al. Conjunctival and tear film changes after vitamin C and E administration in non-insulin dependent diabetes mellitus. *Med Sci Monit.* 2004 May;10(5):CR213–CR217.

Petersen M, Pedersen H, et al. Effect of fish oil versus corn oil supplementation on LDL and HDL subclasses in type II diabetic patients. *Diabetes Care.* 2002 Oct;25(10):1704–8.

Petlevski R, Hadzija M, et al. Effect of 'antidiabetis' herbal preparation on serum glucose and fructosamine in NOD mice. *J Ethnopharmacol.* 2001 May;75(2–3):181–4.

Petlevski R, Hadzija M, et al. Glutathione S-transferases and malondialdehyde in the liver of NOD mice on short-term treatment with plant mixture extract P-9801091. *Phytother Res.* 2003 Apr;17(4):311–4.

Pitombo C et al. Amelioration of diet-induced diabetes mellitus by removal of visceral fat *J. Endocrinol.* 191(3):699–706.

Playford DA, Watts GF, et al. Combined effect of coenzyme Q10 and fenofibrate on forearm microcirculatory function in type II diabetes. *Atherosclerosis.* 2003 May;168(1):169–79.

Pocoit F, Reimers JL, et al. Nicotinamide: Biological actions and therapeutic potential in diabetes prevention. *Diagn Cytopathol.* 1993;36:574–6.

Pozzilli P, Andreani D. The potential role of nicotinamide in the secondary prevention of IDDM. *Diabetes Metabol Rev.* 1993;9:219–30.

Punkt K, Psinia I, et al. Effects on skeletal muscle fibres of diabetes and Ginkgo biloba extract treatment. *Acta Histochem.* 1999 Feb;101(1):53–69.

Kumar V, Abbas AK, et al, eds. *Robbins and Cotran Pathologic Basis of Disease.* 7th ed. Philadelphia, Pa: Elsevier; 2005.

Rodriguez-Moran M, Guerrero-Romero F. Oral magnesium supplementation improves insulin sensitivity and metabolic control in type II diabetic subjects: A randomized double-blind controlled trial. *Diabetes Care.* 2003 Apr;26(4):1147–52.

Rude RK. Magnesium deficiency: A cause of heterogeneous disease in humans. *J Bone Miner Res* 1998;13:749–58.

Sagara M, Satoh J, Wada R, Yagihashi S, Takahashi K, Fukuzawa M, Muto G, Muto Y, Toyota T Third Department of Internal Medicine, Tohoku University School of Medicine, Sendai, Japan. Diabetologia 1996 Mar;39(3):263-9

Sakurai S, Yonekura H, et al. The AGE-RAGE system and diabetic nephropathy. *J Am Soc Nephrol.* 2003 Aug;14(8 Suppl 3):S259–S263.

Sancetta SM, Ayres PR, et al. The use of vitamin B12 in the management of the neurological manifestations of diabetes mellitus, with notes on the administration of massive doses. *Ann Int Med.* 1951;35:1028–48.

Saris NE, Mervaala E, Karppanen H, Khawaja JA, Lewenstam A. Magnesium: an update on physiological, clinical, and analytical aspects. *Clinica Chimica Acta* 2000;294:1–26.

Sato Y, Nagasaki M, et al. Physical exercise improves glucose metabolism in lifestyle-related diseases. *Exp Biol Med* (Maywood). 2003 Nov;228(10):1208–12.

Sato Y. Diabetes and life-styles: Role of physical exercise for primary prevention. *British Journal of Nutrition.* 2000 Dec;84(6 Suppl 2):187–90.

Scharrer A, Ober M. [Anthocyanosides in the treatment of retinopathies (author's transl)]. *Klin Monatsbl Augenheilkd.* 1981 May;178(5):386–9.

Schmidt AM, Stern DM. RAGE: A new target for the prevention and treatment of the vascular and inflammatory complications of diabetes. *Trends Endocrinol Metab.* 2000 Nov 1;11(9):368–75.

Seddon JM, Christen WG, et al. The use of vitamin supplements and the risk of cataract among US male physicians. *Am J Public Health.* 1994;84:788–92.

Sharifi AM, Darabi R, et al. Investigation of antihypertensive mechanism of garlic in 2K1C hypertensive rat. *J Ethnopharmacol.* 2003 Jun;86(2–3):219–24.

Sheard NF. Moderate changes in weight and physical activity can prevent or delay the development of type II diabetes mellitus in susceptible individuals. *Nutr Rev.* 2003 Feb;61(2):76–9.

Sheard NF, Clark NG, et al. Dietary carbohydrate (amount and type) in the prevention and management of diabetes: A statement by the American Diabetes Association. *Diabetes Care.* 2004 Sep 1;27(9):2266–71.

Shirai N, Suzuki H. Effects of Western, Vegetarian, and Japanese dietary fat model diets with or without green tea extract on the plasma lipids and glucose, and liver lipids in mice. A long-term feeding experiment. National Food Research Institute, Kannondai, Tsukuba, Ibaraki, Japan. nshinya@ nfri.affrc.go.jp. *Ann Nutr Metab.* 2004;48(2):95–102. Epub 2004 Feb 25.

Silagy CA, Neil HA. A meta-analysis of the effect of garlic on blood pressure. *J Hypertens.* 1994 Apr;12(4):463–8.

Singh RB, Kumar A, Niaz MA, et al. Randomized, double-blind, placebo controlled trial of coenzyme Q10 in patients with end-stage renal failure. *J Nutr Environ Med.* 2003 Mar;13(1):13–22.

Song EK, Hur H, et al. Epigallocatechin gallate prevents autoimmune diabetes induced by multiple low doses of streptozotocin in mice. *Arch Pharm Res.* 2003 Jul;26(7):559–63.

Song KH, Lee WJ, et al. Alpha-lipoic acid prevents diabetes mellitus in diabetes-prone obese rats. *Biochem Biophys Res Commun.* 2005 Jan 7;326(1):197–202.

Soto C, Mena R, et al. Silymarin induces recovery of pancreatic function after alloxan damage in rats. *Life Sci.* 2004 Sep 17;75(18):2167–80.

Steiner M, Khan AH, et al. A double-blind crossover study in moderately hypercholesterolemic men that compared the effect of aged garlic extract and placebo administration on blood lipids. *Am J Clin Nutr.* 1996 Dec;64(6):866–70.

Stitt A, Gardiner TA, Alderson NL, et al. The AGE inhibitor pyridoxamine inhibits development of retinopathy in experimental diabetes. *Diabetes.* 2002 Sep;51(9):2826–32.

Stratton IM, Adler AI, et al. Association of glycaemia with macrovascular and microvascular complications of type II diabetes (UKPDS 35): Prospective observational study. *BMJ.* 2000 Aug 12;321(7258):405–12.

Superko HR, Krauss RM. Garlic powder, effect on plasma lipids, postprandial lipemia, low-density lipoprotein particle size, high-density lipoprotein subclass distribution and lipoprotein(a). *J Am Coll Cardiol.* 2000 Feb;35(2):321–6.

Suzuki YJ, Tsuchiya M, et al. Lipoate prevents glucose-induced protein modifications. Free Radic Res Commun. 1992;17(3):211–7.

Tanaka S, Han LK, et al. [Effects of the flavonoid fraction from Ginkgo biloba extract on the postprandial blood glucose elevation in rats]. *Yakugaku Zasshi.* 2004 Sep;124(9):605–11.

Tosiello L. Hypomagnesemia and diabetes mellitus: A review of clinical implications. *Arch Intern Med.* 1996 Jun 10;156(11):1143–8.

Tran TT, Naigamwalla D, et al. Hyperinsulinemia, but not other factors associated with insulin resistance, acutely enhances colorectal epithelial proliferation in vivo. *Endocrinology.* 2006 Jan 12, Vol. 147:4, 1830–1837.

Turgut F, Bayrak O, Catal F, et al. Antioxidant and protective effects of silymarin on ischemia and reperfusion injury in the kidney tissues of rats. *Int Urol Nephrol.* 2008 Mar 27.

Turner B, Molgaard C, et al. Effect of garlic (Allium sativum) powder tablets on serum lipids, blood pressure and arterial stiffness in normo-lipidaemic volunteers: A randomised, double-blind, placebo-controlled trial. *Br J Nutr.* 2004 Oct;92(4):701–6.

Turpeinen AK, Kuikka J, et al. Long-term effect of acetyl-L-carnitine on myocardial 123I-M IBG uptake in patients with diabetes. *Clin Auton Res.* 2005;10:13–6.

Tutuncu NB, Bayraktar M, et al. Reversal of defective nerve conduction with vitamin E supplementation in type II diabetes: A preliminary study. *Diabetes Care.* 1998 Nov;21(11):1915–8.

Velussi M, Cernigoi AM, et al. Long-term (12 months) treatment with an anti-oxidant drug (silymarin) is effective on hyperinsulinemia, exogenous insulin need and malondialdehyde levels in cirrhotic diabetic patients. *J Hepatol.* 1997 Apr;26(4):871–9.

Vincent AM, McLean LL, et al. Short-term hyperglycemia produces oxidative damage and apoptosis in neurons. *FASEB J.* 2005 Apr;19(6):638–40.

Vormann J. Magnesium: nutrition and metabolism. *Molecular Aspects of Medicine* 2003:24:27–37.

Warshafsky S, Kamer RS, et al. Effect of garlic on total serum cholesterol: A meta-analysis. *Ann Intern Med.* 1993 Oct 1;119(7 Pt 1):599–605.

Watts GF, Playford DA, et al. Coenzyme Q(10) improves endothelial dysfunction of the brachial artery in Type II diabetes mellitus. *Diabetologia.* 2002 Mar;45(3):420–6.

Wester PO. Magnesium. *Am J Clin Nutr* 1987;45:1305–12.

Wilburn AJ, King DS, et al. The natural treatment of hypertension. *J Clin Hypertens* (Greenwich). 2004 May;6(5):242–8.

Will JC, Byers T. Does diabetes mellitus increase the requirement for vitamin C? *Nutr Rev.* 1996 Jul;54(7):193–202.

Wright E Jr., Scism-Bacon JL, et al. Oxidative stress in type II diabetes: the role of fasting and postprandial glycaemia. *Int J Clin Pract.* 2006 Mar;60(3):308–14.

Xia Z, Nagareddy PR, et al. Antioxidant N-acetylcysteine restores systemic nitric oxide availability and corrects depressions in arterial blood pressure and heart rate in diabetic rats. *Free Radic Res.* 2006 Feb;40(2):175–84.

Yamashita R, Saito T, et al. Effects of dehydroepiandrosterone on gluconeogenic enzymes and glucose uptake in human hepatoma cell line, HepG2. *Endocr J.* 2005 Dec;52(6):727–33.

Yan H, Harding JJ. Carnosine protects against the inactivation of esterase induced by glycation and a steroid. *Biochim Biophys Acta.* 2005 Jun 30;1741(1–2):120–6.

Zhang H, Osada K, et al. A high biotin diet improves the impaired glucose tolerance of long-term spontaneously hyperglycemic rats with noninsulin-dependent diabetes mellitus. *J Nutr Sci Vitaminol* (Tokyo). 1996 Dec;42(6):517–26.

Ziegler D, Gries FA. Alpha-lipoic acid in the treatment of diabetic peripheral and cardiac autonomic neuropathy. *Diabetes.* 1997a Sep;46 Suppl 2:S62–S66.

Ziegler D, Schatz H, et al. Effects of treatment with the antioxidant alpha-lipoic acid on cardiac autonomic neuropathy in NIDDM patients: A 4-month randomized controlled multicenter trial (DEKAN Study). Deutsche Kardiale Autonome Neuropathie. *Diabetes Care.* 1997b Mar;20(3):369–73.

Chapter 6—"It's Not Your Fault You're Fat"

American Academy Of Dermatology (2007, April 18). Psoriasis Linked To Diabetes And Serious Cardiovascular Condition. *ScienceDaily.*

American Academy of Neurology (2008, April 10). Diabetes In Mid-life Linked To Increased Risk Of Alzheimer's Disease. *ScienceDaily.* Retrieved December 17, 2009, from http://www.sciencedaily.com / releases/2008/04/080409170343. htm.

American Academy of Neurology (2009, October 28). Does Diabetes Speed Up Memory Loss In Alzheimer's Disease? *ScienceDaily.* Retrieved December 17, 2009, from http://www.sciencedaily.com / releases/2009/10/091027161521. htm.

American Cancer Society (2009, January 6). Obesity Linked To Elevated Risk Of Ovarian Cancer. *ScienceDaily.* Retrieved December 17, 2009, from http:// www.sciencedaily.com/ releases/2009/01/090105090841.htm.

American Chemical Society 2008 Jan 16. Once Irrelevant Compound May Have Medical Role In Preventing Diabetes Complications. From *www. sciencedaily.com/releases/2008.*

American Heart Association. 2009 November 18. Some Obese People Perceive Body Size as OK, Dismiss Need to Lose Weight. From http://www.sciencedaily.com/ releases/2009.

American Physiological Society (2007 August 13). The Female Advantage in Kidney Disease Does not Extend to Diabetic Women. *ScienceDaily,* From http://www.sciencedaily.com/releases/2007/08/070809103728

American Physiological Society (2008, October 19). Fructose Sets Table For Weight Gain Without Warning. *ScienceDaily.* Retrieved December 16, 2009.

American Society of Nephrology (2008, March 21). Uric Acid May Provide Early Clues To Diabetic Kidney Disease. *ScienceDaily.* Retrieved December 21, 2009, from http://www.sciencedaily.com / releases/2008/03/080318104217.htm.

Andaluu B. et al. Effect of mulberry leaves in streptozotocin diabetic rats. Clin Chim Acta. 2003 Dec; 338 (1–2): 3–10; Sharma R. et al. Mulberry moracins: scavengers of UV stress generated free radicals. *Biosci Biotechnol Biochem.* 2001 June; 65 (6): 1402–5

Anderson JW, Randles KM, et al. Carbohydrate and fiber recommendations for individuals with diabetes: A quantitative assessment and meta-analysis of the evidence. *J Am Coll Nutr.* 2004 Feb;23(1):5–17

Astrup A. et al. Failure to increase lipid oxidation in response to increasing dietary fat content in formerly obese women. *American Journal of Physiology.* 1994 April; 0193–1849/94.

BioMed Central (2007, August 16). Diabetes During Pregnancy Linked To Pancreatic Cancer Later. *ScienceDaily.* Retrieved December 17, 2009, from http://www.sciencedaily.com / releases/2007/08/070816091013.htm.

Boston University Medical Center (2009, December 14). Discovery of new gene called Brd2 that regulates obesity and diabetes. *ScienceDaily*. Retrieved December 16, 2009, from http://www.sciencedaily.com / releases/2009/12/091214201007.htm.

Boutelle, et al. Weight control strategies of overweight adolescents who successfully lost weight. *Journal of the American Diabetic Association*, 2009; 109 (12):2029.

Burnham Institute (2009, February 22). Stem Cell Research Uncovers Mechanism For Type II Diabetes. *ScienceDaily*. Retrieved December 21, 2009, from http://www.sciencedaily.com / releases/2009/02/090212171947.htm.

Brownell, K.D., & Horgen, K.B. (2004). *Food Fight: The Inside Story of the Food Industry, America's Obesity Crisis, and What We Can Do About It*. New York: McGraw-Hill.

Cardiovascular Rehabilitation in Patients with Diabetes. Mourot L, Boussuges A, Maunier S, Chopra S, Rivière F, Debussche X, Blanc P. *J Cardiopulm Rehabil Prev*. 2009 Dec 25.

Cell Press (2009, February 12). New Clues To Pancreatic Cells' Destruction In Diabetes. *ScienceDaily*. Retrieved December 21, 2009, from http:// www. sciencedaily.com /releases/2009/02/090203120716.htm.

Center for the Advancement of Health. "Poor Children More Likely To Develop Diabetes As Adults." *ScienceDaily* 22 June 2008. 31 December 2009 http:// www.sciencedaily.com / releases/2008/06/080619151917.htm

Challem J et al. *Syndrome X*. New York: John Wiley and Sons; 2000.

Chandalia M. et al. Beneficial effects of high dietary fiber intake in patients with type II diabetes mellitus. *New England Journal of Medicine*. 2000 May; 342(19): 1392–8

Chen et al. Psoriasis Independently Associated With Hyperleptinemia Contributing to Metabolic Syndrome. *Archives of Dermatology*, 2008; 144 (12).

Children's Hospital of Philadelphia. 2008 December 23. Overweight Siblings of Children with Type II Diabetes Likely to Have Abnormal Blood Sugar Levels, as reported by Sciencedaily.com/releases/2008.

Children's Hospital of Philadelphia (2009, December 14). Type II diabetes gene predisposes children to obesity. *Science Daily*. Retrieved December 17, 2009, from http://www.sciencedaily.com / releases/2009/12/091207123801.htm.

Columbia University's Mailman School of Public Health (2008, August 8). Periodontal Disease Independently Predicts New Onset Diabetes. *ScienceDaily*. Retrieved December 22, 2009, from http://www.sciencedaily.com/releases/2008/08/080806184905.htm.

Columbia University Medical Center (2006, February 10). Diabetes Can Lead To Gum Disease In Childhood; Onset Is Younger Than Previously Recognized. *ScienceDaily*. Retrieved December 21, 2009, from http://www. sciencedaily.com /releases/2006/02/060210092648.htm.

Cornell University (2009, June 7). Key Regulator Of Fat Cell Development Discovered. *ScienceDaily*. Retrieved December 17, 2009, from http://www. sciencedaily.com /releases/2009/06/090603110150.htm.

Diabetes Prevention Program Research Group. The Diabetes Prevention Program: Baseline characteristics of the randomized cohort. *Diabetes Care*. 2000 Nov 1;23(11):1619–29.

Diabetes Prevention Program Research Group. Reduction in the incidence of type II diabetes with lifestyle intervention or metformin. *N Engl J Med*. 2002 Feb 7;346(6):393–403.

Diabetes Prevention Program Research Group. Within-trial cost-effectiveness of lifestyle intervention or metformin for the primary prevention of type II diabetes. *Diabetes Care*. 2003 Sep 1;26(9):2518–23.

Doolen, et al. Parental disconnect between perceived and actual weight status of children. A metasynthesis of the current research. *Journal of the American Academy of Nurse Practitioners*, 2009; 21(3):160–166.

Duke University Medical Center (2007, March 11). Diabetes, Depression Together Increase Risk For Heart Patients. *ScienceDaily*. Retrieved December 17, 2009, from http://www.sciencedaily.com / releases/2007/03/070309141140.htm.

Eating Disorders. As reported in *www.sciencedaily.com/releases/2009*.

Endocrine Society (2009, December 7). Cardiovascular risk in youth with type I diabetes linked primarily to insulin resistance. *ScienceDaily*. Retrieved December 17, 2009, from http://www.sciencedaily.com/releases /2009/12/091201084207.htm.

Endocrine Society 2007 Nov 15. Family Ties Raise Risk of Diabetes Complications: Risk Greater for Women, from *sciencedaily.com/releases/2007*.

Endocrine Society (2009, October 9). Future Diabetes Treatment May Use Resveratrol To Target The Brain. *ScienceDaily*. Retrieved

December 22, 2009, from http://www.sciencedaily.com/releases/2009/10/091006093341.htm.

Endocrine Society (2008, June 17). Red Wine's Resveratrol May Help Battle Obesity. *ScienceDaily*. Retrieved December 22, 2009, from http://www.sciencedaily.com /releases/2008/06/080616115850.htm.

European Society of Cardiology (2008, April 13). Low Birth Weight And Excessive Weight Gain Linked To Heart Problems In Later Life. *ScienceDaily*. Retrieved December 17, 2009, from http://www.sciencedaily.com/releases/2008/04/0804092050848.htm.

European Society of Cardiology (2009, June 4). Obesity And Diabetes Double Risk Of Heart Failure: Patients With Both Conditions 'Very Difficult' To Treat. *ScienceDaily*. Retrieved December 17, 2009, from http://www.sciencedaily.com/releases/2009/05/090530094510.htm.

Faloon W. What you don't know about blood sugar. *Life Extension Magazine*. January 2004: 11–20.

Fishel MA et al. Hyperinslinemia provokes synchronous increases in central inflammation and beta amyloid in normal adults. *Arch Neurol*. 2005 Oct; 62(10): 1539–44.

Forbes JM, Cooper ME, et al. Role of advanced glycation end products in diabetic nephropathy. *J Am Soc Nephrol*. 2003 Aug;14(8 Suppl 3).

Forbes JM et al 2003; Sakurai S, Yonekura H, et al. The AGE-RAGE system and diabetic nephropathy. *J Am Soc Nephrol*. 2003 Aug;14(8 Suppl 3):S259– S263.

Haffner SM et al. Incidence of type II diabetes in Mexican Americans predicted by fasting insulin and glucose levels, obesity, and body fat distribution. *Diabetes*. 1990 Mar: 39(3): 283–89.

Harvard Medical School (2006, July 12). Type II Diabetes Increases The Risk Of Glaucoma In Women. *ScienceDaily*. Retrieved December 21, 2009, from http://www.sciencedaily.com/releases/2006/07/060712074528.htm.

Helibronn LK, et al. Energy restriction and weight loss on very low fat diets reduce C reactive protein concentrations in obese healthy women. *Arterioscler Thromb Vasc Biol*. 2001 June; 21(6): 968–70.

Institute of Food Technologists (2009, August 13). Black Tea May Fight Diabetes. *ScienceDaily*. Retrieved December 17, 2009, from http://www.sciencedaily. com /releases/2009/07/090728172604.htm.

JAMA and Archives Journals (2007, July 17). Diabetics Experience More Complications Following Trauma. *ScienceDaily*. Retrieved

December 21, 2009, from http://www.sciencedaily.com/releases/2007/07/070716190925.htm.

JAMA and Archives Journals (2007, April 10). Diabetes May Be Associated With Increased Risk Of Mild Cognitive Impairment. *ScienceDaily*. Retrieved December 21, 2009, from http://www.sciencedaily.com/releases/2007/04/070409164906.htm.

Journal of Clinical Investigation (2008, August 6). A Mechanism For The Development Of Obesity-associated Conditions. *ScienceDaily*. Retrieved December 21, 2009, from http://www.sciencedaily.com/releases/2008/08/080802061914. htm.

Journal of Clinical Investigation (2007, August 6). Identifying The Mechanism Behind A Genetic Susceptibility To Type II Diabetes. *ScienceDaily*. Retrieved December 21, 2009, from http://www.sciencedaily.com/releases/2007/08/070802182122.htm.

Journal of Clinical Investigation 2008 June 9. New Molecular Link Between Diabetes and Kidney Failure, from www.sciencedaily.com/releases/2008.

Journal of Clinical Investigation (2007, October 22). Type II Diabetes: What Determines Susceptibility? *ScienceDaily*. Retrieved December 21, 2009, from http://www.sciencedaily.com/releases/2007/10/071018171445.htm.

Journal of the National Cancer Institute (2008, December 31). High Insulin Level Is An Independent Risk Factor For Breast Cancer. *ScienceDaily*. Retrieved December 17, 2009, from http://www.sciencedaily.com /releases/2008/12/081231113031.htm.

Khaw KT, Barrett-Connor E. Dietary potassium and blood pressure in a population. *Am J Clin Nutr*. 1984 Jun;39(6):963–8.

Knolwer WC et al. Reduction in the incidence of type II diabetes with lifestyle intervention or metformin. *New England Journal of Medicine*. 2002. Feb; 346(6): 393–403

Kohn RR, Cerami A, et al. Collagen aging in vitro by nonenzymatic glycosylation and browning. Diabetes. 1984 Jan;33(1):57–9; Monnier VM, Kohn RR, et al. Accelerated age-related browning of human collagen in diabetes mellitus. *Proc Natl Acad Sci* USA. 1984 Jan;81(2):583–7.

Kumar V, Abbas AK, et al, eds. Robbins and Cotran Pathologic Basis of Disease. 7th ed. Philadelphia, Pa: Elsevier; 2005.

Life Extensions Magazine, June 2004, Diabetes: understanding and preventing the next health care epidemic; by Lyle MacWilliam, BSc, MSc, FP.

Life Extensions Magazine December 2006, "The deadly connection between Alzheimer's and diabetes" by Edward R. Rosick, DO, MPH, DABHM.

Luchsinger, JA et al. Hyperinsulinemia and the risk of Alzheimer disease. *Neurology.* 2004 October 12; 63(7): 1187–92.

Lum H, Roebuck KA. Oxidant stress and endothelial cell dysfunction. *Am J Physiol Cell Physiol.* 2001 Apr;280(4):C719–C741.

Luque RM, Kineman RD. Impact of Obesity on the Growth Hormone (GH) Axis: Evidence for a Direct Inhibitory Effect of Hyperinsulinemia on Pituitary Function. *Endocrinology.* 2006 Mar 2.

Mackey et al. Does this make me look fat? Peer crowd and peer contributions to adolescents weight control behaviors. *Journal of Youth and Adolescents,* 2008; DOI: 10.1007/s10964–008–9299–2.

McGarry JD. Banting Lecture 2001: deregulation of fatty acid metabolism in the etiology of type II diabetes. *Diabetes.* 2002 Jan: 51 (1): 7–18.

Mensink M, Blaak EE, et al. Lifestyle intervention according to general recommendations improves glucose tolerance. *Obes Res.* 2003 Dec;11(12):1588–96

Mokdad AH et al. Prevalence of obesity, diabetes, and obesity-related health risk factors, 2001. *JAMA,* 2003 Jan; 289(1): 76–9.

Monash University (2009, July 9). Critical Link Between Obesity And Diabetes Discovered. *ScienceDaily.* Retrieved December 16, 2009, from http://www.sciencedaily.com/releases/2009/07/090708090917.htm.

Mreira PL et al. Oxidative stress and neuro-degeneration. *Ann NY Acad Sci.* 2005 June; 1043: 545–52.

Muniyappa R, El-Atat F, et al. The Diabetes Prevention Program. *Curr Diab Rep.* 2003 Jun;3(3):221–2.

New York University (2009, April 6). New Evidence Of Periodontal Disease Leading To Gestational Diabetes. *ScienceDaily.* Retrieved December 22, 2009, from http://www.sciencedaily.com/releases/2009/04/090404164115.htm.

Nieman DC. *Fitness and Sports Medicine.* 3rd ed. Palo Alto, CA: Bull Publishing, 1995; Diabetes Type II and the Syndrome X Connection. Life Extensions Foundation website *www.lef.org.*

Norbiato G, Bevilacqua M, et al. Effects of potassium supplementation on insulin binding and insulin action in human obesity: Protein-modified fast and refeeding. *Eur J Clin Invest*. 1984 Dec;14(6):414–9.

Opara EC. Oxidative stress, micronutrients, diabetes mellitus and its components. JR Soc Health 2002 March; 122 (1): 28–34.; Houstis N. et al. Reactive oxygen species have a causal role in multiple forms of insulin resistance. *Nature*. 2006 April 13; 440 (7086): 944–48.

Oregon Health & Science University. "Obesity Causes Breakdown In System Which Regulates Appetite And Weight." *ScienceDaily*. 8 March 2007. 28 December 2009, http://www.sciencedaily.com/releases/2007/03/070307075719. htm.

Ott A. et al. Diabetes mellitus and the risk of dementia: The Rotterdam Study. *Neurology*. 1999 Dec 10; 53 (9): 1937–42.

Peninsula College of Medicine and Dentistry (2008, March 20). Grape Skin Compound Fights The Complications Of Diabetes. *ScienceDaily*. Retrieved December 22, 2009, from http://www.sciencedaily.com/releases/2008/03/080318094514.htm.

Penn State. 2008 July 29. Inheritance of hormonal disorder marked by excessive insulin in daughters. *The Journal of Clinical Endocrinology and Metabolism*. Reported in *sciencedaily.com/releases/2008*.

Pyorala M. et al. Plasma insulin and all cause, cardiovascular and non-cardiovascular mortality: the 22 year follow up results of the Helsinki Policemen Study. *Diabetes Care*. 2000 Aug; 23 (8): 1097–102.

Roberts et al. Association of Duration and Severity of Diabetes Mellitus With Mild Cognitive Impairment. *Archives of Neurology*, 2008; 65 (8): 1066.

Rosenbloom A, et al. Type II diabetes in children and adolescents. *Diabetes Care*. 2000 Mar; 23 (3): 381–9.

Saaddine et al. Projection of Diabetic Retinopathy and Other Major Eye Diseases Among People With Diabetes Mellitus: United States, 2005–2050. *Archives of Ophthalmology*, 2008; 126 (12): 1740.

Salmeron J et al. Dietary fat intake and risk of type II diabetes in women. *American Journal of Clinical Nutrition*, 2001 June; 73(6): 1019–26.

Sato Y. Diabetes and life-styles: Role of physical exercise for primary prevention. *British Journal of Nutrition*. 2000 Dec;84(6 Suppl 2):187–90.

Sato Y, Nagasaki M, et al. Physical exercise improves glucose metabolism in lifestyle-related diseases. *Exp Biol Med* (Maywood). 2003 Nov;228(10):1208–12.

Sattar N. et al. Metabolic syndrome with and without C-reactive protein as a predictor of coronary heart disease and diabetes in the West of Scotland Coronary Prevention Study. *Circulation.* 2003 Jul:108(4): 414–19.

Schmidt AM, Stern DM. RAGE: A new target for the prevention and treatment of the vascular and inflammatory complications of diabetes. *Trends Endocrinol Metab.* 2000 Nov 1;11(9):368–75.

Sheard NF. Moderate changes in weight and physical activity can prevent or delay the development of type II diabetes mellitus in susceptible individuals. *Nutr Rev.* 2003 Feb;61(2):76–9.

Simon GE, et al. Association between obesity and depression in middle-aged women. *Gen Hosp Psychiatry.* 2008; 32–39.

Society for the Study of Ingestive Behavior. "Weight Loss Improves Mood In Depressed People, New Research Shows." *ScienceDaily* 29 July 2009. 28 December 2009, http://www.sciencedaily.com/releases/2009/07/090727102028. htm.

Sonestedt, Emily, et al. Fat and carbohydrate intake modify the association between genetic variation in the FTO genotype and obesity. *American Journal of Clinical Nutrition,* 2009; DOI 10.3945/ajcn.2009.27958

Strauss, Shiela M., Stefanie Russell, Alla Wheeler, Robert Norman, Luisa N. Borrell, David Rindskopf. The dental office visit as a potential opportunity for diabetes screening: an analysis using NHANES 2003–2004 data: Opportunity for diabetes screening. *Journal of Public Health Dentistry* 2010.

Srjdan Prodanovich; Robert S. Kirsner; Jeffrey D. Kravetz; Fangchao Ma; Lisa Martinez; Daniel G. Federman. Association of Psoriasis with Coronary Artery, Cerebrovascular, and Peripheral Vascular Diseases and Mortality. *Arch Dermatol.,* 2009; 145(6): 700–03.

Stratton IM, Adler AI, et al. Association of glycaemia with macrovascular and microvascular complications of type II diabetes (UKPDS 35): Prospective observational study. *BMJ.* 2000 Aug 12;321(7258):405–12.

Time Magazine, Lifelong Effects of Childhood Obesity, Tiffany Sharples, Dec. 6, 2007.

Tran TT, Naigamwalla D, et al. Hyperinsulinemia, But Not Other Factors Associated with Insulin Resistance, Acutely Enhances Colorectal Epithelial Proliferation In Vivo. *Endocrinology*. 2006 Jan 12.

Translational Genomics Research Institute. 2009 December 16. Analysis identifies biomarkers for diabetic kidney failure, from *sciencedaily. com/ releases/2009*.

University of Alberta. 2006 March 10. Insulin levels in African American Children worsen through puberty. *The Journal of Pediatrics* as reported by *sciencedaily.com/releases/2006*.

University Of Florida (2007, May 22). Watch What You Put In That Sippy Cup, Experts Warn. *ScienceDaily*. Retrieved December 16, 2009, from http:// www.sciencedaily.com /releases/2007/05/070518155859.htm.

University of Gothenburg (2009, November 25). Fat around the middle increases the risk of dementia. *ScienceDaily*. Retrieved December 17, 2009, from http://www.sciencedaily.com/ releases/2009/11/091123114803.htm.

University of Melbourne (2008, July 9). Overweight, Insulin Resistant Women At Greater Risk Of Advanced Breast Cancer Diagnosis, Says Study. *ScienceDaily*. Retrieved December 17, 2009, from http:// www.sciencedaily.com /releases/2008/07/080707161416.htm.

University of Michigan Health System (2008, July 12). Coming Epidemic Of Type II Diabetes In Young Adults. *ScienceDaily*. Retrieved December 16, 2009, from http://www.sciencedaily.com/ releases/2008/07/080708193249. htm.

University of Southern California, 2009 Jan 28. Getting Diabetes before 65 More than Doubles Risk for Alzheimer's Disease. From www. sciencedaily. com/releases/2009/01/090127152835.htm.

Vincent AM, McLean LL, et al. Short-term hyperglycemia produces oxidative damage and apoptosis in neurons. *FASEB J*. 2005 Apr;19(6):638–40.

Wiley-Blackwell. "Major Study Highlights Weight Differences Among 3–19 Year Olds With Type I and 2 Diabetes." *ScienceDaily* 22 June 2009 From Sciencedaily.com/releases/2009.

Wiley-Blackwell. "Psychotherapy Offers Obesity Prevention for 'at Risk' Teenage Girls." *ScienceDaily* 17 December 2009. 3 March 2010 http://www. sciencedaily.com /releases/2009/12/091215121055.htm.

WHO. Total of People with Diabetes. WHO website. October 31, 2003.

World Journal of Gastroenterology (2009, November 18). Is type II diabetes mellitus a risk factor for gallbladder, biliary and pancreatic cancer? *ScienceDaily*. Retrieved December 17, 2009, from http://www.sciencedaily.com / releases/2009/11/091119101213.htm.

Wright E Jr., Scism-Bacon JL, et al. Oxidative stress in type II diabetes: the role of fasting and postprandial glycaemia. *Int J Clin Pract*. 2006 Mar;60(3):308–14.

Zhang et al. The Economic Costs of Undiagnosed Diabetes. *Population Health Management*, 2009; 12 (2): 95.

Chapter 7—"Sweet Suicide"

Adair, L.S. and P. Gordon-Larsen. Maturational timing and overweight prevalence in US adolescent girls. *Am J Public Health* 2001 Apr;91(4):642–4.

American University, TED Case Studies, "Philippine Sugar and Environment," January 11, 1997, http://www.american.edu/TED/PHILSUG.HTM

Anderson, G.H., et al. Inverse association between the effect of carbohydrates on blood glucose and subsequent short-term food intake in young men. *Am J Clin Nutr* 2002 Nov 76(5):1023–30.

Aylsworth, J. Sugar and Hyperactivity. Winter 1990 *Priorities*; 31–33.

Bartley, G. Neural systems for reinforcement and inhibition of behavior: relevance to eating, addiction, and depression. *Well-being: Foundations of Hedonic Psychology* 1999 pp. 558–572.

Beckles, H. "Sugar and Slavery, 1644–1692," in H. Beckles, *A History of Barbados from Amerindian Settlement to Nation State*. Cambridge Univ. Press: Cambridge, 1990.

Behar, D., et al. Diet and Hyperactivity. *Nutr Behav* 1984; 1:279–288.

Bellisle, F., et al. How sugar-containing drinks might increase adiposity in children. *Lancet* 2001 Feb 17;357(9255):490–1.

Boyle, J.P., et al. Projection of diabetes burden through 2050: impact of changing demography and disease prevalence in the US *Diabetes Care* 2001 Nov;24(11):1936–40.

Bruckdorfer, KR, et al. Insulin sensitivity of adipose tissue of rats fed with various carbohydrates. *Proc Nutr Sci* 1974;33:3A,46–53.

Burfoot, A. Sugar and cardiovascular disease, and other health issues. *Runner's World Website*, 2003; http://www.runnersworld.com/home/0,1300,1-53-84-3623,00.html.

The American Heart Association Report "Sugar and Cardiovascular Disease" is located at http://circ.ahajournals.org/cgi/content/full/106/4/523.

Chardon, R.E. "Sugar Plantations in the Dominican Republic, 1770–1844," *Geographical Review*, 74, 4 (1984).

Cichelli, M, and M Lewis. Naloxone nonselective suppression of drinking of ethanol, sucrose, saccharin, and water by rats. *Pharmacol Biochem Behav* 2002 Jun; 72(3):699–705.

Cleave, T.L. *The Saccharine Disease*, John Wright & Sons. Bristol, 1974, pp. 7, 83.

Cohen, A.M., et al. Experimental Models in Diabetes. In *Sugars in Nutrition*; San Francisco, Academic Press, 1974, p 483–511.

Colantuoni. C., et al. Evidence that intermittent, excessive sugar intake causes endogenous opioid dependence. *Obes Res* 2002 Jun 10(6):478–88.

Cox, Peter, "Sweetness and plight: Slavery on sugar plantations is a thing of the past. Or is it?" *New Internationalist Magazine*, Oxford, England, Issue 189 (November 1988), http://www.newint.org/issue189/plight.htm

Crook, W., Sugar and children's behavior. *New England Journal of Medicine* 1994 June 30;330(26):1901–1904.

Curtin, P.D., "The Sugar Revolution and the Settlement of the Carribean," in *The Rise and Fall of the Plantation Complex: Essays in Atlantic History*. Cambridge Univ. Press: Cambridge, 1990.

Czachowski, C.L., Independent ethanol and sucrose-maintained responding on a multiple schedule of reinforcement. *Alcohol Clin Exp Res* 1999 Mar 23(3):398–403.

Donders, G.G. Lower Genital Tract Infections in Diabetic Women. *Curr Infect Dis Rep* 2002 Dec;4(6):536–539.

Dr. Charles Jacobs, "Slavery: Worldwide Evil, From India to Indiana, more people are enslaved today than ever before," © 2001 Abolish.com, the Anti-Slavery Portal, http://www.iabolish.com/today/background/worldwide-evil.htm.

Elliott, S.S., et al. Fructose, weight gain, and the insulin resistance syndrome. *Am J Clin Nutr* 2002 Nov;76(5):911–22.

Epidemiology, November, 2000; 11: 689–694.

Falco, M.A. The lifetime impact of sugar excess and nutrient depletion on oral health. *Gen Dent* 2001 Nov-Dec;49(6):591–5.

Files, F.J., et al. Sucrose, ethanol, and sucrose/ethanol reinforced responding under variable-interval schedules of reinforcement. *Alcohol Clin Exp Res* 1995 Oct 19(5):1271–8.

Flegal, K.M., et al. Prevalence and trends in obesity among US adults, 1999–2000. *JAMA* 2002 Oct 9;288(14):1723–7.

Freedman, D.S., et al. Trends and correlates of class 3 obesity in the United States from 1990 through 2000. *JAMA* 2002 Oct 9;288(14):1758–61.

Frisina, P, and A Sclafani. Naltrexone suppresses the late but not early licking response to a palatable sweet solution: opioid hedonic hypothesis reconsidered. *Pharmacol Biochem Behav*, 2002 Dec; 74(1):163l, 760–765.

General Internal Medicine. January 2002;17:1–7.

George Mateljan Foundation. Low Fat Diet, "Nutrition Excesses/ Deficiencies," © 2002 http://www.whfoods.com/genpage. php?tname=diet&dbid=11, citing USDA's 1995 Continuing Survey of Food Intakes by Individuals.

Graves, F., July-Aug l984: Common Cause, p 25. Wolraich, R., et al. J Pediatr; l985, 106:675–682.31.

Grimm, J.W., et al. Effect of cocaine and sucrose withdrawal period on extinction behavior, cue-induced reinstatement, and protein levels of the dopamine transporter and tyrosine hydroxylase in limbic and cortical areas in rats, *Behav Pharmacol* 2002 Sep 13(5–6):379–88.

Hellinger, Daniel and Dennis Brooks. *The Democratic Façade*. Cole Publishing Co, 1991, p 233–241; http://www.thirdworldtraveler. com/Democracy_America/Exporting_Facade_TDF.html

Hill, J.O. and C.J. Billington. Obesity: its time has come. *Am J Hypertens* 2002 Jul;15(7 Pt 1):655–6.

Hoogwerf, B.J., et al. Blood glucose concentrations < or = 125 mg/dl and coronary heart disease risk. *Am J Cardiol* 2002 Mar 1;89(5):596–9.

Howard, B.V. and J. Wylie-Rosett. Sugar and cardiovascular disease: A statement for healthcare professionals from the Committee on Nutrition of the Council on Nutrition, Physical Activity, and Metabolism of the American Heart Association. *Circulation* 2002 Jul 23;106(4):523–7. American Heart Association Report at: http://circ.ahajournals.org/cgi/content/full/106/4/523.

Huumonen, S. L. Tjaderhane, T. Backman, E.L. Hietala, E. Pekkala, and M. Larmas. High-sucrose diet reduces defensive reactions of the pulpodentinal complex to dentinal caries in young rats. *Acta Odontol Scand* 2001 Apr;59(2):83–7.

Jacobson, M. Liquid Candy: How Soft Drinks Are Harming Americans' Health. Center for Science in the Public Interest Website, 1998 October. http://www. cspinet.org/sodapop/liquid_candy.htm

Jensen, D, "The New Slavery: an Interview with Kevin Bales," © 2001, *The Sun Magazine*, Chapel Hill, NC, http://www.thesunmagazine. org/slavery. html.

Johnson, R.K. and C. Frary. Choose beverages and foods to moderate your intake of sugars: the 2000 dietary guidelines for Americans—what's all the fuss about? *J Nutr* 2001 Oct;131(10):2766S-2771S.

Jones, C., K. Woods, G. Whittle, H. Worthington, and G. Taylor. Sugar, drinks, deprivation and dental caries in 14-year-old children in the northwest of England in 1995. *Community Dent Health* 1999 Jun 16(2):68–71.

Journal of Hensley, T., and M. Sones. Major Increase in Diabetes Among Adults Occurred Nationwide Between 1990 and 1998. National Center for Chronic Disease Prevention and Health Promotion, Diabetes Public Health Resource, News & Information.

Klein, Herbert; *African Slavery in Latin America and the Caribbean*; 1990, pp.45–47.

Kretchmer, Norman and Claire B. Hollenbeck. Sugars and Sweeteners, CRC Press, June 27, 1991, Preface, p v.

Levine, A.S., et al. Naltrexone infusion inhibits the development of preference for a high-sucrose diet. *Am J Physiol Regul Integr Comp Physiol* 2002 Nov 283(5):R1149–54.

Levine, R. Monosaccharides in Health and Disease. 1986, *Ann Rev Nutr* 6:221–24.

Levine, R.S. Caries experience and bedtime consumption of sugar-sweetened food and drinks—a survey of 600 children. *Community Dent Health* 2001 Dec;18(4):228–31.

Lord, R. Agricultural Outlook Forum Tuesday, February 24, 1998. US SUGAR OUTLOOK, *Ron Lord Agricultural Economist*, USDA. http://jan.mannlib. cornell.edu/reports/erssor/specialty/sss-bb/1998/ sss223f.asc.

Ludwig, D.S., K.E. Peterson, and S.L. Gortmaker. Relation between consumption of sugar-sweetened drinks and childhood obesity: a prospective, observational analysis. *Lancet* 2001 Feb 17;357(9255):505–8.

Matthews, D.B., et al. Effects of sweetened ethanol solutions on ethanol self-administration and blood ethanol levels. *Pharmacol Biochem Behav* 2001 Jan 68(1):13–21.

McGill Jr., H.C., et al. Obesity accelerates the progression of coronary atherosclerosis in young men; *Circulation* 2002 Jun 11;105(23):2712–8.

Melnik, T.A., et al. Overweight school children in New York City: prevalence estimates and characteristics. *Int J Obes Relat Metab Disord* 1998 Jan;22(1):7–13.

Melton, L. AGE breakers, Rupturing the body's sugar-protein bonds might turn back the clock. *Sci Am.* 2000 Jul 283(1):16. See also. Cerami, A., H. Vlassara, and M. Brownlee. Glucose and Aging. *Scientific American* May 1987: 90.

Michaud, D.S., et al. Dietary sugar, glycemic load, and pancreatic cancer risk in a prospective study. *J Natl Cancer Inst* 2002 Sep 4 94(17):1293–300.

Michaud, D.S., et al. Physical activity, obesity, height, and the risk of pancreatic cancer. *JAMA* 2001 Aug 22–29 286(8):921–9.

Moerman, C.J., et al. Dietary sugar intake in the aetiology of biliary tract cancer. *Int J Epidemiol* 1993 Apr 22(2):207–14.

Mohanty, P., et al. Glucose challenge stimulates reactive oxygen species (ROS) generation by leucocytes. *J Clin Endocrinol Metab* 2000 Aug;85(8):2970–3.

Mokdad, A.H., et al. The continuing epidemics of obesity and diabetes in the United States. *JAMA* 2001 Sep 12;286(10):1195–200.

Mokdad, A.H., et al. The continuing increase of diabetes in the US. *Diabetes Care* 2001 Feb;24(2):412.

Mokdad, A.H., et al. The spread of the obesity epidemic in the United States, 1991–1998. *JAMA* 1999 Oct 27;282(16):1519–22.

Nobre Dos Santos, M., L. Melo Dos Santos, S.B. Francisco, J.A. Cury. Relationship among Dental Plaque Composition, Daily Sugar Exposure and Caries in the Primary Dentition. *Caries Res* 2002 Sep-Oct;36(5):347–52.

Norhammar, A., et al. Glucose metabolism in patients with acute myocardial infarction and no previous diagnosis of diabetes mellitus: a prospective study. *Lancet* 2002 Jun 22;359(9324):2140–4.

Ogden, C.L., et al. Prevalence and trends in overweight among US children and adolescents, 1999–2000. *JAMA* 2002 Oct 9;288(14):1728–32.

Olson, G.A., et al. Naloxone and fluid consumption in rats: dose-response relationships for 15 days. *Pharmacol Biochem Behav* 1985 Dec, 23(6):1065–8.

Parajas, I.L. Sugar content of commonly eaten snack foods of school children in relation to their dental health status. *J Philipp Dent Assoc* 1999 Jun-Aug 51(1):4–21.

Further resources:

Abidov M, Ramazanov A, Jimenez Del RM, Chkhikvishvili I. Effect of Blueberin on fasting glucose, C-reactive protein and plasma aminotransferases, in female volunteers with diabetes type II: double-blind, placebo controlled clinical study. *Georgian Med News*. 2006 Dec;(141):66–72.

Anderson JW, Major AW. Pulses and lipaemia, short and long-term effect: potential in the prevention of cardiovascular disease. *Br J Nutr*. (2002) 88 Suppl 3:S263–271.

Anderson JW, Johnstone BM, Cook-Newell ME. Meta-analysis of the effects of soy protein intake on serum lipids. *N Engl J Med*. (1995) 333(5):276–282.

Anderson RA, Roussel AM, Zouari N, Mahjoub S, Matheau JM, Kerkeni A. Potential antioxidant effects of zinc and chromium supplementation in people with type II diabetes mellitus. *J Am Coll Nutr*. 2001 Jun;20(3):212–8.

Anderson RA. Nutritional factors influencing the glucose/insulin system: chromium. *J Am Coll Nutr*.1997 Oct;16(5):404–10.

Anuradha CV, Balakrishnan SD. Taurine attenuates hypertension and improves insulin sensitivity in the fructose-fed rat, an animal model of insulin resistance. *Can J Physiol Pharmacol.* 1999 Oct;77(10):749–54.

Apostolidis E, Kwon YI, Shetty K. Potential of cranberry-based herbal synergies for diabetes and hypertension management. *Asia Pac J Clin Nutr.* 2006;15(3):433–41.

Ataie-Jafari, A.; Hosseini, S.; Karimi, F.; Pajouhi, M. Effects of sour cherry juice on blood glucose and some cardiovascular risk factors improvements in diabetic women. *Nutrition and Food Science* (2008) 38 (4) 355–360.

Barbagallo M, Dominguez LJ, Tagliamonte MR, Resnick LM, Paolisso G. Effects of vitamin E and glutathione on glucose metabolism: role of magnesium. *Hypertension.* 1999 Oct;34(4 Pt 2):1002–6.

Battell ML, Delgatty HL, McNeill JH. Sodium selenate corrects glucose tolerance and heart function in STZ diabetic rats. *Mol Cell Biochem.* 1998 Feb;179(1–2):27–34.

Besnard, M.; Megard, D.; Rousseau, I.; Zaragoza, M. C.; Martinez, N.; Mitjavila, M. T.; Inisan, C. Polyphenolic apple extract: characterisation, safety and potential effect on human glucose metabolism. *Agro Food Industry hi-tech* (2008) 19 (4) 16–19.

Blostein-Fujii A, DiSilvestro RA, Frid D, Katz C, Maladey W. Short-term zinc supplementation in women with non-insulin-dependent diabetes mellitus: effects on plasma 5-nucleotidase activities insulin-like growth factor I concentrations and lysoprotein oxidation rates in vitro. *Am K Clin Nutr.* 1997; 66(3):639–642.

Bwititi P, Musabayane CT, Nhachi CF. Effects of *Opuntia megacantha* on blood glucose and kidney function in streptozotocin diabetic rats. *J Ethnopharmacol.* 2000;69(3):247–252.

Chambers BK, Camire ME. Can cranberry supplementation benefit adults with type II diabetes? *Diabetes Care.* 2003 Sep;26(9):2695–6. 390:

Christensen RL, Shade DL, Graves CB, McDonald JM. Evidence that protein kinase C is involved in regulating glucose transport in the adipocyte. *Int J Biochem.* 1987;19(3):259–65.

Classen JB. Discontinuation of BCG vaccination precedes significant drop in type II diabetes in Japanese children. Role of inflammation and cortisol activity as a cause of type II diabetes. *Open Endocrinology Journal* (2008) 2:1–4.

Classen JB. Type I versus type II diabetes/metabolic syndrome, opposite extremes of an immune spectrum disorder induced by vaccines. *Open Endocrinology Journal* (2008) 2:9–15.

Classen JB, Classen DC. Vaccines and the risk of insulin dependent diabetes (IDDM), potential mechanism of action. *Medical Hypotheses* (2001) 57: 532–8.

Cunningham JJ. The glucose/insulin system and vitamin C: implications in insulin-dependent diabetes mellitus. *J Am Coll Nutr.* 1998 Apr;17(4):105–8.

Dong Hua-Qiang; Ning Zheng-Xiang. Phloridzin and prevention and cure of diabetes mellitus. *Food Science and Technology* (2006) No. 12 192–194.

El-Alfy AT, Ahmed AA, Fatani AJ. Protective effect of red grape seeds proanthocyanidins against induction of diabetes by alloxan in rats. *Pharmacol Res.* 2005;52:264–270.

Facchini F, Coulston AM, Reaven GM. Relation between dietary vitamin intake and resistance to insulin-mediated glucose disposal in healthy volunteers. *Am J Clin Nutr.* 1996 Jun;63(6):946–9.

Frati-Munari A, Fernández-Harp JA, Bañales-Ham M, Ariza-Andraca CR. Decreased blood glucose and insulin by nopal (*Opuntia* sp.). *Arch Invest Med (Mex).* 1983;14(3):269–274.

Frey AB. Rao TD. 7 NKT cell cytokine imbalance in murine diabetes mellitus. *Autoimmunity.* (1999) 29(3):201–14.

Fujioka K, Greenway F, Sheard J, Ying Y. The effects of grapefruit on weight and insulin resistance: relationship to the metabolic syndrome. *J Med Food.* 2006 Spring;9(1):49–54.

Fukai, Y.; Matsuzawa, T.; Keizo, S. The study on the prophylactic effects of agricultural products on lifestyle related diseases: Adipocyte functions and the insulin sensitivity of extracts from 5 fruits including peach, apple, plum, grape (Kyoho) and apricot. *Journal of the Japanese Society for Food Science and Technology* (Nippon Shokuhin Kagaku Kogaku Kaishi) (2000) 47 (2) 92–96

Han DH, Hansen PA, Chen MM, Holloszy JO. DHEA treatment reduces fat accumulation and protects against insulin resistance in male rats. *J Gerontol A Biol Sci Med Sci.* 1998 Jan;53(1):B19–24.

Hannan, J M A, Marenah, Lamin, Ali, Liaquat, Rokeya, Begum, Flatt, Peter R, Abdel-Wahab, Yasser H. Insulin secretory actions of extracts of

Asparagus racemosus root in perfused pancreas, isolated islets and clonal pancreatic {beta}-cells *J. Endocrinol.* 2007 192: 159–168

Ho E, Chen G, Bray TM. Supplementation of N-acetylcysteine inhibits NFkappaB activation and protects against alloxan-induced diabetes in CD-1 mice. *FASEB J.* 1999 Oct;13(13):1845–54.

Hozawa A, Jacobs DR Jr, Steffes MW, Gross M.D., Steffen LM, Lee DH. Associations of serum carotenoid concentrations with the development of diabetes and with insulin concentration: interaction with smoking: the Coronary Artery Risk Development in Young Adults (CARDIA) study. *Am J Epidemiol.* 2006 May 15;163(10):929–37.

Jayaprakasam, B.; Olson, L. K.; Schutzki, R. E.; Mei-Hui Tai; Nair, M. G. Amelioration of obesity and glucose intolerance in high-fat-fed C57BL/6 mice by anthocyanins and ursolic acid in Cornelian cherry (Cornus mas). *Journal of Agricultural and Food Chemistry* (2006) 54 (1) 243–248

Kaneto H, Kajimoto Y, Miyagawa J, et al. Beneficial effects of antioxidants in diabetes: possible protection of pancreatic beta-cells against glucose toxicity. *Diabetes.* 1999 Dec;48(12):2398–406.

Karvonen M, Cepaitis Z, Tuomilehto J. Association between type I diabetes and *Haemophilus influenzae* type b vaccination: birth cohort study. *British Medical Journal* (1999) 318: 1169–1172

Kashiwagi, A. (Patent assignee(s):Spirulina Biological Lab Ltd; Yamada Yakken KK; Kusatsu Ichi; Kusatsushi Nogyo Kyodo Kumiai) [Diabetes preventive food.] (2008) *Japanese Patent Application* JP 2008104399 A

Krishnan S, Rosenberg L, Singer M, et al. Glycemic index, glycemic load, and cereal fiber intake and risk of type II diabetes in US black women. *Arch Intern Med.* (2007) 167(21):2304–2309.

Kwon YI, Vattem DA, Shetty K. Evaluation of clonal herbs of Lamiaceae species for management of diabetes and hypertension. *Asia Pac J Clin Nutr.* 2006;15(1):107–18.

Lans CA. Ethnomedicines used in Trinidad and Tobago for urinary problems and diabetes mellitus. *J Ethnobiol Ethnomed.* 2006 Oct 13;2:45.

Lopez-Ridaura R, Willett WC, Rimm EB, et al. Magnesium intake and risk of type II diabetes in men and women. *Diabetes Care.* 2004 Jan;27(1):134–40.

Martini Betty, Dropping Like Flies: Poisoned by Aspartame, Mission Possible International/Sepp Hassberger webpage, 2003, http://www.newmediaexplorer.org/sepp/2003/09/26/dropping_like_flies_poisoned_by_aspartame. htm

McCarty MF. High-dose biotin, an inducer of glucokinase expression may synergize with chromium picolinate to enable a definitive nutritional therapy for type II diabetes. *Med Hypotheses.* 1999 May;52(5):401–6.

Murase T, Haramizu S, Shimotoyodome A, Tokimitsu I. Reduction of diet-induced obesity by a combination of tea-catechin intake and regular swimming. *Int J Obes* (Lond). 2006 Mar; 30(3):561–8.

Nair AR, Biju MP, Paulose CS. Effect of pyridoxine and insulin administration on brain glutamate dehydrogenase activity and blood glucose control in streptozotocin-induced diabetic rats. *Biochim Biophys Acta.* 1998 Aug 24;1381(3):351–4.

Naito Y, Uchiyama K, Aoi W, et al. Prevention of diabetic nephropathy by treatment with astaxanthin in diabetic db/db mice. *Biofactors.* 2004;20(1):49–59.

Nettleton, J. A.; Harnack, L. J.; Scrafford, C. G.; Mink, P. J.; Barraj, L. M.; Jacobs, D. R. Dietary flavonoids and flavonoid-rich foods are not associated with risk of type II diabetes in postmenopausal women. *Journal of Nutrition* (2006) 136 (12) 3039–3045.

Nikander E, Tiitinen A, Laitinen K, Tikkanen M, Ylikorkala O. Effects of isolated isoflavonoids on lipids, lipoproteins, insulin sensitivity, and ghrelin in postmenopausal women. *J Clin Endocrinol Metab.* (2004) 89(7):3567–3572.

Nothlings U, Schulze MB, Weikert C, et al. Intake of vegetables, legumes, and fruit, and risk for all-cause, cardiovascular, and cancer mortality in a European diabetic population. *J Nutr.* (2008) 138(4):775–781.

Parikh P, Mani U, Iyer U. Role of spirulina in the control of glycemia and lipidemia in type II diabetes mellitus. *J Med Food.* 2001;4(4):193–199.

Patel AV, McCullough ML, Pavluck AL, Jacobs EJ, Thun MJ, Calle EE. Glycemic load, glycemic index, and carbohydrate intake in relation to pancreatic cancer risk in a large US cohort. *Cancer Causes Control.* (2007) 18(3):287–294.

Pinent M, Blay M, Blade MC, Salvado MJ, Arola L, Ardevol A. Grape-seed-derived procyanidins have an antihyperglycemic effect in streptozotocin-induced diabetic rats and insulinomimetic activity in insulin-sensitive cell lines. *Endocrinology.* 2004 Nov;145(11):4985–90.

Pippin, J. Artificial Sweetener Studies Underscore Risk of Relying on Animal Testing, *The Charleston Gazette,* April 23, 2006,

Preuss HG. Effects of glucose/insulin perturbations on aging and chronic disorders of aging: the evidence. *J Am Coll Nutr.* 1997 Oct;16(5):397–403.

Romero-Navarro G, Cabrera-Valladares G, German MS, et al. Biotin regulation of pancreatic glucokinase and insulin in primary cultured rat islets and in biotin-deficient rats. *Endocrinology.* 1999 Oct;140(10):4595–4600.

Rudich A, Tirosh A, Potashnik R, Khamaisi M, Bashan N. Lipoic acid protects against oxidative stress induced impairment in insulin stimulation of protein kinase B and glucose transport in 3T3-L1 adipocytes. *Diabetologia.* 1999 Aug;42(8):949–57.

Salmeron J, Manson JE, Stampfer MJ, Colditz GA, Wing AL, Willett WC. Dietary fiber, glycemic load, and risk of non-insulin-dependent diabetes mellitus in women. *JAMA.* (1997) 277(6):472–477.

Sanchez, D.; Muguerza, B.; Moulay, L.; Hernandez, R.; Miguel, M.; Aleixandre, A. Highly methoxylated pectin improves insulin resistance and other cardiometabolic risk factors in zucker fatty rats. *Journal of Agricultural and Food Chemistry* 5(2008) 6 (10) 3574–3581.

Sarkar S, Pranava M, Marita R. Demonstration of the hypoglycemic action of Momardica charantia in a validated animal model of diabetes. *Pharmacol Res.* 1996 Jan;33(1):1–4.

Schoen RE, Tangen CM, et al. Increased blood glucose and insulin, body size, and incident colorectal cancer. *J Natl Cancer Inst.* 1999 Jul 7;91(13):1147–54.

Shanmugasundaram ER, Rajeswari G, Baskaran K, et al. Use of Gymnema sylvestre leaf extract in the control of blood glucose in insulin-dependent diabetes mellitus. *J Ethnopharmacol.* 1990 Oct;30(3):281–94.

Song Y, Manson JE, Buring JE, Liu S. Dietary magnesium intake in relation to plasma insulin levels and risk of type II diabetes in women. *Diabetes Care.* 2004 Jan;27(1):59–65.

Talpur N, Echard BW, Yasmin T, Bagchi D, Preuss HG. Effects of niacin-bound chromium, Maitake mushroom fraction SX and (-)

hydroxycitric acid on the metabolic syndrome in aged diabetic Zucker fatty rats. *Mol Cell Biochem*. 2003 Oct;252(1–2):369–77.

Teachey MK, Taylor ZC, Maier T, et al. Interactions of conjugated linoleic acid and lipoic acid on insulin action in the obese Zucker rat. *Metabolism*. 2003 Sep;52(9):1167–74.

Thirunavukkarasu M, Penumathsa SV, Koneru S, et al. Resveratrol alleviates cardiac dysfunction in streptozotocin-induced diabetes: Role of nitric oxide, thioredoxin, and heme oxygenase. *Free Radic Biol Med*. 2007 Sep 1;43(5):720–9.

Trejo-González A, Gabriel-Ortiz G, Puebla-Pérez AM, et al. A purified extract from prickly pear cactus (*Opuntia fuliginosa*) controls experimentally induced diabetes in rats. *J Ethnopharmacol*. 1996;55(1):27–33.

Uchiyama K, Naito Y, Hasegawa G, et al. Astaxanthin protects beta-cells against glucose toxicity in diabetic db/db mice. *Redox Rep*. 2002;7(5):290–3.

Villegas R, Gao YT, Yang G, et al. Legume and soy food intake and the incidence of type II diabetes in the Shanghai Women's Health Study. *Am J Clin Nutr*. (2008) 87(1):162–167.

Weggemans RM, Trautwein EA. Relation between soy-associated isoflavones and LDL and HDL cholesterol concentrations in humans: a meta-analysis. *Eur J Clin Nutr*. (2003) 57(8):940–946.

Willett W, Manson J, Liu S. Glycemic index, glycemic load, and risk of type II diabetes. *Am J Clin Nutr*. (2002) 76(1):274S–280S.

Xue, Mingzhan; Qian, Qingwen; Adaikalakoteswari, Antonysunil; Rabbani, Naila, Babaei-Jadidi, Roya; and Paul J. Thornalley. Activation of NF-E2– Related Factor-2 Reverses Biochemical Dysfunction of Endothelial Cells Induced by Hyperglycemia Linked to Vascular Disease Diabetes. October 2008, 57: 2809–2817.

Yeh GY, Eisenberg DM, Kaptchuk TJ, Phillips RS. Systematic review of herbs and dietary supplements for glycemic control in diabetes. *Diabetes Care*. 2003;26(4):1277–1294.

Zhang J. Resveratrol inhibits insulin responses in a SirT1-independent pathway. *Biochem J*. 2006 Aug 1;397(3):519–27.

Index